Journal of Inherited Metabolic Disease

This review issue is also available separately, price Dfl.130.– [ISBN 0-7923-8947-6].
Orders should be sent to: Kluwer Academic Publishers Group, PO Box 322, 3300 AH Dordrecht, The Netherlands, or at PO Box 358, Accord Station, Hingham, MA 02018-0358, USA, or to your local specialist bookseller.

J. Inher. Metab. Dis. 13 (1990) 393–394

Preface

MUNICH 1989–LECTURES, WORKSHOP AND POSTERS

The articles printed in this volume represent the main lectures of the 27th Annual SSIEM meeting in Munich 1989 which was dedicated to "Inherited Disorders of Carbohydrate and Glycoprotein Metabolism" and was preceded by a workshop on "Maternal Phenylketonuria".

It is 60 years since glycogen storage disease (GSD) type I was described by von Gierke (1929), a pathologist from Karlsruhe, Germany, and much progress in our understanding of glycogen biosynthesis and breakdown and the many different types of GSD has been made. However many open questions remain, especially concerning molecular biology, genetic heterogeneity and treatment of glycogen storage disease.

Generally dietary measures have little influence on the natural course of the disease. However Dr G. P. A. Smit from Groningen reviewed promising data from several centres on treatment of glycogen storage disease type I with uncooked starch and nocturnal gastric drip feeding using oligosaccharides.

Dr Y.-T. Chen, Durham, Dr Inge van den Berg, Groningen, and Dr M. W. Kilimann, Bochum, showed the first results of molecular cloning for amylo-1,6-glucosidase and phosphorylase-b-kinase. Several speakers demonstrated examples of the clinical heterogeneity of glycogen storage disease, in the case of glycogen storage disease type III even in correlation with gene cloning results. The diagnosis of glycogen storage disease using biopsy tissues as well as peripheral blood cells was critically reviewed by Dr Yoon S. Shin from Munich. Non-invasive methods for the study of glycogen storage disease and hereditary fructose intolerance using magnetic resonance spectroscopy were presented by Dr R. Oberhänsli from Basel and Dr Aviva Lapidot from Rehovot.

Many of us are anxious about the "clouds over galactosaemia" (Editorial, 1982). Disorders of galactose metabolism were reviewed by Dr J. Holton from Bristol, and Dr S. Segal from Philadelphia gave insights into the regulation of galactose metabolism. Dr N. Buist from Portland presented the discouraging results of the international galactosaemia survey. It has recently become evident that galactose restriction from the first weeks of life will not always result in a normal outcome indicating the need for further research on pathogenetic mechanisms of galactosaemia. Lowered uridine diphosphate galactose in red blood cells of galactosaemia patients was reported by Shin *et al.* in 1985, and confirmed by Ng and colleagues. (1987; 1989). Dr Francine Kaufman and coworkers from Los Angeles showed normalisation of red blood cell UDP galactose levels by oral uridine treatment in four galactosaemia patients and improved neuropsychologic function in two of them. Controlled studies to evaluate this therapy are clearly needed.

In a short session mechanisms and disorders leading to cataract were reviewed. In most cataract patients a metabolic cause can be ruled out. A new and inexplicable finding by Dr C. Jakobs, Amsterdam, was elevated plasma galactitol and/or sorbitol levels in some cataract patients with quite normal activities of the galactose-degrading enzymes and sorbitol dehydrogenase in RBC.

Inherited disorders of glycoprotein metabolism were reviewed by Dr M. Cantz, Heidelberg, followed by detailed presentations on selected disorders.

The meeting was closed by two exciting lectures, given by Dr J. R. Hobbs, London, and Dr F. Ledley, Houston, on the outcome of bone marrow transplantation and on future aspects of gene therapy in patients with inborn errors of metabolism.

Each year the 'Mini' Symposium preceding the main topics attracts increasing numbers and in Munich more than half of the 281 active participants also attended the highly interesting workshop on "Maternal Phenylketonuria", organized by Dr D. Brenton, London. This four-hour workshop included international practical experiences in the treatment of maternal phenylketonuria as well as the results of amino acid transport and animal experiments.

The organizing committee is most grateful to Dr Yoon Shin for her efforts in organizing the large poster exhibition which again contributed largely to the success of the Symposium. 178 posters were presented and 10 were rejected due to more than one poster being submitted by the same author. An innovation at our meetings was the introduction of attended poster demonstrations with chairpersons moderating the discussions in groups of approximately ten posters of related topics. Hopefully this can be continued at future meetings as a better way to stimulate otherwise taciturn people and to acknowledge the considerable efforts in preparation of posters.

As agreed at this year's Annual General Meeting, the SSIEM Award will be judged on Short Communications to be published in the *Journal of Inherited Metabolic Disease.*

We are very grateful to the team in Munich, namely Dr Yoon Shin, Kristin Endres, Dr H. Ibel and Professor A. Roscher, for their enormous efforts in organizing the meeting.

The personal and financial support of our meeting by many persons and companies has been acknowledged in detail in the programme.

W. Endres

The papers listed below were also presented at the meeting. Scripts were not available by the time of publication. 1. The use of ^{31}P magnetic resonance spectroscopy in patients with carbohydrate disorders. R. Oberhänsli, Basel. 2. Sialic acid storage diseases. M. Renlund, Helsinki.

REFERENCES

Editorial. Clouds over galactosaemia. *Lancet* 2 (1982) 1379–1380

Ng, W. G., Xu, Y. K., Kaufman, F. and Donell, G. N. Deficit of uridine diphosphate galactose (UDPGal) in galactosemia (Abstract). *Am. J. Hum. Genet.* **41**, Suppl. 3 (1987) A12

Ng. W. G., Xu, Y. K., Kaufman, F. and Donell, G. N. Deficit of uridine diphosphate galactose in galactosemia. *J. Inher. Metab. Dis.* **12** (1989) 257–266

Shin, Y. S., Rieth, M., Hoyer, S., Endres, W., Böhles, H. and Jakobs, C. Uridine diphosphogalactose, galactose-1-phosphate and galactitol concentration in patients with classical galactosemia. Proceedings of the SSIEM 1985; Liverpool: p-35

von Gierke, E. Hepato-Nephromegalia glykogenica. *Beitr. Pathol. Anat.* **82** (1929) 497–513

J. Inher. Metab. Dis. 13 (1990) 395–410

Mechanisms of Blood Glucose Homeostasis

H.-G. HERS
Laboratoire de Chimie Physiologique, Université Catholique de Louvain and International Institute of Cellular and Molecular Pathology, Brussels B-1200, Belgium

Summary: The mechanisms by which glycogen metabolism, glycolysis and gluconeogenesis are controlled in the liver both by hormones and by the concentration of glucose are reviewed. The control of glycogen metabolism occurs by phosphorylation and dephosphorylation of both glycogen phosphorylase and glycogen synthase catalysed by various protein kinases and protein phosphatases. The hormonal effect is to stimulate glycogenolysis by the intermediary of cyclic AMP, which activates directly or indirectly the protein kinases. The glucose effect is to activate the protein phosphatase system; this occurs by the direct binding of glucose to glycogen phosphorylase which is then a better substrate for phosphorylase phosphatase and is inactivated. Since phosphorylase *a* is a strong inhibitor of synthase phosphatase, its disappearance allows the activation of glycogen synthase and the initiation of glycogen synthesis. When glycogen synthesis is intense, the concentrations of UDPG and of glucose 6-phosphate in the liver decrease, allowing a net glucose uptake by the liver. Glucose uptake is indeed the difference between the activities of glucokinase and glucose 6-phosphatase. Since the K_m of the latter enzyme is far above the physiological concentration of its substrate, the decrease in glucose 6-phosphate concentration proportionally reduces its activity.

The control of glycolysis and of gluconeogenesis occurs mostly at the level of the interconversion of fructose 6-phosphate and fructose 1,6-bisphosphate under the action of phosphofructokinase 1 and fructose 1,6-bisphosphatase. Fructose 2,6-bisphosphate is a potent stimulator of the first of these two enzymes and an inhibitor of the second. It is formed from fructose 6-phosphate and ATP by phosphofructokinase 2 and hydrolysed by a fructose 2,6-bisphosphatase. These two enzymes are part of a single bifunctional protein which is a substrate for cyclic AMP-dependent protein kinase. Its phosphorylation causes the inactivation of phosphofructokinase 2 and the activation of fructose 2,6-bisphosphatase, resulting in the disappearance of fructose 2,6-bisphosphate. The other major effector of these two enzymes is fructose 6-phosphate, which is the substrate of phosphofructokinase 2 and a potent inhibitor of fructose 2,6-bisphosphatase; these properties allow the formation of fructose 2,6-bisphosphate when the level of glycaemia and secondarily that of fructose 6-phosphate is high.

One important function of the liver is to control the level of glycaemia. When this level is elevated, as is the case after a meal, the liver takes up glucose and converts it mostly to glycogen but also, through glycolysis, to pyruvate, which is then in great part converted to fatty acids and exported as very low density lipoprotein. Little of this glucose is utilized for the energy needs of the liver, which consumes mostly fatty acids. When the level of glycaemia is low, as for instance during fasting, the liver delivers a large amount of glucose to the blood to the benefit of the brain, erythrocytes and other tissues. This glucose is provided by the breakdown of glycogen and by gluconeogenesis.

Soskin (1940) emphasized that the concentration of glucose in the blood is the primary stimulus which controls glucose uptake or glucose output by the liver and he compared this homeostatic control of the level of glycaemia to a thermostat-furnace arrangement. He defined the hepatic threshold to glucose as the glucose concentration at which the liver is converted from an organ of glucose output to an organ of glucose uptake. This threshold corresponds to the level of glycaemia which the animal usually maintains and may vary according to the endocrinological conditions. The purpose of this review is to describe the biochemical mechanisms by which these homeostatic and hormonal controls occur.

THE CONTROL OF GLYCOGEN METABOLISM IN THE LIVER

The basic mechanism of control

The sequence of reactions by which glycogen is synthesized and degraded in the liver is shown in Figure 1. As explained in detail in other review articles (Hers, 1976; Hers *et al.*, 1989), where additional information and references to original work can be found, the rate-limiting steps of glycogen synthesis and breakdown are catalysed by glycogen synthase (EC 2.4.1.11) and glycogen phosphorylase (EC 2.4.1.1) respectively. Each of these enzymes exists in two forms: *a*, which is active and *b*, which is inactive in the ionic conditions prevailing in the cell. The *a* and *b* forms are interconvertible through phosphorylation by protein kinases and dephosphorylation by protein phosphatases as indicated in Figure 2, which also shows the point of control by cyclic AMP and glucose. Some control is also exerted at the level of UDPG pyrophosphorylase (EC 2.7.7.9) (see Figure 1).

Glycogen phosphorylase and its converter enzymes: Glycogen phosphorylase catalyses the transfer of a glucose unit from the non-reducing end of the polysaccharide onto inorganic phosphate. The equilibrium is reached when the ratio glucose 1-phosphate/P_i is close to 3 at neutral pH. The reaction is therefore easily reversible *in vitro*, but not *in vivo*, as the concentration of inorganic phosphate is usually 100-fold that of glucose 1-phosphate in cells. The reaction proceeds from the non-reducing ends until about four glucose residues remain on each external chain. The resulting polysaccharide, called a phosphorylase limit dextrin, is the substrate of amylo-1,6-glucosidase (EC 3.2.1.33), also called debranching enzyme, and can be further degraded by phosphorolysis only after the removal of the branching point by the latter enzyme.

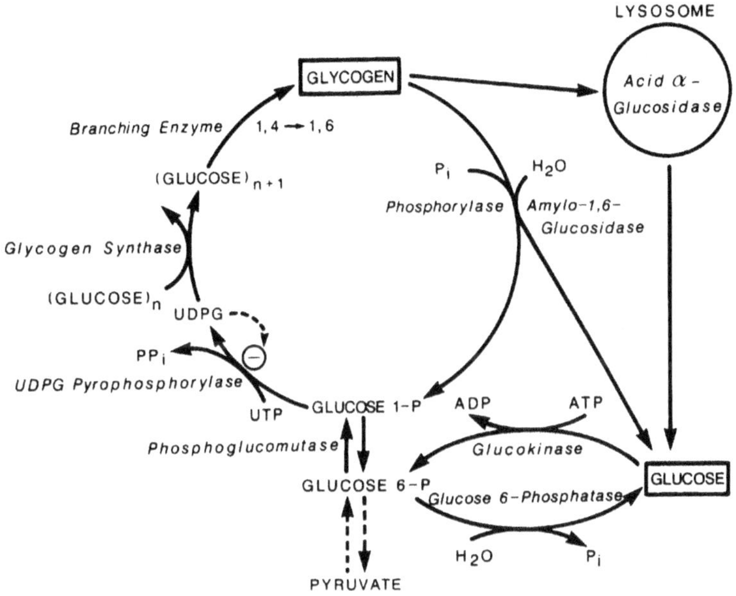

Figure 1 The path of glycogen metabolism in the liver.

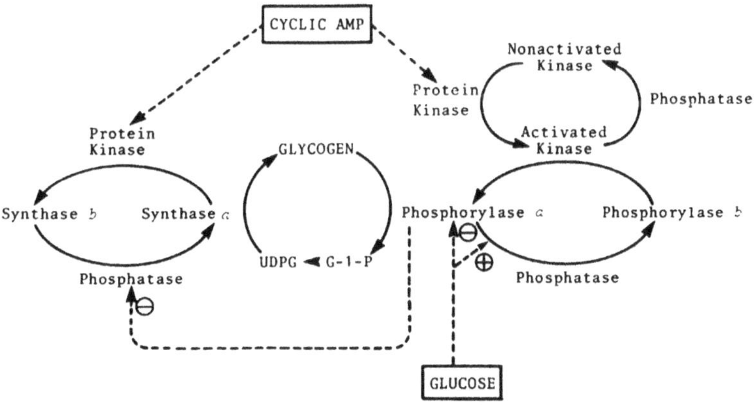

Figure 2 The control of glycogen metabolism in the liver (modified from Hers, 1976).

Phosphorylase *a* bears a phosphate group on the hydroxyl group of the serine residue in position 14. Phosphorylase *b* is the inactive dephosphoenzyme, which may be activated by non-physiological concentrations of AMP. These enzymes are dimers or tetramers of a subunit with a molecular weight close to 100 000 to which one essential pyridoxal phosphate is bound as a Schiff base to a lysine residue close to the active site.

Phosphorylase *b* kinase (EC 2.7.1.38) allows the conversion of phosphorylase *b* into phosphorylase *a* by the transfer of the terminal phosphate of ATP to a serine group in position 14. Phosphorylase *b* kinase itself exists as a phosphorylated active and a non-phosphorylated less active form. The latter is only active in the presence of calcium ($K_a = 10^{-6}$ mol/L), a property which is of importance in the liver submitted to calcium-mediated hormonal actions. The phosphorylation of phosphorylase *b* kinase is catalysed by a cyclic AMP-dependent protein kinase (EC 2.7.1.37). It activates the enzyme 15–20-fold at saturating calcium concentrations and decreases the K_a for calcium 15-fold. Phosphorylase *b* kinase is a large protein of molecular weight 1 300 000 with the structure $(\alpha\beta\gamma\delta)_4$. The α and β subunits are the components phosphorylated by cyclic AMP-dependent protein kinase and the γ-peptide appears to be the catalytic subunit. The δ-subunit is identical to caldmodulin.

The dephosphorylation and resulting inactivation of phosphorylase is catalysed by phosphorylase phosphatase (EC 3.1.3.17). The activity of this enzyme in the liver is increased several fold in the presence of glucose and this effect is counteracted by AMP. The action of these effectors is explained by their association with the substrate of the reaction, phosphorylase *a*. These compounds effect a change in the spatial configuration of phosphorylase *a*, the effect of glucose being to expose the serine phosphate group to the action of the phosphatase.

Glycogen synthase and its converter enzymes: Glycogen synthase catalyses the reaction:

$$(\text{glucose})_n + \text{UDPG} \rightarrow (\text{glucose})_{n+1} + \text{UDP}$$

The greater activity of the *a* form of the liver enzyme is related to its higher affinity for UDPG. The enzyme consists of two subunits of molecular weight close to 85 000. Several protein kinases can phosphorylate glycogen synthase, causing its inactivation. The predominant one is cyclic AMP-dependent protein kinase (EC 2.7.1.37).

Synthase phosphatase (EC 3.1.3.42) catalyses the dephosphorylation of glycogen synthase simultaneously with its activation. The main regulatory property of the liver enzyme is to be strongly inhibited by phosphorylase *a*. The enzyme is composed of two components: a G-component, which binds tightly to glycogen particles, and a cytosolic S-component; the co-operation of the two components is required to allow synthase activation. The G-component is responsible for the inhibitory effects of phosphorylase *a* (reviewed by Stalmans *et al.*, 1987).

UDPG pyrophosphorylase: As shown in Figure 1, UDPG pyrophosphorylase catalyses the formation of UDPG and inorganic pyrophosphate from UTP and glucose 1-phosphate. An interesting property of this enzyme is that it is inhibited by UDPG, a reaction product, competitively with UTP (Tsuboi *et al.*, 1969; Roach *et al.*, 1975). The rate of reaction is therefore controlled by the removal of its product, UDPG, itself dependent on the activity of glycogen synthase. This property is important because it counters the hypothesis that the rate of glycogen synthesis would be controlled by a 'push' given to the pathway by an increase in the concentration of glucose 6-phosphate.

The control by hormones

Glucagon is the principal hormone which controls glycogen metabolism in the liver and its action is easily explained by its ability to activate adenylate cyclase (EC 4.6.1.1) and to increase the concentration of cyclic AMP in the liver. Cyclic AMP-dependent protein kinase can then phosphorylate phosphorylase *b* kinase, which in turn activates phosphorylase and initiates glycogen degradation. Simultaneously, cyclic AMP-dependent protein kinase phosphorylates glycogen synthase, causing its inactivation and the arrest of glycogen synthesis (see upper part of Figure 2). The most reproducible effect of insulin on glycogen metabolism in the liver is to counteract the action of low concentrations of glucagon.

Vasopressin, angiotensin and α-adrenergic agonists induce glycogenolysis in the liver by a cyclic AMP-independent mechanism. These agents appear to generate two intracellular messengers: calcium and diacylglycerol. The initial event (Berridge, 1987) is the breakdown of phosphatidylinositol bisphosphate into inositol trisphosphate, which causes the release of free calcium from intracellular stores, and diacylglycerol, which activates protein kinase C (Nishizuka, 1984). The stimulation of phosphorylase *b* kinase by calcium explains the activation of phosphorylase. The same hormones also cause a substantial inactivation of glycogen synthase (see Mvumbi *et al.*, 1985), an effect which appears to be mediated by the inhibition of synthase phosphatase by phosphorylase *a* (Strickland *et al.*, 1983).

The control by glucose: a pull mechanism

As illustrated in the lower part of Figure 2, the control of liver glycogen metabolism by glucose can be explained by the binding of the hexose to phosphorylase *a*, which is the glucose receptor of the liver. When bound to glucose, phosphorylase *a* is somewhat less active and, more important, is now a much better substrate for phosphorylase phosphatase. The effect of a high glucose concentration is, therefore, to cause the conversion of phosphorylase *a* into phosphorylase *b* and to arrest glycogenolysis. Furthermore, since phosphorylase *a* is a potent inhibitor of synthase phosphatase, its disappearance allows the latter enzyme to activate glycogen synthase, and in doing so to initiate glycogen synthesis. An important observation is that the activation of glycogen synthase by glucose *in vivo* as well as in isolated hepatocytes or in a cell-free system is preceded by a lag period. This lag corresponds precisely to the time required for the nearly complete inactivation of phosphorylase, since activation of the synthase will start only when approximately 90% of phosphorylase is in the *b* form (see Figure 3).

A rise in glucose concentration in the liver is also expected to increase the activity of glucokinase (EC 2.7.1.12) and, secondarily, the concentration of glucose 6-phosphate. Contrary to this expectation, the concentrations of glucose 6-phosphate and of UDPG are not increased but decreased, at least in normally fed animals, because these intermediary metabolites are used rapidly for synthesis of glycogen.

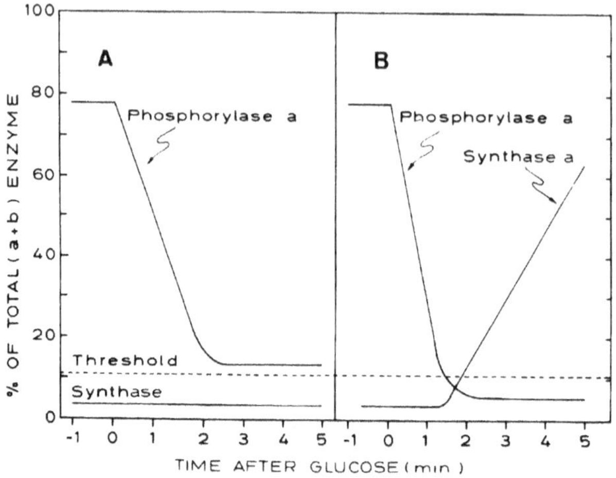

Figure 3 Sequential inactivation of glycogen phosphorylase and activation of glycogen synthase in the liver of fed rats. This schematic representation illustrates that glycogen synthase starts to be activated only if and when the concentration of phosphorylase *a* is lowered below a threshold value (dotted line), approximately equal to 10% of total (*a* + *b*) phosphorylase. This sequence has been observed in cell-free extracts, in isolated hepatocytes and *in vivo* (modified from Hers, 1976).

The decrease in the concentration of UDPG, an inhibitor of UDPG pyrophosphorylase, allows that enzyme automatically to keep up with the increased rate of synthesis; the decrease in the concentration of glucose 6-phosphate causes a proportional decrease in the activity of glucose 6-phosphatase as well as a deinhibition of glucokinase (see below), allowing glucose uptake by the liver. This so-called 'pull mechanism' is currently opposed to the 'push hypothesis' (Nordlie *et al.*, 1980; Youn *et al.*, 1986) in which an increase in the concentration of the precursor metabolites, glucose and hexose phosphates, would sequentially increase the activity of UDPG pyrophosphorylase, the concentration of UDPG and the rate of synthase reaction. The latter hypothesis is incompatible with the property of UDPG pyrophosphorylase to be inhibited by UDPG and is in contradiction with the observed changes in the concentration of UDGP and, under many conditions, of glucose 6-phosphate.

THE CONTROL OF GLYCOLYSIS AND OF GLUCONEOGENESIS

The rôle of glycolysis in the liver is to convert to pyruvate and lactate the glucose which is in excess of the amount that can be converted to glycogen; after decarboxylation to acetyl-CoA, most of the pyruvate is used for the biosynthesis of fatty acids, which are then exported as VLDL to the peripheral tissues.

As shown in Figure 4, a series of enzymes catalysing freely reversible reactions are common to glycolysis and glyconeogenesis. At three levels, however, which are the potential points of regulation, different enzymes are used by glycolysis and by

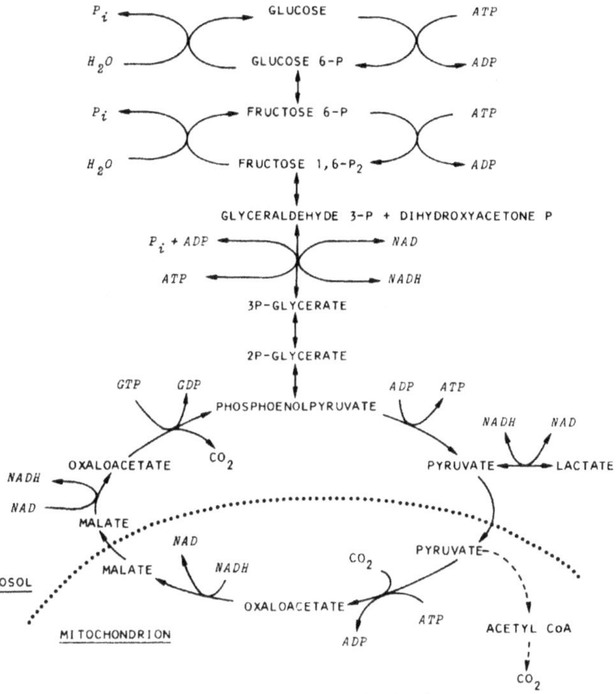

Figure 4 The path of glycolysis and gluconeogenesis in the liver.

gluconeogenesis. These enzymes catalyse irreversible reactions and at least one of them consumes ATP, therefore their simultaneous operation causes what is called a 'futile cycle', i.e. a series of reactions the net balance of which is the hydrolysis of ATP into ADP and P_i. The three levels at which such a futile cycle can occur and which will be discussed in this review are the interconversions of glucose and glucose 6-phosphate, of fructose 6-phosphate and fructose 1,6-bisphosphate and of pyruvate and phosphoenolpyruvate. The first of these interconversions is common to glycogen metabolism and will be discussed separately in the next section (see control of the glucose uptake and output by the liver). Additional information on the control of glycolysis and gluconeogenesis in the liver and references to original work can be found in recent reviews (Hers and Hue, 1983; Pilkis *et al.*, 1988).

The fructose 6-phosphate/fructose 1,6-bisphosphate interconversion

The control by fructose 2,6-bisphosphate: The phosphorylation of fructose 6-phosphate into fructose 1,6-bisphosphate is catalysed by a 6-phosphofructo 1-kinase also called phosphofructokinase 1, the activity of which can be modified by the concentration of its substrates and of various effectors. The control of phosphofructokinase 1 can be summarized by saying that one of its substrates, ATP, acts as a negative allosteric effector, which induces marked co-operativity for the second substrate, fructose 6-phosphate. The latter acts as a positive effector which relieves the inhibition by ATP. Several other substances have an allosteric effect similar to and usually synergistic with those of ATP or fructose 6-phosphate. Citrate and H^+ are negative effectors. The most important positive effectors are AMP and the newly discovered fructose 2,6-bisphosphate (reviewed by Van Schaftingen, 1987), which greatly increases the affinity of the enzyme for fructose 6-phosphate and decreases inhibition by ATP (see Figure 5). It has been calculated that, at the concentrations of substrates and effectors normally present in the cell, phosphofructokinase 1 would be completely inactive in the absence of fructose 2,6-bisphosphate. AMP acts synergistically with fructose 2,6-bisphosphate and seems to play a major rôle in the stimulation of glycolysis under anaerobic conditions but undergoes little variation in the presence of oxygen.

The hydrolysis of fructose 1,6-bisphosphate into fructose 6-phosphate and P_i is catalysed by fructose 1,6-bisphosphatase. This enzyme is stongly inhibited by fructose 2,6-bisphosphate. The main characteristics of this inhibition are (a) to be competitive with fructose 1,6-bisphosphate; (b) to be synergistic with AMP; and (c) to convert the saturation curve for fructose 1,6-bisphosphate from hyperbolic to sigmoidal (see Figure 6).

From the properties of phosphofructokinase 1 and of fructose 1,6-bisphosphatase described above, it appears that the interconversion of fructose 6-phosphate and fructose 1,6-bisphosphate is essentially controlled by the concentration of fructose 2,6-bisphosphate. The mechanism by which this effector is synthesized and degraded

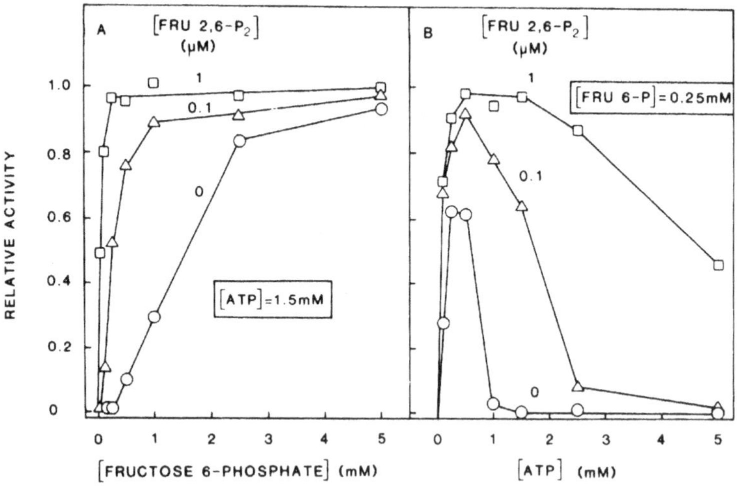

Figure 5 The effect of fructose 2,6-bisphosphate on (a) the affinity of phosphofructokinase 1 for fructose 6-phosphate and (b) the inhibition of the enzyme by ATP (from Van Schaftingen *et al.*, 1981).

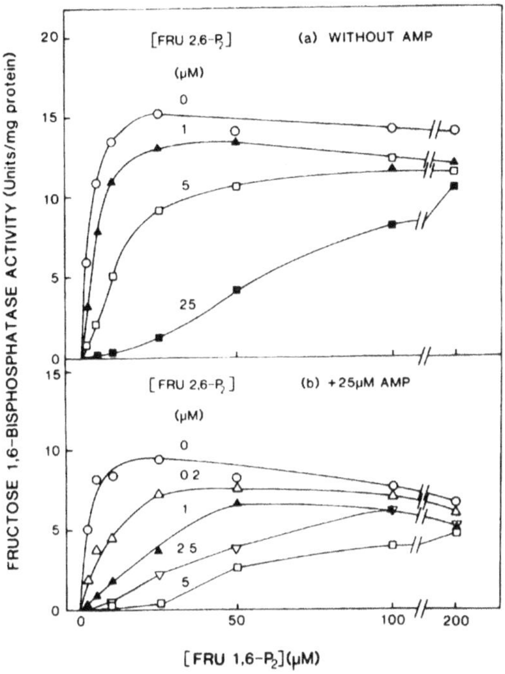

Figure 6 Inhibition of fructose 1,6-bisphosphatase by fructose 2,6-bisphosphate at various concentrations of substrate in the absence (a) and in the presence (b) of 20 μmol/L AMP (from Van Schaftingen and Hers, 1981).

in the liver is shown in Figure 7. It can be seen that fructose 2,6-bisphosphate is formed from fructose 6-phosphate and ATP by a 6-phosphofructo 2-kinase also called phosphofructokinase 2, and that it is degraded back to fructose 6-phosphate and P_i by a fructose 2,6-bisphosphatase. The concentration of fructose 2,6-bisphosphate in the liver is, therefore, controlled by the relative activities of phosphofructokinase 2 and of fructose 2,6-bisphosphatase. These two enzymes have the remarkable property that they are part of a single bifunctional protein (phosphofructokinase 2/fructose 2,6-bisphosphatase), which is a substrate for cyclic AMP-dependent protein kinase. When this bifunctional protein is phosphorylated, phosphofructokinase 2 becomes inactive and fructose 2,6-bisphosphatase is activated, causing the disappearance of fructose 2,6-bisphosphate. This occurs under the stimulus of glucagon during fasting, explaining the arrest of glycolysis and the initiation of gluconeogenesis under this condition.

The activities of phosphofructokinase 2 and of fructose 2,6-bisphosphatase are also controlled by the concentration of their substrates and of various effectors. The most important one is fructose 6-phosphate, which is the substrate of phosphofructokinase 2 and a potent non-competitive inhibitor of fructose 2,6-bisphosphatase. Glycerol 3-phosphate and phosphoenolpyruvate have an opposite effect. As a result of this, the

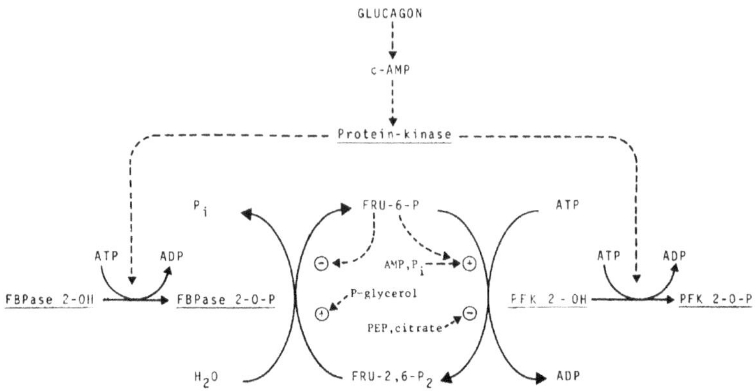

Figure 7 Biosynthesis and biodegradation of fructose 2,6-bisphosphate in the liver and their control by glucagon and metabolites (modified from Hers and Van Schaftingen, 1982).

concentration of fructose 2,6-bisphosphate is high when that of the hexose 6-phosphates is elevated, whereas it is low when the concentration of the three carbon metabolites is increased.

The sequence of events after refeeding: It is well established that the concentration of fructose 2,6-bisphosphate is elevated in the livers of fed rats and also in hepatocytes isolated from fasted rats incubated in the presence of a high concentration of glucose. It is therefore remarkable that Kuwajima *et al.* (1984) have reported that, when fasted rats are refed, the concentration of fructose 2,6-bisphosphate in their livers increases only after a delay of several hours (see Figure 8). This sequence of events, which had been predicted by Hers and Van Schaftingen (1982), is in agreement with the properties of the regulatory mechanisms which govern glycogen synthesis and glycolysis, as described above. An important point is that, as long as glycogen synthesis is intense, as occurs soon after refeeding, the concentration of hexose 6-

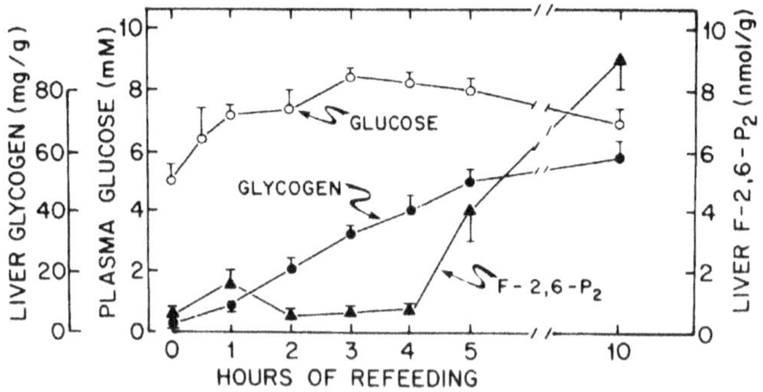

Figure 8 Effects of refeeding in fasted rats (modified from Kuwajima *et al.*, 1984).

phosphates and therefore that of fructose 2,6-bisphosphate remain low. It is only when the rate of glycogen synthesis decreases, because the glycogen stores are replete, that the concentrations of hexose 6-phosphates and secondarily that of fructose 2,6-bisphosphate increase. Such a situation is not observed in isolated hepatocytes in which, for various reasons, the rate of glycogen synthesis is much slower than *in vivo*. This situation indicates the existence of two levels of sensitivity to glucose in the liver. The disposal of glucose as glycogen is the primary function, which is initiated as soon as the level of glycaemia rises, whereas glycolysis and lipogenesis will only later consume the glucose in excess of that which is needed for glycogen synthesis (Hers and Van Schaftingen, 1982).

The significance of the futile recycling between fructose 6-phosphate and fructose 1,6-bisphosphate: The recycling between fructose 6-phosphate and fructose 1,6-bisphosphate is controlled by what could be called an incomplete on/off mechanism. As discussed by Hers and Hue (1983), the system oscillates between two extreme conditions. During fasting, because of the low concentration of fructose 2,6-bisphosphate, phosphofructokinase 1 is inactive and the flux of metabolites is unidirectionally gluconeogenic. In contrast, in the fed state, fructose 2,6-bisphosphate is present and it activates phosphofructokinase 1 as well as inhibiting fructose 1,6-bisphosphatase, at least in the first stage (on/off mechanism). Under these conditions, futile recycling would be avoided. The experimental evidence indicates, however, that in the fed state, as much as 30% of fructose 1,6-bisphosphate formed by phosphofructokinase 1 is converted back to glucose. There is then an up to tenfold increase in the concentration of fructose 1,6-bisphosphate, which is explained by the greater capacity of phosphofructokinase 1 relative to the enzymatic systems able to utilize fructose 1,6-bisphosphate. Because of the competitive aspect of the inhibition of fructose 1,6-bisphosphatase by fructose 2,6-bisphosphate, the increased concentration of substrate reactivates the enzyme and allows a substantial part of the metabolites to be converted back to fructose 6-phosphate. Because the saturation curve for fructose 1,6-bisphosphate is sigmoidal in the presence of fructose 2,6-bisphosphate, recycling occurs only at relatively high concentrations of substrate.

From the above considerations it appears that the futile recycling of metabolites between fructose 6-phosphate and fructose 1,6-bisphosphate in the liver results from an overflow of fructose 1,6-bisphosphate when this compound is formed by phosphofructokinase in excess of the glycolytic capacity of the cell. It has the advantage of preventing a deleterious accumulation of fructose 1,6-bisphosphate, as well as of lactic acid, in excess of the lipogenic capacity of the liver.

The pyruvate/phosphoenolpyruvate interconversion

This cycle is made up of three reactions. One, catalysed by the pyruvate kinase, forms 1 ATP; the two others, controlled by pyruvate carboxylase and phosphoenolpyruvate carboxykinase, each consume 1 ATP. The net balance is the hydrolysis of 1 ATP into ADP and P_i. There is good evidence that recycling is continuously operating and is more intense in the fed than in the fasted state.

One important property of the cycle is the compartmentation of its constituent enzymes. Pyruvate kinase is cytosolic and highly regulated, mostly by phosphorylation and simultaneous inactivation under the action of cyclic AMP-dependent protein kinase. Pyruvate carboxylase is mitochondrial, and thus not accessible to control by cyclic AMP-dependent protein kinase. Phosphoenolpyruvate carboxykinase is both cytosolic and mitochondrial, with a variable distribution from species to species. A purely cytosolic or purely mitochondrial control would, therefore, be of limited efficiency. The activity of this enzyme is mostly controlled by protein synthesis. One concludes, therefore, that the two gluconeogenic enzymes of the cycle are apparently not submitted to short term regulation, rendering futile recycling inescapable under glycolytic conditions. The long term decrease in the amount of phosphoenolypyruvate carboxykinase in the fed state and of pyruvate kinase during fasting is a means of decreasing recycling severalfold. When gluconeogenesis is predominant, the intensity of cycling is controlled by cyclic AMP-dependent inactivation of pyruvate kinase. This inactivation is, however, incomplete even under maximal hormonal stimulation. The pyruvate/phosphoenolpyruvate futile cycle therefore appears to be inherent to the location of its two gluconeogenic enzymes (Hers and Hue, 1983).

THE CONTROL OF GLUCOSE UPTAKE AND OUTPUT BY THE LIVER

The uptake of glucose by the liver occurs under the action of glucokinase. Glucose output occurs for the greatest part by hydrolysis of glucose 6-phosphate by glucose-6-phosphatase and for a minor part by the activity of amylo-1,6-glucosidase at the branching points of glycogen, and also of the lysosomal acid α-glucosidase during the process of autophagy. The two latter enzymes will not be considered here.

Glucokinase

General properties: Most cells possess one or several low (10^{-7}–10^{-6} mol/L) K_m hexokinases, which form glucose 6-phosphate from glucose and ATP, and also act similarly, but with a lower affinity, on mannose and fructose. These enzymes are inhibited by glucose 6-phosphate (K_i: 0.5 mmol/L), an effect which allows the control of glucose phosphorylation by the removal of hexose 6-phosphates under the action of phosphofructokinase 1.

The hepatocyte differs from other cells by the low affinity of its hexokinase for its sugar substrates and inhibitor. This liver enzyme is called glucokinase, because glucose is the only sugar that it phosphorylates under physiological conditions. Its K_m for glucose is close to 10 mmol/L and therefore the rate of glucose phosphorylation in the liver is affected by the level of glycaemia, although not by the level of glucose 6-phosphate (K_i: 60 mmol/L). The saturation curve for glucose is slightly sigmoidal (Hill coefficient = 1.6), allowing the reaction to be most sensitive to a small change in glucose concentration in the physiological range of 5–10 mmol/L. The short term control is therefore essentially by substrate concentration. Long term control occurs at the level of protein synthesis, since the concentration of glucokinase in rat liver (3 units per g) is decreased by about 50% with prolonged fasting or in diabetes.

Inhibition by fructose 6-phosphate and deinhibition by fructose 1-phosphate: It has been recently observed that the phosphorylation of glucose by a liver extract is inhibited by as much as 70% by physiological concentrations of fructose 6-phosphate and that this inhibition is competitively released by fructose 1-phosphate. These effects, which are due to modifications of the affinity of the enzyme for glucose, are, however, not observed with purified glucokinase, unless another protein, called the regulatory protein, is also present (Van Schaftingen, 1989). This regulatory protein has been purified to near homogeneity (Van Schaftingen and Vandercammen, personal communication). Figure 9 shows the inhibition of purified glucokinase by millimolar concentrations of fructose 6-phosphate when incubated in the presence of the regulatory protein, and the competitive release of this inhibition by fructose 1-phosphate. The effective concentrations of fructose 1-phosphate are those reached in the liver in the presence of very low fructose concentrations.

The inhibition by fructose 6-phosphate (which is always in equilibrium with glucose 6-phosphate due to the action of glucose 6-phosphate isomerase), although incomplete, confers on glucokinase the property of product inhibition common to the other hexokinases. It results in a decrease in glucose uptake during the course of glycogenolysis and of intense gluconeogenesis, allowing an indirect control of glucokinase by cyclic AMP and fructose 2,6-bisphosphate. This inhibition also explains the fact that the K_m of glucokinase for glucose is about twice as large when measured in isolated hepatocytes (15–20 mmol/L) than with the purified enzyme (10 mmol/L).

The deinhibition by fructose 1-phosphate explains the long-standing observation that fructose favours glucose utilization (Hers, 1957; Seglen, 1974). Figure 10 shows that this effect of fructose is actually on the phosphorylation of glucose as measured

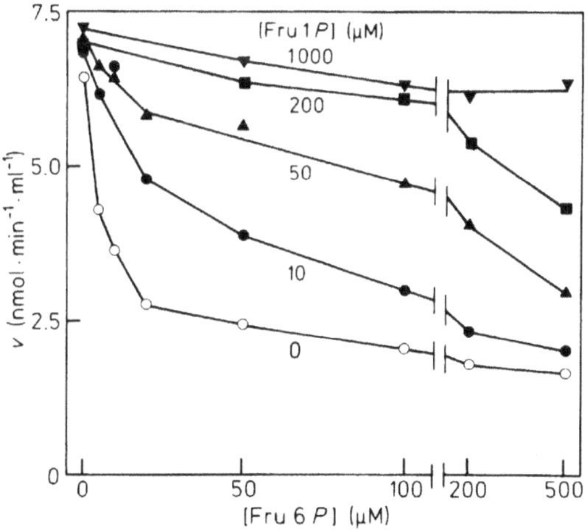

Figure 9 The effect of fructose 1-phosphate on the inhibition exerted on purified glucokinase by fructose 6-phosphate in the presence of the regulatory protein (from Van Schaftingen, 1989).

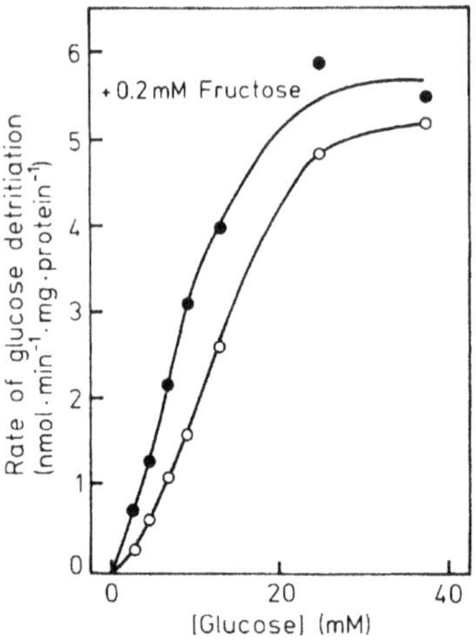

Figure 10 The effect of 0.2 mmol/L fructose on the affinity of glucokinase for glucose in hepatocytes isolated from an overnight fasted rat. The activity of glucokinase was measured by the formation of ^3H_2O from [2-^{3}H]glucose (from Van Schaftingen and Vandercammen, 1989).

in isolated hepatocytes by the release of [^3H_2O] from [2-^{3}H]glucose (Van Schaftingen and Vandercammen, 1989)).

Glucose 6-phosphatase

This enzyme catalyses the hydrolysis of glucose 6-phosphate into glucose and P_i. It plays a primary rôle in animal physiology because, with the exception of the small amount of glucose liberated by amylo-1,6-glucosidase and acid α-glucosidase, it is entirely responsible for the formation of endogenous glucose originating from gluconeogenesis and from glycogenolysis. Glucose 6-phosphatase is present in liver and kidney, and also in some species (including man) in the intestinal mucosa. It is bound to the endoplasmic reticulum and is therefore recovered in the microsomal fraction in the course of differential centrifugation. According to Arion *et al.* (1975; 1980), the hydrolysis of glucose 6-phosphate by the endoplasmic reticulum requires three components: (a) a glucose 6-phosphate specific transporter, called T_1, which mediates penetration of its substrate into the microsomal cisternae; (b) a phosphohydrolase localized on the luminal site of the reticulum network; and (c) a second translocase, called T_2, controlling the permeability of microsomes to P_i.

The liver of normally fed rats contains about 10 units of glucose 6-phosphatase per g and this amount is doubled by an overnight fast. The K_m of the undisrupted enzyme for glucose 6-phosphate is around 2 mmol/L, i.e. about 10-fold greater than the usual concentration of glucose 6-phosphate in the liver. The hydrolysis of glucose 6-phosphate is, therefore, a first order reaction, essentially controlled by substrate concentration.

Glucose uptake and output

As there is apparently no on/off mechanism of control of glucokinase and of glucose 6-phosphatase, these two enzymes are always simultaneously in operation in the liver. In such a recycling system, glucose uptake and output are the difference between the activities of glucokinase and of glucose 6-phosphatase. It has been calculated that, at a level of glycaemia equal to 5.7 mmol/L, the two activities would be equal to 0.9 μmol of substrate converted per minute per gram of liver and would balance each other, so that there is no net flux of metabolite through the system. Since the two enzymic activities are controlled by the concentration of their substrate, a net uptake occurs when the concentration of glucose is increased or/and when that of glucose 6-phosphate is decreased, as occurs for instance when glycogen synthesis is intense and exerts a pull on the concentration of the intermediary metabolites, UDPG and glucose 6-phosphate. Conversely, the large increase in glucose 6-phosphate concentration which occurs when glycogenolysis is stimulated greatly increases glucose output. The advantage of the system is that it allows very large changes of flux, controlled only by substrate concentration.

CONCLUSION

From the mechanisms which have been described in this paper, it appears that the primary function of the liver in the control of glucose homeostasis is to store glucose as glycogen. It is indeed only when the glycogen stores have been refilled that the liver converts the excess glucose to fatty acids which are exported as VLDL. This sequence of events occurs thanks to the low concentrations of hexose 6-phosphates which are maintained as long as glycogen synthesis is intense and which prevent the formation of fructose 2,6-bisphosphate and therefore glycolysis.

REFERENCES

Arion, W. J., Wallin, B. K., Lange, A. J. and Ballas, L. M. On the involvement of a glucose 6-phosphate transport system in the function of microsomal glucose 6-phosphatase. *Mol. Cell. Biochem.* 6 (1975) 75–83

Arion, W. J., Lange, A. J., Walls, H. E. and Ballas L. M. Evidence for the participation of independent translocases for phosphate and glucose 6-phosphate in the microsomal glucose-6-phosphatase system. *J. Biol. Chem.* 255 (1980) 10396–10406

Berridge, M. J. Inositol trisphosphate and diacylglycerol: two interacting second messengers. *Annu. Rev. Biochem.* 56 (1987) 159–193

Hers, H. G. Le Métabolisme du Fructose. *Editions Arsia*, Bruxelles (1957) pp. 200

Hers, H. G. The control of glycogen metabolism in the liver. *Annu. Rev. Biochem.* 45 (1976) 167–89

Hers, H. G. and Van Schaftingen, E. Fructose 2,6-bisphosphate. Two years after its discovery. *Biochem. J.* 206 (1982) 1–12

Hers, H. G. and Hue, L. Gluconeogenesis and related aspects of glycolysis. *Annu. Rev. Biochem.* 52 (1983) 617–653

Hers, H. G., Van Hoof, F. and de Barsy, T. The glycogen storage diseases. In: Scriver, C. R., Beaudet, A. L., Sly W. S. and Valle, D. (eds.), *The Metabolic Basis of Inherited Disease*, 6th edn., McGraw-Hill, New York, Vol. 1, 1989, 425–452

Kuwajima, M., Newgard, C., Foster, D. W. and McGarry, D. Time course and significance of changes in hepatic fructose 2,6-bisphosphate levels during refeeding of fasted rats. *J. Clin. Invest.* 74 (1984) 1108–1111

Mvumbi, L., Bollen, M., and Stalmans, W. Calcium ions and glycogen act synergistically as inhibitors of hepatic glycogen-synthase phosphatase. *Biochem. J.* 232 (1985) 697–704

Nishizuka, Y. The role of protein kinase C in cell surface signal transduction and tumour promotion. *Nature* 308 (1984) 693–698

Nordlie, R. C., Sukalski, A. and Alvarez, F. L. Responses of glucose 6-phosphate levels to varied glucose loads in the isolated perfused rat liver. *J. Biol. Chem.* 255 (1980) 1834–1838

Pilkis, S. J., El-Maghrabi, M. R. and Claus, T. H. Hormonal regulation of hepatic gluconeogenesis and glycolysis. *Annu. Rev. Biochem.* 57 (1988) 755–783

Roach, P. J., Warren, K. R. and Atkinson, D. E. Uridine diphosphate glucose synthase from calf liver: determinants of enzyme activity *in vitro*. *Biochemistry* 14 (1975) 544–5450

Seglen, P. O. Autoregulation of glycolysis, respiration, gluconeogenesis and glycogen synthesis in isolated parenchymal rat liver cells under aerobic and anaerobic conditions. *Biochem. Biophys. Acta* 338 (1974) 317–336

Soskin, S. The liver and carbohydate metabolism. *Endocrinology* 26 (1940) 297–308

Stalmans, W., Bollen, M., and Mvumbi, L. Control of glycogen synthesis in health and disease. *Diabetes/Metab. Rev.* 3 (1987) 127–161

Strickland, W. G., Imazu, M., Chrisman, T. D. and Exton, J. H. Regulation of rat liver glycogen synthase. Roles of Ca^{2+}, phosphorylase kinase and phosphorylase *a*. *J. Biol. Chem.* 258 (1983) 5490–5497

Tsuboi, K. K., Fukunaga, K. and Petricciani, J. C. Purification and specific kinetic properties of erythrocyte uridine diphosphate glucose pyrophosphorylase. *J. Biol. Chem.* 244 (1969) 1008–1015

Van Schaftingen, E. Fructose 2,6-bisphosphate. *Adv. Enzymol. Relat. Areas Mol. Biol.* 59 (1987) 315–395

Van Schaftingen, E. A protein from rat liver confers to glucokinase the property of being antagonistically regulated by fructose 6-phosphate and by fructose 1-phosphate. *Eur. J. Biochem.* 179 (1989) 179–184

Van Schaftingen, E. and Hers, H. G. Inhibition of fructose-1,6-bisphosphatase by fructose 2,6-bisphosphate. *Biochemistry* 78 (1981) 2861–2863

Van Schaftingen, E. and Vandercammen, A. Stimulation of glucose phosphorylation by fructose in isolated hepatocyte. *Eur. J. Biochem.* 179 (1989) 173–177

Van Schaftingen, E., Jett, M. F., Hue, L. and Hers, H. G. Control of liver 6-phosphofructokinase by fructose 2,6-bisphosphate and other effectors. *Biochemisty* 78 (1981) 3483–3486

Youn, J. H., Youn, M. S. and Bergman, R. N. Synergism of glucose and fructose in net glycogen synthesis in perfused rat livers. *J. Biol. Chem.* 261 (1986) 15960–15969

J. Inher. Metab. Dis. 13 (1990) 411–418

The Long-term Outcome of Patients with Glycogen Storage Diseases

G. P. A. Smit[1], J. Fernandes[1], J. V. Leonard[2], E. E. Matthews[2], S. W. Moses[3], M. Odievre[4] and K. Ullrich[5]
[1]*Department of Paediatrics, University Hospital of the University of Groningen, Oostersingel 59, 9713 EZ Groningen, The Netherlands;* [2]*Institute of Child Health, London, UK;* [3]*Department of Paediatrics, Soroko Medical Centre, Beer Sheba, Israel;* [4]*Service de Pédiatrie, Hôpital Antoine Beclere Clamart, France;* [5]*Klinik für Kinderheilkunde, Westfälische Wilhelms-Universität Münster, FRG*

Summary: In this retrospective study from five centres, 139 patients over 10 years of age with glycogen storage disease types I, III, VI and IX are described. Almost half of the patients with glycogen storage disease type Ia had retarded growth and most had hyperlipidaemia. One-third of the patients had adenomas, although none of these showed malignant transformations. With increasing age the growth, liver size and hyperlipidaemia of patients with glycogen storage disease type III improve. However, there was a high incidence of myopathy and cardiomyopathy. Patients with glycogen storage disease types VI and IX had a normal growth pattern after childhood. Hepatomegaly and hypercholesterolaemia, however, were still present in half of the patients.

As only limited information is available at present about the long-term outcome of patients with glycogen storage diseases (Huijing and Fernandes, 1969; Fernandes, 1975; Hers *et al.*, 1989) we reviewed all the patients with the more common types of glycogen storage disease who were under our care and over 10 years of age. We studied the growth and the complications in patients with glycogen storage disease type I (glucose-6-phosphatase deficiency), glycogen storage disease type III (debranching enzyme deficiency), glycogen storage disease type VI (phosphorylase deficiency) and glycogen storage disease type IX (phosphorylase-*b*-kinase deficiency).

Since the therapeutic approach to patients with the different types of glycogen storage disease is generally similar in the participating metabolic centres (Fernandes *et al.*, 1988) and specific information on treatment of individuals was not available, treatment is not discussed in detail.

PATIENTS AND METHODS

139 patients over 10 years of age with glycogen storage disease were included in this study: 41 patients with glycogen storage disease type 1a (16 females / 25 males), 5

patients with glycogen storage disease type Ib (4 females / 1 male), 50 patients with glycogen storage disease type III (25 females / 25 males), and 43 patients with glycogen storage disease types VI and IX (6 females / 37 males). Patients were diagnosed by enzyme assay of either liver biopsy or leukocytes. Since the two disorders of the phosphorylase system show very similar clinical and biochemical abnormalities they were combined.

Glycogen storage disease type 1a, glucose-6-phosphatase deficiency: This glycogen storage disease is the most severe type because both gluconeogenesis and glycogenolysis are impaired. Patients with this glycogen storage disease are characterized clinically by short stature, hepatomegaly, and enlarged kidneys. As the patients become older they may develop liver adenoma and glomerular sclerosis. Biochemically the patients often have marked hypoglycaemia together with hyperlactacidaemia, hyperlipidaemia and hyperuricaemia (Hers *et al.*, 1989).

Glycogen storage disease type Ib, glucose-6-phosphatase translocase deficiency: The majority of the clinical and biochemical symptoms of this glycogen storage disease are identical to those of glycogen storage disease type Ia, but the susceptibility to bacterial infections due to neutropenia and impaired neutrophil function reduces the number of patients who survive to older age. From the small number of patients reported in this study it is not possible to assess the long-term outcome which may reflect the poor long-term prognosis of this glycogen storage disease (Schaub and Heyne, 1983; Hers *et al.*, 1989).

Glycogen storage disease type III, debranching enzyme deficiency: Usually the clinical findings in this glycogen storage disease are less severe than in glycogen storage disease type I. Hepatomegaly, growth retardation and the propensity for hypoglycaemia seem to be age-related and become less severe with increasing age. Myopathy and cardiomyopathy, however, may become more clinically apparent (Hers *et al.*, 1989).

Glycogen storage disease types VI and IX, deficiencies of the liver phosphorylase system: Because of the similarity in clinical and biochemical parameters these two glycogen storage diseases were combined. Hepatomegaly and growth retardation usually resolve before puberty. In most patients hypoglycaemia is only seen during infections or prolonged fasting (Huijing and Fernandes, 1969; Fernandes, 1975; Hers *et al.*, 1989).

The definitions used in the study were as follows:

(1) Growth: patients's centiles were calculated for their own country and those below the 3rd centile were considered to have retarded growth.

(2) Hepatomegaly: a liver palpable more than 2 cm below the costal margin in the mid-clavicular line.

(3) Liver adenoma: detected by ultrasound investigation and/or computer tomography.

(4) Myopathy: clinical symptoms of myopathy defined by exercise intolerance and/or muscle wasting.

(5) Cardiomyopathy: defined by either clinical signs and/or abnormal ECG/echocardiogram.

(6) Mental development: regarded as 'normal' when patients were able to attend normal school.

(7) Hypoglycaemia: attacks of drowsiness, excessive sweating, hunger or diminished consciousness, with or without documented hypoglycaemia (blood glucose < 2.0 mmol/L).

(8) Hypercholesterolaemia: blood cholesterol concentration > 5.0 mmol/L.

(9) Hypertriglyceridaemia: blood triglyceride concentration > 2.0 mmol/L.

(10) Hyperuricaemia: when patients were on allopurinol treatment and/or blood uric acid concentration was < 0.36 mmol/L.

RESULTS

Glycogen storage disease type Ia

19 out of the 41 patients (16 females and 25 males) studied were below the 3rd centile and there was no apparent improvement with age (Figure 1). Hypoglycaemia was reported in only 6 out of 41 patients, but hepatomegaly was still present in 39 out of 40 patients on whom information was available, and 11 out of the 27 patients with quantitative measurement had marked hepatomegaly (greater than 10 cm in the mid-clavicular line).

Adenomas were detected in 11 out of 39 patients investigated by ultrasound or computer tomography. α1-Fetoprotein was reported to be within normal limits in a total of 22 patients, of whom 6 had liver adenomas.

Blood cholesterol concentration was elevated in 31 out of 38 reported patients and in 7 of these, the concentration was more than 10.0 mmol/L. Blood triglyceride concentration was also elevated in 29 out of 34 patients, of whom 18 had concentrations $\geqslant 4.0$ mmol/L. Blood uric acid concentration was found to be elevated in 19 out of 35 patients studied, and 12 of these patients were being treated with allopurinol.

Mental development was reported to be normal in 32 out of 37 patients.

Renal function was not investigated systematically in all centres. Unpublished data available from one centre, however, on glomerular filtration rates and renal plasma flow rates showed that virtually all patients had elevated values of both.

Limited information on treatment is available for 39 patients. Of these, 33 have or did receive nocturnal gastric drip feeding; the remaining 6 patients are on a frequent meal regimen. No differences could be detected between the two treatment groups.

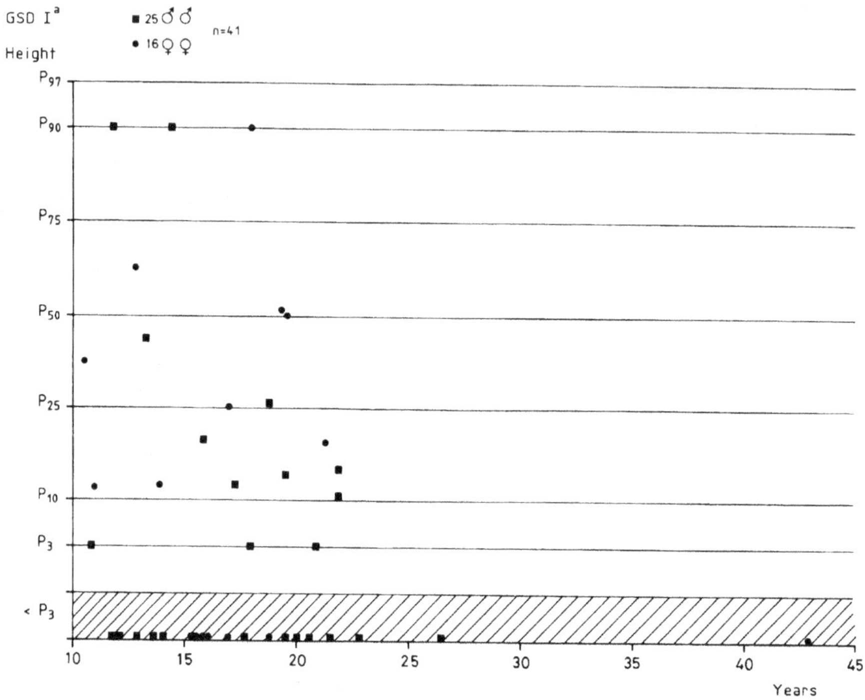

Figure 1 Height in centiles in GSD Ia patients over 10 years of age.

Glycogen storage disease type Ib

Four out of 5 reported patients were below the 3rd centile in height (Figure 2). However, it is not possible from the small number of patients to assess the long-term outcome.

Glycogen storage disease type III

Of the 50 patients (25 females and 25 males) reported, 18 were below the 3rd centile (Figure 3). An improvement in the growth in height with increasing age was apparent.

Hypoglycaemia was reported in only 4 out of the 50 patients.

Hepatomegaly was detected in 34 out of 50 patients, of whom 5 patients had a very large liver (⩾ 10 cm in the mid-clavicular line). The remaining 16 patients had a normal liver size; these patients were all over 15 years of age. Liver adenomas were reported in 3 out of 30 investigated patients.

Myopathy was diagnosed in 26 out of 41 reported patients and in 17 of these 26 patients cardiomyopathy was also present. Cardiomyopathy was diagnosed in a total

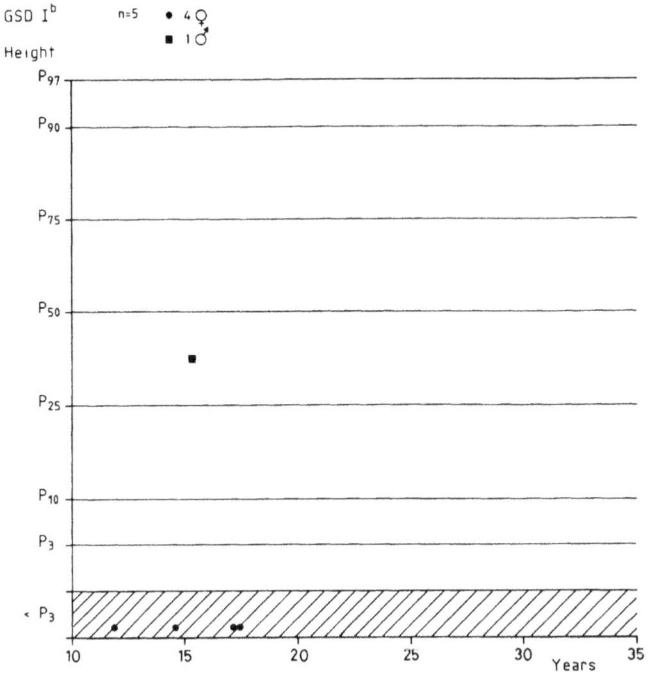

Figure 2 Height in centiles in GSD Ib patients over 10 years of age.

of 22 out of 44 reported patients. There was no correlation with age for either the myopathy or the cardiomyopathy.

Hypercholesterolaemia was present in 17 out of 44 reported patients and was seen mainly in patients below 20 years of age. Hypertriglyceridaemia was present in 14 out of 38 patients but there was no correlation with age. Mental development was reported to be normal in 41 out of 44 patients.

Glycogen storage disease types VI and IX

Four out of the 43 reported patients had growth retardation (Figure 4). The patients in this group had the most pronounced age-related improvement in height of all the types studied.

Hypoglycaemia was not reported. Hepatomegaly was present in 18 of the 43 patients, with no correlation with age.

Hypercholesterolaemia was present in 22 of the reported 41 patients and hypertriglyceridaemia in 7 out of 35. There was no correlation with age for either of the blood lipid concentrations.

Mental development was normal in all 42 reported patients.

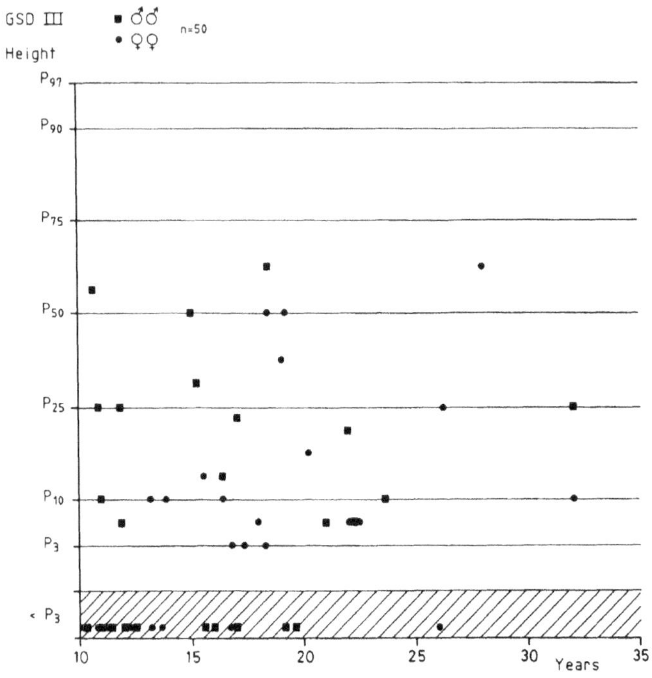

Figure 3 Height in centiles in GSD III patients over 10 years of age.

DISCUSSION

Glycogen storage disease type Ia

With increasing age hypoglycaemia becomes less of a problem. This improvement probably reflects the natural decrease in metabolic rate, and therefore glucose consumption expressed in kg bodyweight, rather than any real improvement in metabolic control. Cholesterol and triglyceride concentrations remain elevated in most patients, and may even become worse with increasing age, which suggests that despite the improvement metabolic control remains unsatisfactory. This is also reflected in the large number of patients who show retarded growth and have developed adenomas. Fortunately none of the patients with adenomas have developed elevated α1-fetoprotein concentrations or hepatocellular carcinoma, although this may still be a possible future threat (Coire *et al.*, 1987).

Another potential problem is the progressive glomerular injury leading to focal glomerulosclerosis (Chen *et al.*, 1988; Baker *et al.*, 1989), the prognosis and treatment of which needs further study in order to identify reliable and predictive indicators of future renal function and to develop possible long-term treatment.

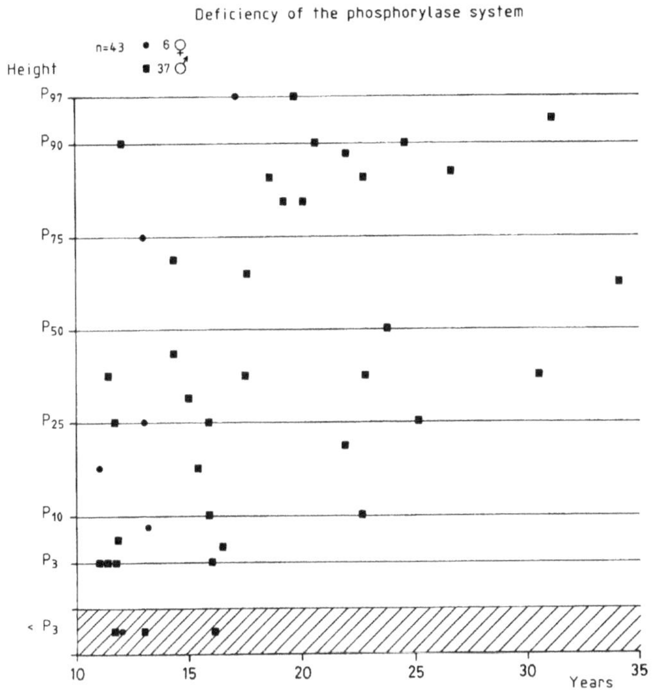

Figure 4 Height in centiles in GSD VI and IX patients over 10 years of age.

Glycogen storage disease type III

An age-related improvement was seen in this glycogen storage disease with respect to height, liver size and cholesterol concentration. However, there is a high incidence of cardiomyopathy, the importance of which in terms of long-term prognosis remains to be determined.

Glycogen storage disease types VI and IX

Virtually all patients with these glycogen storage disease types have normal growth patterns after childhood. Despite this improvement, however, in about half of the patients the liver remains palpable and the serum cholesterol concentration elevated.

CONCLUSION

From this retrospective study glycogen storage disease types VI and IX clearly have the best long-term follow-up results, and patients with glycogen storage disease type

Table 1 Long-term follow-up results for patients with different types of glycogen storage disease

	Type of glycogen storage disease		
	Ia (%)	*III* (%)	*VI/IX* (%)
Height < P3	46	36	9
Hepatomegaly	98	68	42
Hepatomegaly > 10 cm	41	10	0
Adenoma	28	10	0
Hypoglycaemia	15	8	0
Cholesterol > 5.0 mmol/L	82	39	54
Cholesterol > 10.0 mmol/L	18	0	0
Triglycerides > 2.0 mmol/L	85	37	20
Triglycerides > 4.0 mmol/L	53	13	0
Uric acid > 0.36 mmol/L	54		
Normal mental development	85	93	100

Ib, as expected, have the worst (Table 1). The high incidences of both adenoma and (probably) hyperfiltration were impressive and unexpected. The long-term prognosis for these types of glycogen storage disease must remain guarded.

REFERENCES

Baker, L., Dahlem, S., Godfarb, S., Kern, E. F. O., Stanley, C. A., Egler, J. and Heymans, S. Hyperfiltration and renal disease in glycogen storage disease, type I. *Kidney Int.* 35 (1989) 1345–1350

Chen, Y.-T., Coleman, R. A., Scheinmann, J. I., Kolbeck, P. C. and Sidbury, J. B. Renal disease in type I glycogen storage disease. *N. Engl. J. Med.* 318 (1988) 7–11

Coire, C. I., Qizilbash, A. H. and Castelli, M. F. Hepatic adenomata in type Ia glycogen storage disease. *Arch. Pathol. Lab. Med.* 111 (1987) 166–169

Fernandes, J. Hepatic glycogen storage disease. In: Raine, D. N. (ed.) *The Treatment of Metabolic Disease*, MTP Press, Lancaster, 1975, pp. 115–149

Fernandes, J., Leonard, J. V., Moses, S. W., Odievre, M., di Rocco, M., Schaub, J., Smit, G. P. A., Ullrich, K. and Durand, P. Glycogen storage disease: recommendations for treatment (review). *Eur. J. Pediatr.* 147 (1988) 226–228

Hers, H.-G., Van Hoof, F. and De Barsy, T. Glycogen storage diseases. In: Scriver, C. R., Beaudet, A. L., Sly, W. S. and Valle, D. (eds.) *The Metabolic Basis of Inherited Disease, 6th Edn.*, McGraw Hill, New York 1989 pp. 425–452

Huijing, F. and Fernandes, J. F. X-chromosomal inheritance of liver glycogenosis with phosphorylase kinase deficiency. *Am. J. Hum. Genet.* 21 (1969) 275–284

Schaub, J. and Heyne, K. Glycogen storage disease type Ib (review). *Eur. J. Pediatr.* 140 (1983) 283–288

J. Inher. Metab. Dis. 13 (1990) 419–434

Diagnosis of Glycogen Storage Disease

Y. S. SHIN
Children's Hospital, University of Munich, FRG

Summary: Glycogen storage diseases are associated with more than 15 different enzyme deficiencies and can be clinically divided mainly into two groups, those that affect primarily the liver and those that affect principally the muscle. In this report each glycogenosis has been clinically and biochemically documented and possibilities for an accurate and prompt diagnosis of the various types have been summarized. Most of the patients suffering from type II, type III, type IV and type VIa can easily be diagnosed by analysis of peripheral blood cells without the need for tissue biopsies. First trimester diagnosis using chorionic villi is feasible for severe forms of the glycogenoses, type IIa, type IIIa and type IV.

Glycogen storage disease comprises a group of inherited disorders characterized by abnormal glycogen metabolism. More than ten different types of the glycogenoses associated with an enzyme deficiency in glycogen metabolism have been identified to date (Figure 1 and Table 1). Type I glycogen storage disease (von Gierke's disease) was actually the first inborn error of metabolism in which the enzyme deficiency was demonstrated (Cori and Cori, 1954).

Clinically the glycogenoses can be divided into two main groups, one primarily affecting liver and the other muscle. There is also a third type of glycogen storage disease affecting only the heart muscle in which only a heart type isozyme of phosphorylase *b* kinase is apparently absent (Mitzuta *et al.*, 1984; Servidei *et al.*, 1988). It is not always easy to recognize heritable diseases by the clinical symptoms alone, especially in the glycogenoses where discrimination becomes complicated since there are not only different types but also different forms and subtypes with various degrees of symptoms involved. For an accurate diagnosis of these diseases it is obligatory to investigate the affected organs, i.e. liver or muscle, by determination of glycogen content and enzyme assays in biopsied samples. There are, however, many difficulties involved in this procedure. Biopsy is an invasive act, especially that of liver and cardiac muscle. In addition, the tissues to be biopsied should be in good condition without any damage. Furthermore, the assay should be carried out immediately after the tissues are obtained in order to avoid tissue deterioration, especially for the diagnosis of glycogen storage disease types Ib or Ic. The amount of tissue obtained by needle biopsy is often not sufficient for all tests, so that repetition of the biopsy is required in some cases. In order to ensure an easier and more accurate diagnosis of the glycogenoses, we have developed a procedure in which

Table 1 Various types of glycogen storage disease

Type	*Enzyme deficiency*	*Laboratory finding*	*Disturbed organ function*
Ia	Glucose-6-phosphatase	Hypoglycaemia Lactic acidaemia Hyperuricaemia	Hepatomegaly Nephromegaly
Ib	Glucose-6-phosphate translocase (T1)	Hypoglycaemia Lactic acidaemia Hyperuricaemia Neutropenia	Hepatomegaly Nephromegaly Splenomegaly Recurrent infections
Ic	Phosphotranslocase (T2)		Liver enlargement
II			
Infantile	Lysosomal glucosidase	Oligosaccharide excretion	Cardiomegaly
Juvenile	Lysosomal glucosidase	Oligosaccharide excretion	Cardiomegaly(?) Muscular hypotonia
Adult	Lysosomal glucosidase	Oligosaccharide excretion	Muscular hypotonia
III (a–h)	Amyloglucosidase	Hypoglycaemia(?) Lactic acidaemia(?)	Hepatosplenomegaly Cardiomegaly(?) Muscular hypotonia
IV			
Severe	Amylo-1,4:1,6-glucan transferase	Oligosaccharide excretion(?)	Hepatosplenomegaly Fatal liver cirrhosis Muscular hypotonia
Mild	Amylo-1,4:1,6-glucan transferase		Hepatomegaly(?) Muscular hypotonia(?)

continued

Table 1 *continued*

Type	*Enzyme deficiency*	*Laboratory finding*	*Disturbed organ function*
V			
	Phosphorylase (muscle)	Myoglobinuria(?)	Fatigue and cramp during exercise
Fatal form	Phosphorylase (muscle)		Respiratory failure
VI			
	Phosphorylase (liver)	Oligosaccharide in urine(?)	Hepatomegaly
VIa			
	Phosphorylase kinase (X-linked)	Fasting hypoglycaemia	Hepatomegaly Growth retardation(?)
	Phosphorylase kinase (autosomal recessive)	Fasting hypoglycaemia	Hepatomegaly
	Phosphorylase kinase (in heart)		Growth retardation(?) Cardiomyopathy Hepatosplenomegaly(?)
	Phosphorylase kinase (in skeletal muscle)		Muscular hypotonia
VII Mild form	Phosphofructokinase	Haemolysis Hyperuricaemia(?)	Exercise intolerance
Fatal form	Phosphofructokinase		Respiratory failure
0			
	Glycogen synthase	Lactic acidaemia(?) Fasting hypoglycaemia	Hepatomegaly(?)

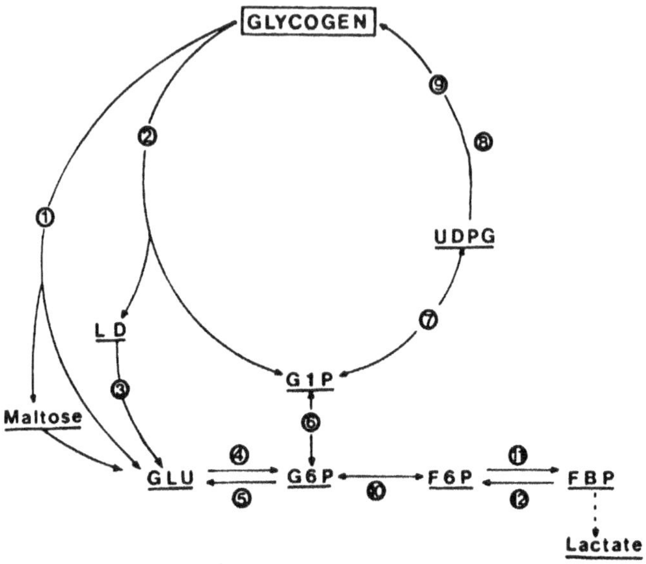

Figure 1 Metabolism of glycogen.
Enzymes: (1) lysosomal 1,4-α-glucosidase; (2) phosphorylase and phosphorylase kinase; (3) amylo-1,6-glucosidase; (4) glucokinase; (5) glucose-6-phosphatase; (6) phosphoglucomutase; (7) pyrophosphorylase; (8) branching enzyme; (9) glycogen synthase; (10) phosphoglucoisomerase; (11) phosphofructokinase; (12) fructose-1,6-bisphosphatase
Abbreviations:
FBP: fructose-1,6-bisphosphate
F6P: fructose-6-phosphate
GLU: glucose or glucosidase
G1P: glucose-1-phosphate
G6P: glucose-6-phosphate
LD: limit dextrin
UDPG: uridine diphosphoglucose

micro-assay techniques are applied using peripheral blood cells to establish the diagnosis.

The first part of this article deals with the diagnostic method for each glycogenosis and the second part describes how one generally proceeds with the investigation of suspected cases of glycogen storage disease.

MATERIALS AND METHODS

Materials: All radiochemicals were obtained from NEN Co., Dreieich, FRG or from Amersham-Buchler, Braunschweig, FRG. Enzyme preparations were from Sigma Chemie GmbH, FRG or from Boehringer-Mannheim, FRG. When not specified the other chemicals were from E. Merck Co., FRG or from Sigma Chemie GmbH, FRG.

Determination of glycogen: 100 μl erythrocytes (0.5 mg liver or 1.0 mg muscle) was added to 200 μl boiling water, heated for 3 min at 95°C, cooled and centrifuged. 50 μl of the supernatant was incubated with amyloglucosidase in 50 μl 0.1 mol/L sodium acetate buffer, pH 4.8 for 30 min at 30°C and the glucose produced was determined by the hexokinase/glucose-6-phosphate dehydrogenase method. The glycogen content was expressed as mg glucose produced per 100 ml for red cells and g glucose per 100 g fresh tissue for liver and muscle.

Glucose-6-phosphatase (EC 3.1.3.9) *assay*: Approximately 4 mg of liver biopsy, which can be kept at 4°C for up to 6 h without significant damage to the microsomal fractions, was carefully hand-homogenized in 500 μl of a 0.25 mol/L sucrose solution containing 2 mmol/L EDTA and centrifuged at 800 g for 3 min to remove debris. Half of the supernatant was treated further by sonification to disrupt microsomes. The glucose-6-phosphatase activity was determined in 20 μl of two different supernatants, one with intact microsomes and the other with disrupted microsomes, by adding 20 μl of the reaction mixture containing 10 mmol/L (^{14}C)glucose-6-phosphate (0.05 μCi), 100 mmol/L cacodylate buffer, pH 6.5 and 2 mmol/L EDTA. The reaction was carried out by incubating at 30°C for 90 min and was terminated by heating at 95°C for 2 min. The separation of the product, (^{14}C)glucose from the substrate, (^{14}C)glucose-6-phosphate was carried out on a mini DEAE-cellulose column as described for galactokinase assay (Shin-Buehring *et al.*, 1977). The non-specific phosphatase activity, the phosphotranslocase activity and the microsomal intactness of the samples was determined as described above for glucose-6-phosphatase using different radioactive substrates, glycerol-3-phosphate, carbamylphosphate and mannose-6-phosphate respectively. (^{14}C)Mannose-6-phosphate was prepared by treating (^{14}C)mannose with hexokinase and was purified by DEAE-cellulose column chromatography (Shin-Buehring *et al.*, 1977).

Determination of glucose transport: 5 ml of heparinized blood, which can be kept for up to 7 h at room temperature without a significant loss of polymorphonuclear-neutrophils, was mixed with 10 ml of 0.154 mmol/L NaCl containing 3% dextran. After 1 h the supernatants were layered on a Ficoll-Paque solution with a ratio of 2 volumes to 1 and centrifuged at 400 *g* for 30 min at 4°C. The red cells in the pellets were disrupted by stirring with 500 μl of cold distilled water for 20 s. The remaining cells were washed twice with saline and suspended in 150 μl of Krebs-Ringer-phosphate solution containing (^{3}H)2-desoxyglucose (0.25 μCi). After 0, 5 and 10 min incubation at 30°C, 20 μl of the mixture was pipetted into a mini-tube containing 500 μl of ice-cold saline, centrifuged at 900 *g* for 2 min, the cells were washed once more with cold saline and the final pellets were sonicated in 100 μl of water. 20 μl of the preparation was used for protein determination and the rest for the radioactivity measurement. The rate of glucose transport was expressed as nmol desoxyglucose taken up by the cells per min per mg protein.

Acid α-1,4,-glucosidase (*EC* 3.2.1.20) *assay*: The enzyme assay was carried out as described by Shin and colleagues (1985) using methylumbelliferylglucose as the substrate. For the enzyme assay in leukocytes and chorionic villi a specific antibody preparation for the enzyme was necessary (Shin *et al.*, 1985; Grubisic *et al.*, 1986).

Measurement of the incorporation rate of radioactive substrates into glycogen: As shown in Table 2, various radioactive substrates were used for different enzyme assays. The separation of glycogen from the substrates was performed by Sephadex G-50 column chromatography (Shin *et al.*, 1984). On a 0.9 × 40 cm column, glycogen eluted in the void volume (5.5–8.5 ml) and the substrates about the total volume with water (Figure 2). The enzyme activity was expressed as nmol substrate incorporated into glycogen per min per mg protein or g Hb.

Table 2 Enzyme assay by Sephadex column chromatography (separation of glycogen from various substrates)

Enzyme	*GSD type*	*Substrate*	*Enzyme added*
Amyloglucosidase	III	Glucose	None
Phosphorylase	V,VI	Glucose-1-phosphate	None
Phosphorylase *b* kinase	VIa	Glucose-1-phosphate	Phosphorylase *b*
Glycogen synthase	0	UDP-glucose	None
Branching enzyme	IV	UDP-glucose	Glycogen synthase

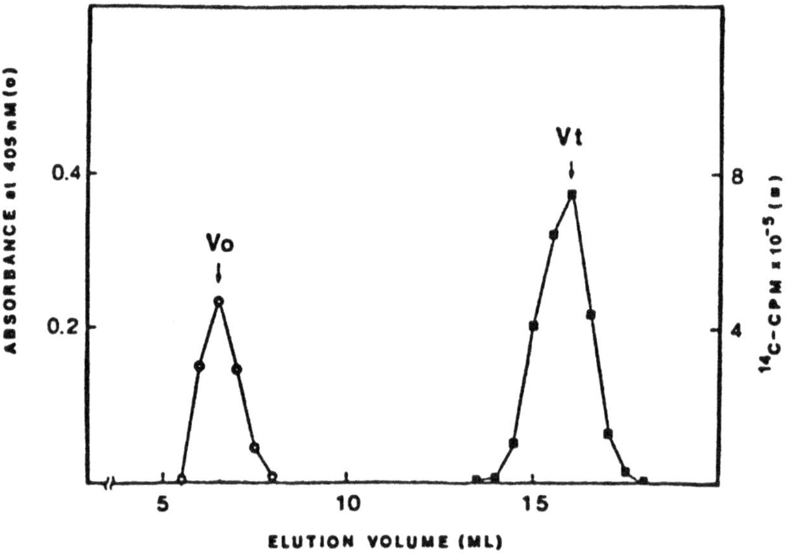

Figure 2 Separation of glycogen from glucose on a Sephadex G-50 column. Column size: 0.7 × 40 cm; elution buffer: distilled water; Vo = void volume; Vt = total volume. (○) = glycogen, (■) = (^{14}C)glucose

Phosphorylase b-kinase assay (*EC* 2.7.1.38): The washed red cells were diluted 4-fold with water. The samples of leukocytes, liver, fibroblasts and chorionic villi were sonicated in water to have protein concentrations of approximately 1.2, 0.5, 0.8 and 0.7 mg/ml. 50 μl samples were incubated in 50 μl of the reaction mixture containing 80 mmol/L tris-β-glycerophosphate buffer, pH 8.2 (for red cells pH 6.8), 12 mmol/L ATP, 20 mmol/L magnesium acetate and 1 U phosphorylase *b*. After 0 and 15 min incubation at 32°C, 20 μl of the mixture was added to 600 μl of ice-cold solution containing 0.1 mol/L NaF and 5 mmol/L EDTA. The measurement of the phosphorylase activity was carried out by incubating 50 μl of the above mixture with 50 μl of the reaction mixture pH 6.1 containing 0.1 mol/L glucose-1-phosphate, 2% glycogen and 1 mol/L NaF for 30 min at 32°C. The activity was expressed as μmol phosphate produced per min per g Hb (or mg protein).

Spectrophotometric method for branching enzyme (*EC* 2.4.1.18) *assay*: Washed red cells were diluted 60-fold and the tissues or the cultured cells were sonicated in water to give a protein concentration between 0.03 and 0.1 mg/ml. The reaction was carried out by incubating 50 μl samples with 50 μl of the reaction mixture pH 6.5 containing 250 mmol/L glucose-1-phosphate, 7 mmol/L AMP and 1.0 U phosphorylase *a*. The blank was prepared by using samples which had been heat-denatured prior to the addition of the reaction mixture. After 30 min incubation at 32°C, the reaction was terminated by heating at 95°C for 3 min. The activity was expressed as μmol phosphate released per min per g Hb or mg protein.

Phosphofructokinase (*EC* 2.7.1.11) *assay*: Washed red cells were diluted 200-fold and the muscle tissue was hand-homogenated in 0.1 mol/L potassium phosphate buffer, pH 7.6 to obtain a protein concentration of 0.1–0.2 mg/ml. The reaction was carried out by incubating 50 μl samples with 50 μl of the reaction mixture containing 0.07 mol/L potassium phosphate buffer pH 7.6, 7 mmol/L $MgCl_2$, 0.7 mmol/L ATP, 0.3 mmol/L EDTA, 3 mmol/L dithiothreitol, 1.4 mmol/L NH_4Cl and 0.7 mmol/L (^{14}C)fructose-6-phosphate (0.05 μCi). After 20 min incubation at 32°C, the reaction was terminated by heating at 95°C for 3 min. The fructose-bisphosphate fraction produced was separated from fructose-6-phosphate by a mini DEAE-cellulose chromatography (Shin-Buehring *et al*., 1977).

RESULTS

Diagnosis of various glycogenoses

Table 3 summarizes the results of glucose-6-phosphatase assay in liver. These data show that a liver biopsy can be transported at 4°C if the laboratory can be reached within 5–6 h. As shown in Figure 3, the rate of desoxyglucose transport is a convenient means of distinguishing type Ib glycogenosis from type Ia. This can easily be used for the confirmation of the diagnosis, e.g. in cases of clinically suspected glycogen storage disease type I with an elevated glycogen content and a normal glucose-6-phosphatase activity in frozen liver. However, the diagnosis using only the

Table 3 The activity of the glucose-6-phosphatase system in liver biopsy[a]

Subject	*Diagnosis*	*Glycogen*	*Phosphatase activity*[b]	
			Glucose-6-phosphate	*Mannose-6-phosphate*
A	GSD Ia	10.5	2.7 (2.2)	2.0 (1.7)
B	GSD Ia	10.3	1.7 (1.5)	1.4 (1.1)
C	GSD Ib	8.1	33.3 (13.4)	37.0 (15.8)
D	GSD Ib	8.2	42.0 (3.9)	31.3 (3.2)
E	GSD Ib	7.9	25.6 (8.8)	22.1 (9.4)
F	GSD VIa	13.8	53.7 (51.8)	38.9 (2.1)
G	FBPase def.[c]	5.3	25.8 (27.6)	18.9 (2.5)

[a]All samples were kept at 4°C for 4–7 h after the biopsy. They were transported from different places in Germany

[b]The values in parentheses are from the homogenate preparation with intact microsomes and all activities are expressed as nmol min^{-1} (mg protein)$^{-1}$

[c]Fructose-1,6-bisphosphatase deficiency

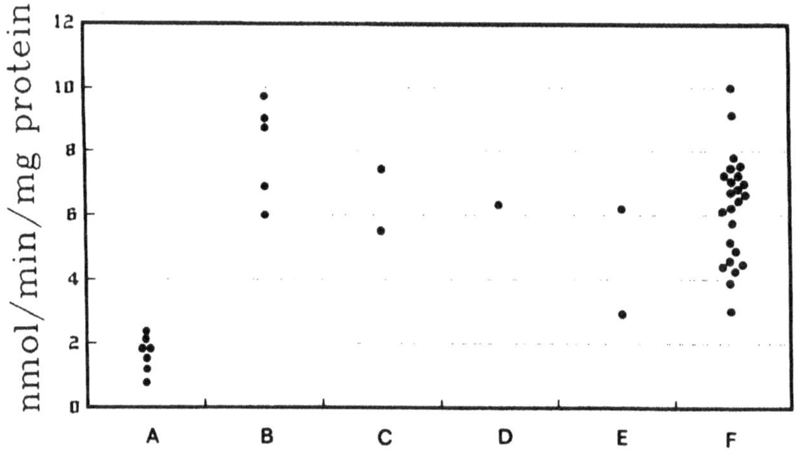

Figure 3 Desoxyglucose transport in polymorphonuclearneutrophils. A = type Ib GSD; B = type Ia GSD; C = heterozygous for type Ib; D = type III GSD; E = type VIa GSD (liver form); F = controls

polymorphonuclear neutrophil study may not be optimal until the mechanisms of the transport system in these cells are completely understood. It would be interesting, however, to study this system in patients with other glycogen storage disease types such as Ic or possibly Id (Nordlie *et al.*, 1983; Burchell *et al.*, 1987). Up to now a fetal liver biopsy has been the only method of prenatal diagnosis of this disease (Golbus *et al.*, 1988), since no enzyme activity has been measured in culture cells or in chorionic villi (Shin *et al.*, 1986a). The identification and study of the gene responsible for this disease may therefore contribute a major step towards achieving the diagnosis in the fetus.

For the diagnosis of different forms of Pompe's disease (infantile, juvenile and adult form), muscle biopsy or fibroblast cultures are commonly used (Reuser *et al.*, 1987). In our experience, crude homogenates of leukocytes and the use of antibody preparations is sufficient to detect the various forms of type II glycogen storage disease as well as the respective heterozygotes (Shin *et al.*, 1985; Figure 4). In Table 4, examples of the diagnosis of type II glycogen storage disease using leukocytes and the confirmation by biopsy samples are shown. Prenatal diagnosis using chorionic villi has become routine (Grubisic, 1986; Shin *et al.*, 1989). It is noteworthy that one can predict heterozygosity reasonably well by measuring the enzyme activity in the chorionic villi (Shin *et al.*, 1989).

Diagnosis of type III glycogen storage disease can be easily established by analysing red cells. In all the cases we have investigated the glycogen content was increased (20–50 mg/dl) and amyloglucosidase activity was absent in red cells of the patients with type III glycogen storage disease. Heterozygotes have an intermediate level of enzyme activity (Shin *et al.*, 1984). However, in view of the numerous biochemical subtypes (van Hoof and Hers, 1967) as well as a type III glycogen storage disease case with normal enzyme activity in red cells (Gutman *et al.*, 1985), it is recommended that other tissues should be investigated in clinically suspected cases which have normal activity in red cells. So far all our cases with this type of glycogen storage disease showed a deficient enzyme activity in red cells but their clinical features were rather variable. In two patients a liver biopsy was analysed to confirm the diagnosis and absent enzyme activity was found in this tissue as well. In another patient deficient activity was also observed in liver, muscle and fibroblasts (Table 4). Prenatal diagnosis is possible by analysis of cultured amniotic fluid cells or direct assay of chorionic villi (Shin *et al.*, 1989).

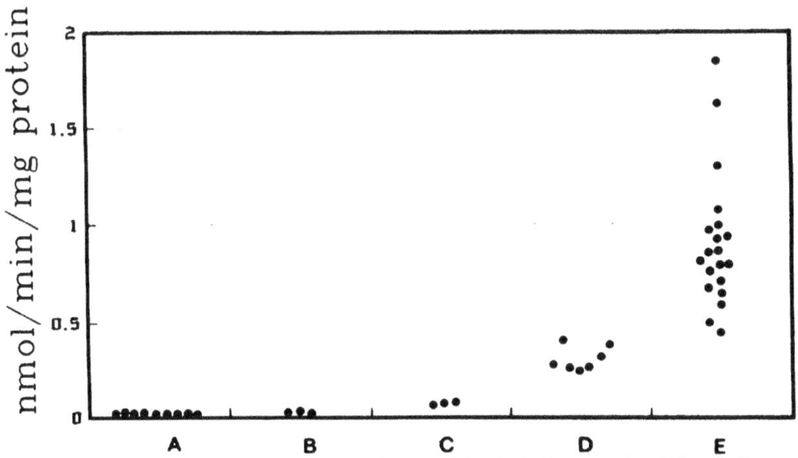

Figure 4 The lysosomal acid 1,4-α-glucosidase activity in leukocytes. A = infantile form of Pompe's disease; B = juvenile form; C = adult form; D = heterozygotes; E = controls

Table 4 Diagnosis of glycogenoses by analysis of blood cells and the confirmation with tissue biopsy samples

Type	*Sample*	*Activity*[a]	*Normal range*
II (infantile)	Leukocytes	0.02	0.5–2.0
	Muscle	0.01	0.3–3.0
II (adult)	Leukocytes	0.09	0.5–2.0
	Fibroblasts	0.10	1.0–7.0
III	Erythrocytes	0, 0	0.6–3.0
	Liver	0.03, 0	1.0–5.0
	Muscle	0.02	0.6–3.5
IV (severe)	Erythrocytes	0.09	5.0–15.0[b]
	Liver	0.01	0.3–2.0[b]
IV (mild)	Erythrocytes	1.66	5.0–15.0[b]
	Fibroblasts	0	0.5–3.0[b]
VI (1)	Erythrocytes	8.9	30–90[c]
	Liver	14.7	30–110[c]
VI (2)	Leukocytes	6.7	20–70[c]
	Liver	8.9	30–110[c]

[a]All activities are expressed per mg protein except for erythrocytes (per g Hb)
[b]By the spectrophotometric method using glucose-1-phosphate as a substrate and phosphorylase *a* as an additional enzyme
[c]Total phosphorylase activity

We have previously shown that in patients with type IV glycogen storage disease the branching enzyme activity is deficient not only in fibroblasts but also in erythrocytes (Shin *et al.*, 1988). As shown in Figure 5, heterozygotes can be distinguished by the erythrocyte enzyme activity. Prenatal diagnosis of this disease

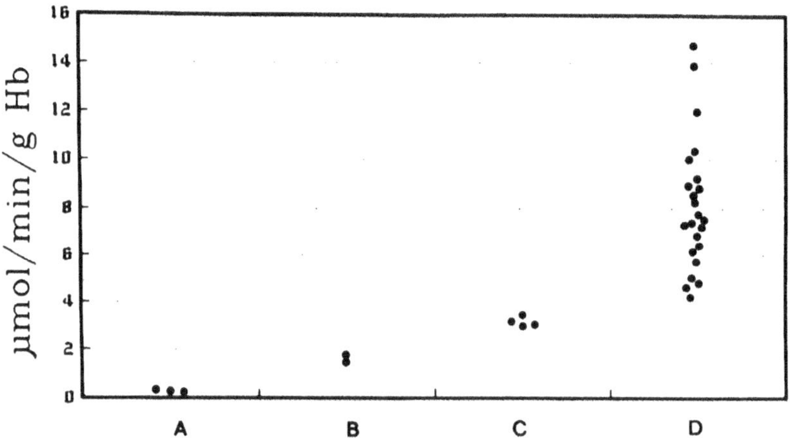

Figure 5 The branching enzyme activity in red blood cells. A = severe form of type IV GSD; B = mild form; C = heterozygotes for the group IA; D = controls

can therefore be performed with cultured amniocytes or chorionic villi (Brown and Brown, 1989). We have found that branching enzyme activity can be determined in uncultured chorionic villi; however, the feasibility of the diagnosis using the direct assay of chorionic villi is still to be tested (Shin *et al.*, 1988).

For the diagnosis of phosphorylase deficiency in skeletal muscle and liver (types V and VI glycogen storage disease, respectively) the use of the specific tissue biopsy is the most secure method. It is known that the phosphorylase activity in peripheral blood cells is the sum of the activities of various isoenzymes and therefore the activity in red cells or in leukocytes is not always representative of that in the liver or muscle (Table 4). Since the clinical symptoms are mild and the prognoses are good, it may not always be necessary to confirm the clinical diagnosis by the respective tissue biopsy. Recent progress in the molecular studies of phosphorylases may soon offer a better and easier method for detection of various phenotypes of types V and VI glycogen storage disease.

Many subgroups of phosphorylase kinase deficiency (designated as types VIa, VIII or IX) have been described (de Barsy and Lederer, 1980; Hug, 1980). In the most common subtype, an X-linked liver phosphorylase *b* kinase deficiency, both the homozygotes and heterozygotes can be easily identified by analysis of erythrocytes (Besley, 1987, Figure 5). The clinical severity of this form correlates well with the elevation of the glycogen content and the amyloglucosidase activity (Shin *et al.*, 1986b; Table 5).

The autosomal recessive form of phosphorylase *b* kinase deficiency often manifests itself with severe clinical disability and can be mistaken for type I glycogen storage disease. Two of our three female patients had been originally suspected of having type I glycogen storage disease. It is interesting to note that the glycogen content in red cells of these patients is relatively low considering the severity of the symptoms (Table 5). In addition, we have recently observed four male patients in a large pedigree of an Austrian family who had deficient phosphorylase *b* kinase activity only in the liver and a decreased activity in leukocytes. In erythrocytes from these patients,

Table 5 Clinical and biochemical variability of the liver form of phosphorylase *b* kinase deficiency

Parameter	*Group*					
	A (n = 6)	*B (n = 4)*	*C (n = 3)*	*D (n = 3)*	*E (n = 3)*	*Controls*
Sex	Male	Male	Male	Male	Female	Both
Clinical severity	±	+	+ + +	+ +	+ + +(+)	None
In erythrocytes						
Phosphorylase *b* kinase	15–25	7–10	≤ 5	70–90	3–5	80–200
Phosphorylase[a]	2–30	14–17	7–15	30–40	21–25	20–80
Amyloglucosidase	2.2–3.8	4.0–4.4	5.9–14	1.5–3.0	4.9–7.8	0.6–3.0
Glycogen	2.0–17	15–20	180–600	8–10	16–30	0–10
In liver						
Phosphorylase *b* kinase	nd[b]	nd	nd	1.0,0,97	0.47	4–24
Glycogen	nd	nd	nd	13.5,15.0	10.5–15.0	2–6

[a]Phosphorylase *a* activity
[b]nd = not determined

however, the glycogen content and the phosphorylase *b* kinase activity were completely normal.

Hepatic phosphorylase *b* kinase deficiency with a normal enzyme activity in leukocytes has been also described (Alvarado *et al.*, 1988), therefore the use of liver biopsy is unavoidable in special situations. Likewise, diagnosis of phosphorylase *b* kinase deficiency in heart (Mitzuta *et al.*, 1984; Servidei *et al.*, 1988) can only be performed at present using cardiac muscle biopsy. In view of the multiple enzyme forms present in the phosphorylase *b* kinase system, it is not entirely surprising to have such a variety of phenotypes for phosphorylase *b* kinase deficiency. Studies of molecular genetics may elaborate phosphorylase *b* kinase deficiency more precisely, so that the differentiation of the various forms becomes easier in the future.

Other types of glycogen storage disease, phosphofructokinase deficiency (type VII), glycogen synthase deficiency (type 0), phosphoglucomutase deficiency and others have not yet been observed in the patients studied in our laboratory. It is known that phosphofructokinase deficiency can be diagnosed by analysing erythrocytes, since the enzyme in red cells consists of a mixture of the liver and the muscle isozymes (Vora *et al.*, 1980). As in the case of muscle phosphorylase deficiency (DiMauro and Hartlage, 1979) a severe form of type VII glycogen storage disease can be fatal (Guibaud *et al.*, 1978). Glycogen synthase deficiency was reported to be detected by the enzyme assay in liver (Aynsley-Green *et al.*, 1977).

A general procedure for the diagnosis of glycogenoses

Table 6 lists the type of peripheral blood cells which can be used for the differential diagnosis of glycogen storage disease. All the investigations can be performed on less than 5 ml whole blood using the microanalytic techniques described above. When the blood is anticoagulated with liquid heparin, all parameters to be determined are stable for at least several days at room temperature so that the samples can be

Table 6 Differential diagnosis of glycogenoses with peripheral blood cells

Type	*Blood cells*	*Determination*	*Heterozygote detection*
Ib Ic(?)	Polymorphonuclear neutrophils	Desoxyglucose transport	No
II	Leukocytes	Acid α-glucosidase	Yes
	Lymphocytes	Acid α- glucosidase	
III	Erythrocytes	Amyloglucosidase	Yes
	Erythrocytes	Glycogen	
IV	Erythrocytes	Branching enzyme	Yes
	Leukocytes	Branching enzyme	
VI	Erythrocytes	Phosphorylase	?
	Leukocytes	Phosphorylase	
VIa	Erythrocytes	Phosphorylase kinase	Yes
	Leukocytes	Glycogen	
		Phosphorylase *a*	
VII	Erythrocytes	Phosphofructokinase	?

Table 7 Distribution of the types of glycogenosis in 111 patients detected in our laboratory (1982–1988)

Type	*Total number*	*Initial detection in*	
		Blood cells	*fetus*
Ia	15	0	0
Ib	15	6	0
II (infantile)	15	8	6
II (juvenile)	3	3	0
II (adult)	3	3	0
III	25	22	1
IV	5	2	1
V	2	0	0
VI	4	2	0
VIa	27	22	0
Total	114	68	8

transported by special mail. Even though a careful examination of clinical symptoms can help a great deal in focusing the biochemical investigation, clinical diagnosis is not always accurate due to the overlapping of diverse clinical expressions between the groups and the subtypes. It is, however, quite time-consuming to do all the analyses. We have therefore devised a simple scheme for the diagnosis, and especially for the exclusion, of many glycogen storage diseases (Figure 6). When the liver is involved in the suspected patients and the glycogen level in red cells is over 10 mg/100 ml, the assay of amyloglucosidase and phosphorylase *b* kinase in erythrocytes will lead to the diagnosis of types III and VIa glycogen storage disease respectively. When the glycogen level in red cells is normal, phosphorylases and branching enzyme should be tested in red and white cells. When all parameters are normal, liver biopsy should be performed in order to detect type I glycogen storage diseases and other atypical liver forms of glycogen storage disease. At this point measurement of the desoxyglucose transport in polymorphonuclearneutrophils (before or after the biopsy) would help in confirming the diagnosis of type Ib. When the glycogen concentration in liver is low, the assay of glycogen synthase may be the next step. In cases with an elevated glycogen level in liver but a normal glucose-6-phosphatase activity, it is advisable to assay phosphorylase and phosphorylase *b* kinase to detect variant forms of types VI or VIa glycogen storage disease.

For the mild forms of muscle glycogen storage disease the following enzymes can be analysed in blood cells: phosphorylases, phosphorylase *b* kinase and acid α-glucosidase in white blood cells and phosphofructokinase in red cells. Various forms of Pompe's disease can easily be detected by the enzyme assay in leukocytes or lymphocytes. For other muscle forms of glycogen storage disease such as type V and muscle deficiency, a muscle biopsy may still be needed for an accurate diagnosis. Except for types III and VIa glycogen storage disease, the diagnostic procedure using the specific tissue biopsy is a direct proof of glycogen storage. However, this procedure of investigating blood cells before tissue biopsy saves a great deal of time and effort in achieving the correct diagnosis. Early diagnosis of glycogen storage diseases,

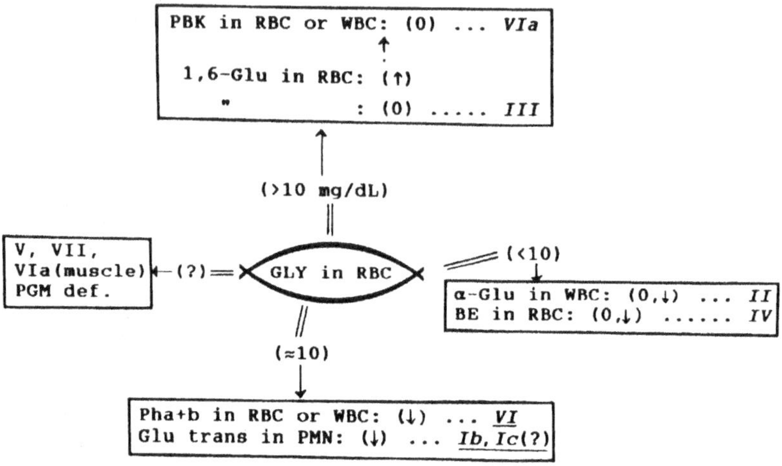

Figure 6 Schematic illustration of the GSD diagnostic procedure. (↑) = elevation; (↓) = decrease; (?) = not known
Abbreviations:
BE: branching enzyme
def.: deficiency
Glu: glucose or glucosidase
GLY: glycogen
PBK: phosphorylase *b* kinase
PGM: phosphoglucomutase
PMN: polymorphonuclearneutrophils
RBC: red blood cells
WBC: white blood cells

especially type I (Burchell *et al.*, 1989), is indeed very important since prompt management of the disease will in some cases save the life of the suffering patients.

ACKNOWLEDGEMENT

This work is supported in part by the Deutsche Forschungsgemeinschaft grant, Sh 17/1-1.

REFERENCES

Alvarado, L. J. F., Gasca-Centeno, E. and Grier, R. E. Hepatic phosphorylase *b* kinase deficiency with normal enzyme activity in leukocytes. *J. Pediatr.* 113 (1988) 865–867

Aynsley-Green, A., Williamson, D. H., Gitzelmann, R. Hepatic glycogen synthetase deficiency. *Arch. Dis. Child.* 52 (1977) 573–575

Bashan, N., Iancu, T. C., Lerner, A., Fraser, D., Potashnik, R. and Moses, S. W. Glycogenosis

due to liver and muscle phosphorylase kinase deficiency. *Pediatr. Res.* 15 (1981) 299–303
Besley, G. T. N. Phosphorylase *b* kinase deficiency in glycogenosis type VIII: Differentiation of different phenotypes and heterozygotes by erythrocyte enzyme assay. *J. Inher. Metab. Dis.* 10 (1987) 115–118
Brown, B. I., Brown, D. H. Branching enzyme activity of cultured amniocytes and chorionic villi: Prenatal testing for type IV glycogen storage disease. *Am. J. Hum. Genet.* 44 (1989) 378–381
Burchell, A., Jung, R. T., Lang, C. C., Bennet, W. and Shepard, A. N. Diagnosis of type Ia and type Ic glycogen storage diseases in adults. *Lancet* 1 (1987) 1059–1062
Burchell, A., Bell, J. E., Busuttil, A. and Hume, R. Hepatic microsomal glucose-6-phosphatase system and sudden infant death syndrome. *Lancet* 2 (1989) 291–294
Cori, G. T. and Cori, C. F. Glucose-6-phosphatase of the liver in glycogen storage disease. *J. Biol. Chem.* 199 (1952 661
De Barsy, T. and Lederer, B. Type VI glycogenosis: identification of subgroups. In Burman, D., Holton, J. B. and Pennock, C. A. (eds.), *Inherited Disorders of Carbohydrate Metabolism*, MTP Press, Lancaster, 1980, pp. 369–380
DiMauro, S. and Hartlage, P. L. Fatal infantile form of muscle phosphorylase deficiency. *Neurology* 29 (1979) 1124
Golbus, M. S., Simpson, T. J., Koresawa, M., Appelman, Z. and Alpers, C. E. The prenatal determination of glucose-6-phosphatase activity by fetal liver biopsy. *Prenatal Diag.* 8 (1988) 401–404
Grubisic, A., Shin, Y. S., Meyer, W., Endres, W., Becker, U. and Wischerath, H. First trimester diagnosis of Pompe's disease (glycogenosis type II) with normal outcome – assay of acid α-glucosidase in chorionic villous biopsy using antibodies. *Clin. Genet.* 30 (1986) 298–302
Guibaud, P., Carrier, H., Mathieu, M., Dorche, C., Parchoux, B., Béthenod, M. and Larbre, F. Observation familiale de dystrophie musculaire congenitale par deficit en phosphofructokinase. *Arch. Fr. Pédiatr.* 35 (1978) 1105-1115
Gutman, A., Barash, V., Schramm, R. J., Deckelbaum, J., Granot, E., Aker, M. and Kohn, G. Incorporation of (^{14}C)glucose into α-1,4 bonds of glycogen by leukocytes and fibroblasts of patients with type III glycogen storage disease. *Pediatr. Res.* 19 (1985) 28–32
Hug, G. Pre- and postnatal diagnosis of glycogen storage disease. In Burman, D., Holton, J. B. and Pennock, C. A. (eds.), *Inherited Disorders of Carbohydrate Metabolism*, MTP Press, Lancaster, 1980, pp. 327-367
Mizuta, K., Kashimoto, E., Tsutou, A., Eishi, Y., Takemura, T., Narisawa, K. and Yamamura, H. A new type of glycogen storage disease caused by deficiency of cardiac phosphorylase kinase. *Biochem. Biophys. Res. Commun.* 119 (1984) 582–587
Nordlie, R. C., Sukalski, K. A., Munoz, J. M. and Baldwin, J. J. Type Ic, a novel glycogenosis. *J. Biol. Chem.* 258 (1983) 9739–9744
Reuser, A. J. J., Kroos, M., Willemsen, R., Swallow, D., Tager, J. M., Galjaard, H. Clinical diversity in glycogenosis type II. *J. Clin. Invest.* 79 (1987) 1689–1699
Servidei, S., Metlay, L. A., Chodosh, J. and DiMauro, S. Fatal infantile cardiopathy caused by phosphorylase *b* kinase deficiency. *J. Pediatr.* 113 (1988) 82–85
Shin, Y. S., Rieth, M., Ungar, R. and Endres, W. A. A simple method for amylo-1,6-glucosidase assay. Detection of heterozygotes for type III glycogenosis in erythrocytes. *Clin. Chem.* 30 (1984) 1717–1718
Shin, Y. S., Endres, W., Unterreithmeier, J., Rieth, M. and Schaub, J. Diagnosis of Pompe's disease using leukocyte preparations. Kinetic and immunological studies of 1,4-α-glucosidase in human fetal and adult tissues and cultured cells. *Clin. Chim. Acta* 148 (1985) 9–21
Shin, Y. S., Friedel, J., Besser, A., Rieth, M., Gerg, J. and Endres, W. Glycogen metabolism in chorionic villous samplings: possibilities for prenatal diagnosis of glycogen storage diseases. *Pediatr. Res.* 20 (1986a) 1058
Shin, Y. S., Rieth, M. and Endres, W. Clinical and biochemical variability phosphorylase *b* kinase deficiency: its differentiation using erythrocyte parameters. *Proc. Soc. Study Inborn Error Metab.* (1986b) p. 87

Shin, Y. S., Steigüber, H., Klemm, P., Endres, W., Schwab, O. and Wolff, G. Branching enzyme in erythrocytes. Detection of type IV glycogenosis homozygotes and heterozygotes. *J. Inher. Metab. Dis.* 11 Suppl. 2 (1988) 252–254

Shin, Y. S., Rieth, M., Tausendfreund, J. and Endres, W. First trimester diagnosis of glycogen storage disease type II and type III. *J. Inher. Metab. Dis.* 12 Suppl. 2 (1989) 289–291

Shin-Buehring, Y. S., Osang, M., Ziegler, R. and Schaub, J. A. Simple assay for galactokinase using DEAE-cellulose column chromatography. *Clin. Chim. Acta* 74 (1977) 1–5

Van Hoof, F. and Hers, H. F. The subgroups of type III glycogenosis. *Eur. J. Biochem.* 2 (1967) 265–269

Vora, S., Seaman, C., Durham, S. and Piomelli, S. Isozymes of human phosphofructokinase: Identification and subunit structural characterization of a new system. *Proc. Natl. Acad. Sci. USA* 77 (1980) 62–66

J. Inher. Metab. Dis. 13 (1990) 435–441

Molecular Genetics of Phosphorylase Kinase: cDNA Cloning, Chromosomal Mapping and Isoform Structure

M. W. Kilimann
Institut für Physiologische Chemie (Abteilung für Biochemie Supramolekularer Systeme), Ruhr-Universität Bochum, Postfach 10 21 48, D-4630 Bochum 1, FRG

Summary: A deficiency in phosphorylase kinase is responsible for several forms of glycogen storage disease which differ in heredity and affected tissues. This is so because phosphorylase kinase consists of four different subunits and has multiple tissue-specific isoforms. To elucidate the molecular basis of phosphorylase kinase deficiencies, the cDNAs encoding the subunits α and β were cloned and sequenced. Each subunit was shown to be encoded by a single gene. The α subunit gene was mapped to chromosome Xq12-q13 and the β subunit gene to chromosome 16q12-q13. Isoform cDNAs reveal differential mRNA splicing. Thus, the stage is set for the molecular characterization of the genes and their deficiency mutations.

Phosphorylase kinase (EC 2.7.1.38) is a key regulatory enzyme of glycogen metabolism. It phosphorylates and activates glycogen phosphorylase, and in this way enhances glycogen breakdown in response to neural or hormonal stimulation (review: Pickett-Gies and Walsh, 1986). A deficiency in phosphorylase kinase is responsible for several forms of glycogen storage disease in humans and animals (Table 1).

The most frequently occurring form of phosphorylase kinase deficiency (ca. 75%) affects primarily the liver and is X-chromosomally transmitted (Huijing and Fernandes, 1969; Schimke *et al.*, 1973). In most patients with autosomally inherited phosphorylase kinase deficiency, both liver and muscle seem to be affected (Lederer *et al.*, 1980; Lerner *et al.*, 1982). Sporadic cases of phosphorylase kinase deficiency confined to either muscle (Abarbanel *et al.*, 1982; Ohtani *et al.*, 1982) or heart (Eishi

Table 1 Glycogen storage diseases caused by phosphorylase kinase deficiency

Species	*Affected tissues*	*Inheritance*
Human	Liver	X-chromosomal
	Muscle and liver	Autosomal
	Muscle	(Autosomal?)
	Heart	(Autosomal?)
Mouse (I strain)	Muscle and heart	X-chromosomal
Rat (*gsd* strain)	Liver	Autosomal

et al., 1985; Servidei *et al.*, 1988) have been reported, all apparently with autosomal inheritance. Residual enzyme activity and clinical severity vary, but the conditions are generally compatible with life. The two infants reported with heart phosphorylase kinase deficiency died from cardiac failure at a few months of age.

There are also animal models. A mouse mutant with an X-chromosomal, muscle- and heart-specific deficiency has been the subject of particularly intensive biochemical and genetic study (Lyon, 1970; Cohen and Cohen, 1981). A rat strain with an autosomal, liver-specific defect is also known (Malthus *et al.*, 1980).

It is not surprising that mutations affecting phosphorylase kinase should give rise to multiple phenotypes, as this is a complex protein consisting of four different subunits and it occurs in several tissue-specific isoforms (Table 2). The catalytic subunit, γ, is regulated by calcium through the subunit δ, which is identical to calmodulin. The two large subunits, α and β, mediate the regulation of the enzyme by phosphorylation. Several tissue-specific isoenzymes can be discriminated by biochemical and genetic criteria (reviewed in Pickett-Gies and Walsh, 1986).

MOLECULAR GENETICS OF PHOSPHORYLASE KINASE

To understand the molecular basis of phosphorylase kinase-dependent glycogen storage diseases, it is necessary to clone the genes for the different subunits, to determine their chromosomal localizations, and to elucidate the molecular nature of isoenzyme diversity. Thus, candidate DNA sequences would be identified where we would expect to find the mutations responsible for the various forms of phosphorylase kinase deficiency.

The δ and γ subunits

The δ subunit is calmodulin. There are several calmodulin genes in the human genome (Fischer *et al.*, 1988), but it appears that there is no specific gene for the

Table 2 Basic data on the structural complexity of phosphorylase kinase. Subunit molecular weights (rounded) are deduced from the amino acid sequences.

Phosphorylase kinase subunit structure: $(\alpha\beta\gamma\delta)_4$		
Subunit	*Molecular weight*	*Function*
α	138 000	Regulatory (phosphorylated)
β	125 000	Regulatory (phosphorylated)
γ	43 000	Catalytic
δ (calmodulin)	17 000	Regulatory (Ca^{2+})
Phosphorylase kinase isoenzymes (biochemical and/or genetic evidence)		
White muscle		
Red muscle		
Heart		
Liver		
Neonatal		

phosphorylase kinase δ subunit: rather, phosphorylase kinase seems to participate in the whole calmodulin and calmodulin mRNA pools of the cell (Bender *et al.*, 1988). Mutations in calmodulin genes (the genes are autosomal: Scambler *et al.*, 1987) are therefore unlikely to cause isolated phosphorylase kinase deficiency; they would be expected to produce more complex and severe phenotypes.

Cloning of the γ subunit cDNA from mouse and rabbit muscle was reported in 1987 by several groups. Its gene was localized on an autosome. Isoforms other than from muscle have not been characterized (Bender and Emerson, 1987; Chamberlain *et al.*, 1987; da Cruz e Silva and Cohen, 1987).

The α and β subunits

My own laboratory undertook to clone the two large subunits, α and β. Using oligonucleotide hybridization probes derived from partial amino acid sequences, we succeeded in isolating full-copy cDNAs encoding the subunits from rabbit muscle (Kilimann *et al.*, 1988; Zander *et al.*, 1988). From their nucleotide sequences, the complete primary structures of both polypeptides could be deduced (Figure 1).

Analysis of the two amino acid sequences revealed that they are unrelated to any other known proteins, but homologous to each other. The two molecules exhibit substantial sequence similarity over most of their length, but each subunit possesses additional short unique sequences. Remarkably, most of the known phosphorylation sites reside in those unique sequences. This is most striking in the α subunit, where all seven known phosphorylation sites cluster in a stretch of only 60 amino acids. This provides an insight into the molecular evolution of the enzyme. Apparently, the α and β subunit genes are derived from a common ancestral gene, and in the course of their divergence each acquired additional exons encoding subunit-specific, phosphorylatable, regulatory domains (Figure 2). The next question was: How many genes are there for each subunit, and what is their chromosomal localization?

The number of genes relates to the problem of tissue-specific isoenzymes. Different isoforms of a polypeptide may be generated from separate genes. This is the case, for example, with the substrate protein of phosphorylase kinase, glycogen phosphorylase. The muscle, liver, and brain isoenzymes of glycogen phosphorylase are encoded by distinct genes (Lebo *et al.*, 1984; Newgard *et al.*, 1987, 1988). Alternatively, isoforms may be generated by differential splicing of the primary transcripts of a single gene. We have found that this is the case with phosphorylase kinase. The α and β subunits of phosphorylase kinase are each encoded by a single gene.

Chromosomal mapping of the human genes was carried out by Uta Francke and her associates at Yale (Francke *et al.*, 1989). In interspecies hybrid cell line panels, the α subunit gene co-segregated with the X chromosome and the β subunit gene with chromosome 16. This was confirmed by *in situ* hybridization of metaphase chromosomes, and the α gene was more accurately mapped to Xq12-q13 and the β gene to 16q12-q13 (Francke *et al.*, 1989). Mapping of α to Xq12-q13 was confirmed in H.H. Ropers' laboratory in Nijmegen using DNA from patients with small deletions or duplications in this region (F.P.M. Cremers and H.H. Ropers, unpublished data; cf. Cremers *et al.*, 1989). In further agreement with these data, genetic mapping of

```
alpha subunit                                                       MRSRSNSGVRLDSYARLVQQTILCHQNPVTGLLPA---SYDQKDAWV   44
                                                                       .:: : ..:  :.:  : : ::: :.    . ::  : .
beta subunit   AGATGLMAEVSWKVLERRARTKRSGSVYEPLKSINLPRPDNETLWDKLDYYYKIVKSTLLLYQSPTTGLFPTKTCGGDQ-TAKI   83
                        [P]                 [P]

RDNVYSILAVWGLGLAYRKNADRDEDKAKAYELEQSVVKLMRGLLHCMIRQVDKVESFKYSQSTKDSLHAKYNTKTCATVVGDDQWGHLQLDATSVYLLF   144
.: .:   . :.:.::::.      :.::... ::: : .: :::.: : .:: :::. ::      .    ::. .: .:    ... ...::::..: :.:::.
HDSLYCAAGAWALALAYRRI---DDDKGRTHELEHSAIKCMRGILYCYMRQADKVQQFKQDPRPTTCLHSLFNVHTGDELLSYEEYGHLQINAVSLYLLY   180

LAQMTASGLHIIHSLDEVNFIQNLVFYIEAAYKTADFGIWERGDKTNQGISELNASSVGMAKAALEALDELDLFGVKGGPQSVIHVLADEVQHCQSILNS   244
: .: .::: ::    ::: :::::: .:   :. .:::.:::: : :.: .:: .::::.:::::::..   .:::   : . ::: :  :  ..    : :
LVEMISSGLQIIYNTDEVSFIQNLVFCVERVYRVPDFGVWERGSKYNNGSTELHSSSVGLAKAALEAINGFNLFGNQGCSWSVIFVDLDAHNRNRQTLCS   280

LLPRASTSKEVDASLLSVISFPAFAVEDSKLVEITKQEIITKLQGRYGCCRFLRDGYKTPKEDPNRLYYEPAELKLFENIECEWPLFWTYFILDGVFSGN   344
:::: : :.. ::.::. ::.::::..:  : . : . .: :: :.::  ::::::.:. ::: : :: :::.:::. ::::.:.:. : ..:::: ::
LLPRESRSHNTDAALLPCISYPAFALDDDVLYNQTLDKVIRKLKGKYGFKRFLRDGYRTSLEDPKRRYYKPAEIKLFDGIECEFPIFFLYMMIDGVFRGN   380

AEQVQEYREALEAVLIKGKNGVPLLPELYSVPPDKVDEEYQNPHTVDRVP-----MGKLPHMWGQSLYILGSLMAEGFLAPGEIDPLNR----------   428
. :: :: . : .::  . .: :..: : ::.: :. :  ::  . : :         :::  .:::.:::.. :.:.  ..: .:::.:
PKQVKEYQDLLTPVLHQTTEGYPVVPKYYYVPADFVEYEKRNPGSQKRFPSNCGRDGKL-FLWGQALYIIAKLLADELISPKDIDPVQRYVPLQNQRNVS   479

-RFST-VP-KPDVVVQVSILAETEEIKAILKDKGINVETIAEVYPIRVQPARILSHIYSSLGCNNRMKLSGRPYRHMGVLGTSKLYDI-RKTIFTFTPQF   524
 :.:   :   :.:: :...::..  .    :    ::. .:  .: :: . :    : . :  :: :... :::: : .: :::::.: :  ::.   . :
MRYSNQGPLENDLVVHVALVAESQRLQVFLNTYGIQTQTPQQVEPIQIWPQQELVKAYFHLGINEKLGLSGRPDRPIGCLGTSKIYRILGKTVVCY-PII   578

                                                                            [FTC]
IDQQQFYLALDNKMIVEMLRTDLSYLCSRWRMTGQPTITFPISQTMLDEDGTSLNSSILAALRKMQDGYFGGARIQTGKLSEFLTTSCCTHLSFMDPGPE   624
 :  .::.. :  .... ..  : ..   :.: : :        : .  .         .:::: :  .: :: ..   .:    ....    : :.  .
FDLSDFYMSQDVLLLIDDIKNALQFIKQYWKMHGRPLFLVLIREDNIRGSRFNPMLDMLAAL-K--NGMIGGVKVHDRLQTLISGAVVEQLDFLRISDT   675
```

```
GKLYSEDYDDNYDELESGDWMDGYNSTSTARCGD-EVARYLD-HLLAHTAPHPKLAPASQKGGLNRFRAAVQTTCDLMSLVTKAKELHVQNVHMYLPTKL   722
EEL-PEFK--SFEELEPPKHSKVKRQSSTSNAPELEQQPEVSVTEWRNKPTHE-----------------------------------------------   725

FQASRPSLNLLDSSHPSQEDQVPTVRVEVHLPRDQSGEVDFQALVLQ-LKETSSLQEQADILYMLYTMKGPDWDTELYEEGSATVRELLTELYGKVG-KI   820
-----------------------------------------------ILQKLNDCSCLASQTILLGILLKREGPNFITQ---EG--TVSDHIERLYRRAGSK-   775

RHWGLIRYISGILRKKVEALDEACTDLLSHQKHLTVGLPPEPREKTISAPLPYEALTRLIEEACEG-DMNISILTQEIMVYLAMYMRTQPGLFAEMFRLR   919
KLWLAVRYGAAFTQKFSSSIAPHITTFLVHGKQVTLGAFGHEEE-VISNPLSPRVIKNIIYYKCNTHDEREAVIQQELVIHIGWIISNNPELFSGMLKIR   874

IGLIIQVMATELAHSLRCSAEEATEGLMNLSPSAMKNLLHHILSGKEFGVERSVRPTDSNVSPAISIHEIGAVGATKTERTGIMQLKSEIKQVEFRRLSI   1019
IGWIIHAMEYELQ--IR-SGDKPAKDLYQLSPSEVKQLLLDILQPQQ-----------------------------------------------------   918

STESQPNGGHSLGADLMSPSFLSPGTSVTPSSGSFPGHHTSKDSRQGQ-WQRRRRLDGALNRVPIGFYQKVWKVLQKC-HGLSVEGFVLPSSTTR-EMTP   1116
---------------------------------------------NGRCWLNKRQIDGSLNRTPTGFYDRVWQILERTPNGIIVAGKHLPQQPTLSDMTM   973

GEIKFSVHVESVLNRVPQPEYRQLLVEAILVLTMLADIEIHSIGSIIAVEKIVHIANDLFLQEQKTLGADDIMLAKDPASGICTLLYDSAPSGRFGTMTY   1216
YEMNFSLLVEDMLGNIDQPKYRQIVVELLMVVSIVLERN-PELEFQDKVD-LDKLVKEAFHEFQK----DESRLKEIEKQDDMTSFYNTPPLGKRGTCSY   1067

LSKAAATYV-Q-EFLPHSI--CAMQ   1237
LTKVVMNLLLEGEVKPSNEDSCLVS   1092
```

Figure 1 Homologous amino acid sequences of the α and β subunits of phosphorylase kinase (Kilimann *et al.*, 1988). A boxed P indicates an autophosphorylation site, a circled P an endogenously phosphorylated site, and a triangle a phosphorylation site for cAMP-dependent protein kinase. Putative calmodulin-binding domains (according to criteria of primary structure) are under- and overlined. See Kilimann *et al.*, 1988, for further details.

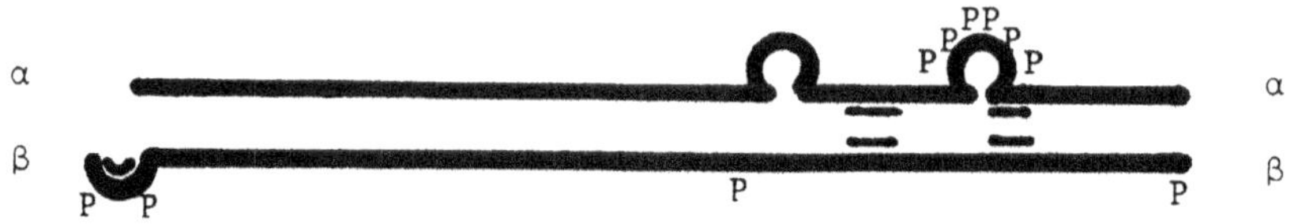

Figure 2 Comparative overall organization of the α and β subunits. Homologous regions are drawn in parallel; subunit-specific domains are drawn as loops. A P indicates a phosphorylation site (the multiphosphorylation domain of α has at least seven phosphorylation sites), and thin parallel lines indicate putative calmodulin binding sites. The relative size of the β subunit-specific N-terminal domain is exaggerated.

the mouse α gene using *M. musculus* × *M. spretus* hybrid backcrosses in Pene Barnard's laboratory at the MRC, Cambridge has located it very close (ca. 1 cM) to the phosphoglycerate kinase gene (Barnard *et al.*, 1990).

We conclude that X-chromosomally transmitted phosphorylase kinase deficiencies are likely to be related to the structural gene of the α subunit, and autosomal deficiencies are likely to be caused by mutations in the β or γ subunit genes. The next step is to characterize the isoenzyme cDNAs and to look for tissue-specifically expressed exons. This would allow us to define those parts of the genes where we can suppose the tissue-specific mutations to be localized. The muscle cDNAs cross-hybridize with mRNA from the other tissues. We have isolated full-copy cDNAs from several tissues (liver, red muscle, heart and brain) and are now in the process of characterizing them. We find that isoforms arise through differential mRNA splicing. In some instances, this affects protein domains of crucial regulatory functions, namely, phosphorylation sites and putative calmodulin binding sites (N.F. Zander, B. Harmann and M.W. Kilimann, unpublished data).

REFERENCES

Abarbanel, J.M., Bashan, N., Potashnik, R., Osimani, A., Moses, S.W. and Herishanu, Y. Adult muscle phosphorylase *b* kinase deficiency. *Neurology* 36 (1986) 560–562

Barnard, P.J., Derry, J.M.J., Ryder-Cook, A.S., Zander, N.F. and Kilimann, M.W. Mapping of the phosphorylase kinase α subunit gene on the mouse X chromosome. *Cytogenet. Cell Genet.*, 1990 in press

Bender, P.K. and Emerson, C.P. Skeletal muscle phosphorylase kinase catalytic subunit mRNAs are expressed in heart tissue but not in liver. *J. Biol. Chem.* 262 (1987) 8799–8805

Bender, P.K., Dedman, J.R. and Emerson, C.P. The abundance of calmodulin mRNAs is regulated in phosphorylase kinase-deficient skeletal muscle. *J. Biol. Chem.* 263 (1988) 9733–9737

Chamberlain, J.S., Van Tuinen, P., Reeves, A.A., Philip, B.A. and Caskey, C.T. Isolation of cDNA clones for the catalytic γ subunit of mouse muscle phosphorylase kinase: expression of mRNA in normal and mutant Phk mice. *Proc. Natl. Acad. Sci. USA* 84 (1987) 2886–2890

Cohen, P.T.W. and Cohen, P. The molecular basis of muscle phosphorylase kinase deficiency in I-strain mice. In Randle, P.J., Steiner, D.F. and Whelan, W.J. (eds.), *Carbohydrate Metabolism and its Disorders, Vol. 3*, Academic Press, London, 1981, pp. 119–138

Cremers, F.P.M., van de Pol, D.J.R., Diergaarde, D.J., Wieringa, B., Nussbaum, R.L., Schwartz, M. and Ropers, H.H. Physical fine mapping of the chorioideremia locus using Xq21 deletions associated with complex syndromes. *Genomics* 4 (1989) 41–46

da Cruz e Silva, E.F. and Cohen, P.T.W. Isolation and sequence analysis of a cDNA clone encoding the entire catalytic subunit of phosphorylase kinase. *FEBS Lett.* 220 (1987) 36–42

Eishi, Y., Takemura, T., Sone, R., Yamamura, H., Narisawa, K., Ichinohasama, R., Tanaka, M. and Hatakeyama, S. Glycogen storage disease confined to the heart with deficient activity of cardiac phosphorylase kinase: A new type of glycogen storage disease. *Hum. Pathol.* 16 (1985) 193–197

Fischer, R., Koller, M., Flura, M., Mathews, S., Strehler-Page, M.-A., Krebs, J., Penniston, J.T., Carafoli, E. and Strehler, E.E. Multiple divergent mRNAs code for a single human calmodulin. *J. Biol. Chem.* 263 (1988) 17055–17062

Francke, U., Darras, B.T., Zander, N.F. and Kilimann, M.W. Assignment of human genes for phosphorylase kinase subunits α (PHKA) to Xq12-q13 and β (PHKB) to 16q12-q13. *Am. J. Hum. Genet.* 45 (1989) 276–282

Huijing, F. and Fernandes, J. X-Chromosomal inheritance of liver glycogenosis with phosphorylase kinase deficiency. *Am. J. Hum. Genet.* 21 (1969) 275–284

Kilimann, M.W., Zander, N.F., Kuhn, C.C., Crabb, J.W., Meyer, H.E. and Heilmeyer, L.M.G. Jr. The α and β subunits of phosphorylase kinase are homologous: cDNA cloning and primary structure of the β subunit. *Proc. Natl. Acad. Sci. USA* 85 (1988) 9381–9385

Lebo, R.V., Gorin, F., Fletterick, F.J., Kao, F.-T., Cheung, M.C., Bruce, B.D. and Kan, Y.W. High-resolution chromosome sorting and DNA spot-blot analysis assign McArdle's syndrome to chromosome 11. *Science* 225 (1984) 57–59

Lederer, G., van de Werve, G., de Barsy, Th. and Hers, H.G. The autosomal form of phosphorylase kinase deficiency in man: Reduced activity of the muscle enzyme. *Biochem. Biophys. Res. Commun.* 92 (1980) 169-174

Lerner, A., Iancu, T.C., Bashan, N., Potashnik, R. and Moses, S. A new variant of glycogen storage disease. *Am. J. Dis. Child* 136 (1982) 406–410

Lyon, J.B. The X chromosome and the enzymes controlling muscle glycogen: phosphorylase kinase. *Biochem. Genet.* 4 (1970) 169–175

Malthus, R., Clark, D.G., Watts, C. and Sneyd, J.G.T. Glycogen storage disease in rats: a genetically determined deficiency of liver phosphorylase kinase. *Biochem. J.* 188 (1980) 99–106

Newgard, C.B., Fletterick, R.J., Anderson, L.A. and Lebo, R.V. The polymorphic locus for glycogen storage disease VI (liver glycogen phosphorylase) maps to chromosome 14. *Am. J. Hum. Genet.* 40 (1987) 351–364

Newgard, C.B., Littmann, D.R., van Genderen, C., Smith, M. and Fletterick, R.J. Human brain glycogen phosphorylase. *J. Biol. Chem.* 263 (1988) 3850–3857

Ohtani, Y., Matsuda, I., Iwamasa, T., Tamari, H., Origuchi, Y. and Miike, T. Infantile glycogen storage myopathy in a girl with phosphorylase kinase deficiency. *Neurology* 32 (1982) 833–838

Pickett-Gies, C.R. and Walsh, D.A. Phosphorylase kinase. In Boyer, P.D. and Krebs, E.G. (eds.), *The Enzymes, Vol. 17*, Academic Press, Orlando, FL, 1986, pp. 395–459

Scambler, P.J., McPherson, M.A., Bates, G., Bradbury, N.A., Dormer, R.L. and Williamson, R. Biochemical and genetic exclusion of calmodulin as the site of the basic defect in cystic fibrosis. *Hum. Genet.* 76 (1987) 278–282

Schimke, R.N., Zakheim, R.M., Corder, R.C. and Hug, G. Glycogen storage disease type IX: benign glycogenosis of liver and hepatic phosphorylase kinase deficiency. *J. Pediatr.* 83 (1973) 1031–1034

Servidei, S., Metlay, L.A., Chodosh, J. and DiMauro, S. Fatal infantile cardiopathy caused by phosphorylase *b* kinase deficiency. *J. Pediatr.* 113 (1988) 82–85

Zander, N.F., Meyer, H.E., Hoffmann-Posorske, E., Crabb, J.W., Heilmeyer, L.M.G. Jr. and Kilimann, M.W. cDNA cloning and complete primary structure of skeletal muscle phosphorylase kinase (α subunit). *Proc. Natl. Acad. Sci. USA* 85 (1988) 2929–2933

J. Inher. Metab. Dis. 13 (1990) 442–451

Phosphorylase b Kinase Deficiency in Man: a Review

I. E. T. van den Berg and R. Berger
University Children's Hospital 'Het Wilhelmina Kinderziekenhuis', Nieuwe Gracht 137, NL-3512 LK Utrecht, The Netherlands

Summary: Phosphorylase b kinase is involved in the activation of glycogen phosphorylase and is thus involved in the breakdown of glycogen. The enzyme exists as several tissue specific isoenzymes of which the muscle enzyme (rabbit) has been most characterized. It is a multimeric protein composed of four subunits, α, β, γ and δ. The four subunits are coded on different chromosomes, the α, β and γ subunit genes being on the X, 16 and 17 chromosomes respectively. The δ subunit is a calmodulin and confers calcium sensitivity on phosphorylase b kinase. Tissue specificity of the enzyme is conferred, at least in some cases, by variation in the γ subunit.

Seven different clinical types of phosphorylase b kinase deficiency have been described. The most common type is X-linked and affects the liver only; other types affect liver, muscle and liver, muscle or heart and have an autosomal recessive mode of inheritance, while in some types the mode of inheritance is not clear. Diagnosis based on the study of erythrocytes or leukocytes can be misleading due to the tissue specific nature of the enzyme, and liver or muscle biopsies may be required.

The breakdown of glycogen in tissues is controlled through the action of several protein kinases and phosphatases (Hems and Whitton, 1980). Glycogen phosphorylase (EC 2.4.1.1), the enzyme directly catalysing the breakdown of the polysaccharide molecule, exists in two different forms: the inactive b form is converted into the active a form by phosphorylation of a serine residue catalysed by the enzyme phosphorylase b kinase (Huijing, 1975). Phosphorylase b kinase (EC 2.7.1.38) from rabbit muscle has been extensively studied. The enzyme is a multimeric protein composed of four different subunits α, β, γ and δ with apparent molecular masses of 145 000, 128 000, 45 000 and 18 000 Da respectively. Furthermore, an isoform of the α subunit has been found in the muscle enzyme α^1, with a molecular mass of 140 000 (Cohen, 1973; Cohen *et al.*, 1978). The molecular weight of the enzyme is 1.28×10^6 Da making the subunit composition $(\alpha\beta\gamma\delta)_4$ or $(\alpha^1\beta\gamma\delta)_4$. The γ subunit carries the catalytic activity (Shuster *et al.*, 1980); the Ca^{2+} sensitivity is conferred by the δ subunit which is a calmodulin (Cohen *et al.*, 1978). The expression of catalytic activity is regulated by the degree of phosphorylation of the α and β subunits (Cohen, 1973).

Although the enzymic properties of the liver enzyme have been investigated

(Vandenheede *et al.*, 1979), little information is available on the size and subunit composition and on the relationship with the corresponding subunits of the enzyme from muscle (Sakai *et al.*, 1979; Chrisman *et al.*, 1982).

Recently the coding parts of the (rabbit muscle) α, β and γ genes have been sequenced and characterized. Moreover, the genes have been assigned to particular chromosomes. A single locus has been found for the α subunit on the X-chromosome (Francke *et al.*, 1989). The complete coding sequence comprises 3711 nucleotides and encodes a protein of 1237 amino acids with a molecular mass of 138 422 Da (Zander *et al.*, 1988). The gene for the β subunit has been assigned to chromosome 16 (Francke *et al.*, 1989). It encodes a protein of 1092 amino acids with a molecular mass of 125 205 Da. The α and β genes from rabbit muscle are highly homologous but unique sequences for both of the subunits have been identified (Kilimann *et al.*, 1988).

The gene encoding the muscle γ subunit has been assigned to chromosome 7 while a pseudogene has been found on chromosome 11 (Chamberlain *et al.*, 1987). cDNA probes for the muscle γ subunit hybridize with mRNA fractions from heart but not from liver (Bender and Emerson, 1987). These findings indicate that at least the γ subunit of phosphorylase b kinase is tissue specific.

In man liver and/or muscle phosphorylase b kinase deficiency has been described. It is the purpose of this paper to review the different phenotypes and genotypes described in the literature and to speculate on the relationship between genetic defect and expression of phosphorylase b kinase deficiency.

PHOSPHORYLASE KINASE DEFICIENCY IN MAN

The first description of a patient with phosphorylase b kinase deficiency (McKusick 30600) was given by Hug and colleagues (1966), who described a four-year-old female patient with glycogen storage in liver but not in muscle, with a low activity of liver phosphorylase. They showed that phosphorylase activity in liver homogenate of this patient could be restored by the addition of phosphorylase b kinase from rabbit muscle. Subsequently many patients with phosphorylase b kinase deficiency have been described and now several different types of the deficiency are recognized.

Phosphorylase b kinase deficiency in man can be divided into four groups depending on the tissue affected. Further distinction can be made based on the mode of inheritance of the disease. The different types of phosphorylase b kinase deficiency are listed in Table 1. The most common variety of phosphorylase b kinase deficiency is the liver type with an X-linked recessive mode of inheritance. It is not clear whether this type of phosphorylase b kinase deficiency is confined to the liver in all cases. Huijing and Fernandes (1969) described two large families with 26 patients with liver phosphorylase b kinase deficiency and clearly showed that there was an X-linked mode of inheritance. A majority of these patients had mild muscle weakness without neurological abnormalities but no muscle biopsies were performed. Only 4 of the 48 patients described in the literature belonging to this group were shown to have normal phosphorylase b kinase activity in muscle.

A small group of patients has liver phosphorylase b kinase deficiency with an

Table 1 Variability in expression of phosphorylase b kinase deficiency

Affected tissue	*Mode of inheritance*	*Number of patients* *Male*	*Female*	*References*	
I. Liver	a. X-linked recessive	32		Huijing *et al.*	(1969)
		2[a]		Schimke *et al.*	(1973)
		7		Lederer *et al.*	(1975)
		2[a]		Lederer *et al.*	(1975)
		2		Goji *et al.*	(1985)
		3		Besley *et al.*	(1987)
	b. Autosomal recessive	2[ab]	3[ab]	Hug *et al.*	(1969)
		1	1	Lederer *et al.*	(1975)
			1[a]	Sovik *et al.*	(1982)
		2	1	Gray *et al.*	(1983)
	c. Unknown		1[ab]	Hug *et al.*	(1966)
		1[a]		Morishita *et al.*	(1973)
		16	1	Baussan *et al.*	(1981)
		1[a]		Tuchman *et al.*	(1986)
		1		Bashan *et al.*	(1987)
		1		Alvarado *et al.*	(1988)
		4		Kikuchi *et al.*	(1988)
		1[a]		Kikuchi *et al.*	(1988)
II. Liver and muscle	a. Autosomal recessive	1[a]	1	Lederer *et al.*	(1980)
		1[a]	2[a]	Bashan *et al.*	(1981)
				Lerner *et al.*	(1982)
	b. Unknown	1[a]		Besley	(1987)
		1[a]		Kikuchi *et al.*	(1988)
III. Muscle	Unknown		1[a]	Ohtani *et al.*	(1982)
			2[a]	Iwamasa *et al.*	(1983)
		1[a]		Abarbanel *et al.*	(1986)
IV. Heart	Unknown	1[a]		Mizuta *et al.*	(1984)
			1[a]	Servidei *et al.*	(1988)

[a]Patients in whom a muscle biopsy was investigated
[b]Phosphorylase kinase activity was not measured directly

apparent autosomal recessive mode of inheritance. Eleven patients with this type of phosphorylase b kinase deficiency have been described in the literature. In five of these patients, phosphorylase b kinase activity has not been measured directly, but other measurements strongly support the diagnosis of liver phosphorylase b kinase deficiency. In five other patients nothing is known about muscle phosphorylase b kinase. Lederer and colleagues (1975) described four patients initially thought to belong to this group but it was found later that two of their patients, a brother and a sister, had diminished activity of phosphorylase b kinase in muscle as well (Lederer *et al.*, 1980). An 11th patient, described by Søvik *et al.* (1982), had almost undetectable liver phosphorylase b kinase activity and low muscle phosphorylase b kinase activity, but all enzymes measured in muscle had lowered activities (35–40% of normal activities) and therefore this patient is incorporated into this group. Autosomal recessive mode of inheritance in this patient was likely because of consanguinity of the parents. The patients with liver phosphorylase b kinase deficiency and unknown mode of inheritance probably belong to groups Ia or Ib (Table 1).

A less common form of phosphorylase b kinase deficiency is the combined deficiency of liver and muscle phosphorylase b kinase. There are eight patients described as belonging to this group: a brother and a sister (Lederer *et al.*, 1980), a brother and two sisters (Bashan *et al.*, 1981; Lerner *et al.*, 1982) and two boys without affected family members (Besley, 1987; Kikuchi *et al.*, 1988) who are classified in group IIb (Table 1).

The other forms of phosphorylase b kinase deficiency are even more rare. Phosphorylase b kinase deficiency confined to muscle has, to our knowledge, been described in five patients, four of whom are shown in Table 1. One of the patients described by Iwamasa and colleagues (1983) is probably the same patient as the one described by Ohtani and colleagues (1982). It is a very heterogenous group of patients. Age of onset of the disease, for instance, is 0, 5 and 35 years. Nothing is known about the mode of inheritance of this type of phosphorylase b kinase deficiency.

Two patients with deficiency of heart phosphorylase b kinase have been described (Mizuta *et al.*, 1984; Servidei *et al.*, 1988). Both patients, a boy and a girl, died within 6 months of birth and were diagnosed at autopsy. Phosphorylase b kinase in liver, muscle and kidney was normal.

DIAGNOSIS OF PHOSPHORYLASE B KINASE DEFICIENCY

Phosphorylase b kinase deficiency of liver and of liver and muscle is in general a mild disease, though more severe forms have been described (Lederer *et al.*, 1975; Søvik *et al.*, 1982; Tuchman *et al.*, 1986). It is not possible to differentiate between liver phosphorylase deficiency, liver phosphorylase b kinase deficiency and combined liver and muscle phosphorylase b kinase deficiency with respect to symptoms, biochemical analysis of serum and glucagon stimulation and galactose tolerance tests. The symptoms vary from patient to patient, even within one family (Gray *et al.*, 1983). The most consistently found symptoms are hepatomegaly, growth retardation, delayed motor development and hyperlipidaemia (Baussan *et al.*, 1981; Willems *et al.*, 1990). In some patients fasting hypoglycaemia or fasting hyperketosis is found.

The galactose tolerance test is normal in some patients (Lederer *et al.*, 1975) and in other patients galactose administration leads to an increase in serum lactate (Søvik *et al.*, 1982; Tuchman *et al.*, 1985; Alvarado *et al.*, 1988).

The glucagon stimulation test is normal in most patients with phosphorylase b kinase deficiency, but some patients show no rise in blood glucose after glucagon injection. Gray and colleagues (1983) found an abnormal response to glucagon in one of their patients and a normal response in her brother who had liver phosphorylase b kinase deficiency as well. Baussan and colleagues (1981) found a normal response to glucagon in ten patients with liver phosphorylase b kinase deficiency and in four patients with liver phosphorylase deficiency. This means that enzyme analysis is necessary to establish the diagnosis of phosphorylase b kinase deficiency.

Huijing (1967) and Huijing and Fernandes (1969) showed that liver phosphorylase b kinase deficiency with X-linked mode of inheritance is expressed in leukocytes. Lederer and colleagues (1975) showed that liver phosphorylase b kinase deficiencies with X-linked mode of inheritance and with autosomal recessive mode of inheritance are expressed in leukocytes and in erythrocytes. They could even distinguish the two forms from each other by measuring phosphorylase b kinase activity in erythrocytes. Since then many authors have measured phosphorylase b kinase activities in erythrocytes, leukocytes and lymphocytes. The figures found in the literature are listed in Table 2. Phosphorylase b kinase activities in erythrocytes have been measured with both endogenous and exogenous phosphorylase as substrate. Except for phosphorylase b kinase deficiency in muscle, all cases listed in Table 2 have diminished phosphorylase b kinase activity in erythrocytes. It is apparently not possible to distinguish the different forms of phosphorylase b kinase deficiency based on the relative amount of phosphorylase b kinase activity measured in erythrocytes. It is possible to establish the diagnosis of deficiency of liver phosphorylase b kinase or of liver and muscle phosphorylase b kinase if a diminished phosphorylase b kinase activity is found in erythrocytes. However, normal phosphorylase b kinase activity in erythrocytes does not rule out liver and/or muscle deficiency. Recently patients have been described with elevated phosphorylase b kinase activity in erythrocytes measured on exogenous phosphorylase and liver phosphorylase b kinase deficiency. When phosphorylase b kinase activity was measured using endogenous phosphorylase as substrate a deficient activity was found in erythrocytes.

In most cases phosphorylase b kinase deficiency is also expressed in leukocytes and in lymphocytes, although it is less pronounced than in erythrocytes and more exceptions are described in the literature. In one case with normal leukocyte phosphorylase b kinase, described by Bashan and colleagues (1987), leukocyte phosphorylase b kinase activity was also measured using endogenous phosphorylase and found to be deficient. It is possible that in other cases with normal leukocyte phosphorylase b kinase activity, diminished activity will be found when measurements are performed with endogenous phosphorylase. It is not clear whether patients with normal leukocyte phosphorylase b kinase activity are separate entities within the various groups of phosphorylase b kinase deficiencies. Such patients are found in the group with liver phosphorylase b kinase deficiency and in the group with combined muscle and liver phosphorylase b kinase deficiency. It is not possible to establish the diagnosis of phosphorylase b kinase deficiency if measurements are performed only on leukocytes; too many patients with normal leukocyte phosphorylase b kinase activity are described in the literature. Erythrocyte and leukocyte phosphorylase b kinase from one patient with muscle phosphorylase b kinase deficiency have been investigated and were found to have normal activity.

Three groups have investigated phosphorylase b kinase activity in fibroblasts of patients with phosphorylase b kinase deficiency. Migeon and Huijing (1974) found deficient activity of fibroblast phosphorylase b kinase in a patient with liver phosphorylase b kinase deficiency and an X-linked mode of inheritance. The relative amount of fibroblast phosphorylase b kinase activity varied from 20 to 55% of control values in various experiments. Tuchman and colleagues (1986) found normal fibroblast phosphorylase b kinase activity in a boy with a severe form of liver phosphorylase b kinase deficiency with unknown mode of inheritance. Besley (1987) measured a fibroblast phosphorylase b kinase activity of 14–19% of control values

Table 2 Expression of phosphorylase b kinase deficiency in blood cells

Affected tissue	Mode of inheritance	*Phosphorylase b kinase activity (% of normal values) in* — Erythrocytes: Activation of endogenous phosphorylase b	Erythrocytes: Activation of exogenous phosphorylase b	Leukocytes: Activation of exogenous phosphorylase b	Lymphocytes: Activation of exogenous phosphorylase b	References	
I. Liver	a. X-linked recessive		0–18 (32)[a]	0–36 (32)[a]		Huijing **et al.**	(1969)
		0–11 (7)	0–7 (9)	16–25 (4)		Lederer *et al.*	(1975)
			6–16 (3)	13–23 (3)	40–44 (3)	Goji *et al.*	(1985)
			5–9 (3)	59–62 (3)		Besley	(1987)
	b. Autosomal recessive	17–23 (2)	30 (2)	20–34 (2)		Lederer *et al.*	(1975)
			5–15 (3)	5–15 (3)		Gray *et al.*	(1983)
	c. Unknown	0–3 (16)	5–13 (16)			Baussan *et al.*	(1981)
		≦3 (1)	25 (1)			Baussan *et al.*	(1981)
		0 (1)	0 (1)	120 (1)		Bashan *et al.*	(1987)
			18 (1)	90 (1)		Alvarado *et al.*	(1988)
			4–10 (4)		22–35 (4)	Kikuchi *et al.*	(1988)
			30 (1)		22 (1)	Kikuchi *et al.*	(1988)
II. Liver and muscle	a. Autosomal recessive		15–19 (2)			Lederer *et al.*	(1975)
			10–30 (3)	13–25 (3)		Lerner *et al.*	(1982)
	b. Unknown		16 (1)	89 (1)		Besley	(1987)
			4 (1)		33 (1)	Kikuchi *et al.*	(1988)
III. Muscle	Unknown		100 (1)	100(1)		Abarbanel *et al.*	(1986)

[a]Patients in whom a muscle biopsy was investigated

in two patients with liver phosphorylase b kinase deficiency and X-linked mode of inheritance. For one patient with the muscle and liver form of phosphorylase b kinase deficiency he found 36% of normal values. Thus two groups found expression of phosphorylase b kinase deficiency in fibroblasts while the third did not. It is too early to explain this on the basis that we are dealing with different forms of phosphorylase b kinase deficiency: further investigations of fibroblast phosphorylase b kinase in the different groups will be necessary.

GENETICS OF PHOSPHORYLASE B KINASE DEFICIENCY

Francke and colleagues (1989) found a single locus for the (muscle) α subunit on the human X-chromosome. They presume that the α isoforms originate from the α gene by tissue specific splicing, thus the α gene is most likely affected in the X-linked form of isolated liver phosphorylase b kinase deficiency. This hypothesis implies that the α subunits of the liver and muscle enzymes are different. However, a difficulty remains in explaining the muscle hypotonia observed in the majority of cases with this type of phosphorylase b kinase deficiency (Willems *et al.*, 1990). Alternatively it may be possible that the α subunits of the two isoenzymes are identical, but that the α^1 isoform is formed by muscle tissue specific splicing. Red fibres containing almost exclusively the α^1 isoform (Lawrence *et al.*, 1986) are not affected, but white fibres, containing the α isoform (Lawrence *et al.*, 1986), could be deficient in enzyme activity.

There is increasing evidence that the γ subunit of phosphorylase b kinase is tissue specific. The electrophoretic mobility in polyacrylamide gel electrophoresis under denaturing and reducing conditions of the liver γ subunit is different from that of the muscle γ subunit (Chrisman *et al.*, 1982). cDNA sequences for the muscle γ subunit do not cross-hybridize with mRNA fractions from liver (Chamberlain *et al.*, 1982), thus the autosomal recessive form of liver phosphorylase b kinase deficiency could be caused by a mutation in the gene encoding the liver γ subunit. Alternatively it was suggested that due to the fact that a single locus has been found for the β gene (Francke *et al.*, 1989), tissue-specific β subunits are produced by differential splicing. In that case mutation occurs in those regions of the gene (exons) retained in the formation of liver β mRNA but removed when muscle β mRNA is formed by splicing.

Mutations leading to the autosomal recessive phosphorylase b kinase deficiency in both liver and muscle must be in the gene coding for a common subunit. The α and γ genes can be ruled out considering the mode of inheritance and tissue specificity respectively. The β gene could be a candidate provided that the mutations occur in the exons common to liver and muscle mRNAs. Isolated muscle phosphorylase b kinase deficiency, in which the mode of inheritance is not known, can be due to mutations in the α or β genes.

Isolated cardiac muscle phosphorylase b kinase deficiency, described in one girl and one boy, is difficult to explain. cDNA probes specific for the muscle γ subunit cross-hybridize with mRNA fractions not only from heart but also from brain. Tissue specific splicing or post-translational modification cannot be ruled out but has not been observed (Chamberlain *et al.*, 1987).

ACKNOWLEDGEMENT

This study was made possible by a grant from the Dutch Liver and Gut Foundation.

REFERENCES

Abarbanel, J. M., Bashan, N., Potashnik, R., Osimani, A., Moses, S. W. and Herishann, Y. Adult muscle phosphorylase 'b' kinase deficiency. *Neurology* 36 (1986) 560–562

Alvarado, L. J. F., Gasca-Centeno, E. and Grier, R. E. Hepatic phosphorylase b kinase deficiency with normal enzyme activity in leukocytes. *J. Pediatr.* 113 (1988) 865–867

Bashan, N., Iancu, T. C., Lerner, A., Fraser, D., Potashnik, R. and Moses, S. W. Glycogenesis due to liver and muscle phosphorylase kinase deficiency. *Pediatr. Res.* 15 (1981) 299–303

Bashan, W., Potashnik, R., Ehrlich, T. and Moses, S. W. Phosphorylase kinase in leukocytes and erythrocytes of a patient with glycogen storage disease type IX. *J. Inher. Metab. Dis.* 10 (1987) 119–127

Baussan, C., Moatti, N., Odievre, M. and Lemmonier, A. Liver glycogenesis caused by a defective phosphorylase system: hemolysate analysis. *Pediatrics* 67 (1981) 107–112

Bender, P. K. and Emerson, C. P. Skeletal muscle phosphorylase kinase catalytic subunit mRNAs are expressed in heart tissue but not in liver. *J. Biol. Chem.* 262 (1987) 8799–8805

Besley, G. T. N. Phosphorylase b kinase deficiency in glycogenosis type VIII: Differentiation of different phenotypes and heterozygotes by erythrocyte enzyme assay. *J. Inher. Metab. Dis.* 10 (1987) 115–118

Chamberlain, J. S., Van Tuinen, P., Reeves, A. A., Philip, B. A. and Caskey, C. T. Isolation of cDNA clones for the catalytic γ subunit of mouse muscle phosphorylase kinase: Expression of mRNA in normal and mutant PhK mice. *Proc. Natl. Acad. Sci. USA* 84 (1987) 2886–2890

Chrisman, T. D., Jordan, J. E. and Exton, J. H. Purification of rat liver phosphorylase b kinase. *J. Biol. Chem.* 257 (1982) 10798–10804

Cohen, P. The subunit structure of rabbit-skeletal muscle phosphorylase b kinase, and the molecular basis for its activation reactions. *Eur. J. Biochem.* 34 (1973) 1–14

Cohen, P., Burchell, A., Foulkes, J. G., Cohen, P. T. W., Vanaman, T. C. and Nairn, A. C. Identification of the Ca^{2+}-dependent modulation protein as the fourth subunit of rabbit skeletal muscle phosphorylase kinase. *FEBS Lett.* 92 (1978) 287–292

Francke, U., Darras, B. T., Zander, N. F. and Kilimann, M. W. Assignment of human genes for phosphorylase kinase subunits β (PHKA) to Xq12–q13 and β (PHKB) to 16q12–q13. *Am. J. Hum. Genet.* 45 (1989) 276–282

Goji, K., Morishita, Y., Kodama, S., Takahashi, T. and Matsuo, T. Lymphocyte phosphorylase kinase activities in the sex-linked form of liver phosphorylase kinase deficiency. *Eur. J. Pediatr.* 143 (1985) 179–182

Gray, R. G. F., Kumar, D. and Whitfield, A. E. Glycogen phosphorylase b kinase deficiency in three siblings. *J. Inher. Metab. Dis.* 6 (1983) 107

Hems, D. A. and Whitton, P. D. Control of hepatic glycogenolysis. *Physiol. Rev.* 60 (1980) 1–50

Hug, G., Schubert, W. K. and Chuck, G. Phosphorylase kinase of the liver: deficiency in a girl with increased hepatic glycogen. *Science* 153 (1966) 1534–1535

Hug, G., Schubert, W. K. and Chuck, G. Deficient activity of diphosphophosphorylase kinase and accumulation of glycogen in the liver. *J. Clin. Invest.* 48 (1969) 704–715

Hug, G., Schubert, W. K. and Chuck, G. Loss of cyclic 3^15^1-AMP dependent kinase and reduction of phosphorylase kinase in skeletal muscle of a girl with deactivated phosphorylase and glycogenosis of liver and muscle. *Biochem. Biophys. Res. Commun.* 40 (1970) 982–988

Huijing, F. Phosphorylase kinase in leucocytes of normal subjects and of patients with glycogen storage disease. *Biochim. Biophys. Acta* 148 (1967) 601–603

Huijing, F. Glycogen storage disease type VIa: low phosphorylase kinase activity caused by a low enzyme-substrate affinity. *Biochim. Biophys. Acta* 206 (1970) 199–201

Huijing, F. Glycogen metabolism and glycogen storage diseases. *Physiol. Rev.* 55 (1975) 609–658

Huijing, F. and Fernandes, J. X-Chromosomal inheritance of liver glycogenosis with phosphorylase kinase deficiency. *Am. J. Hum. Genet.* 21 (1969) 275–284

Iwamasa, T., Fukuda, S., Tokumitsu, S., Ninomiya, N., Matsuda, J. and Osame, M. Myopathy due to glycogen storage disease: Pathological and biochemical studies in relation to glycogenosome formation. *Exp. Mol. Pathol.* 38 (1983) 405–420

Kikuchi, M., Aikawa, J., Ishizawa, S., Igarashi, Y., Narisawa, K. and Tada, K. Enzymatic analysis in lymphocytes and erythrocytes from six patients with different phenotypes of phosphorylase kinase deficiency. *J. Inher. Metab. Dis.* 11 (1988) 315–318

Kilimann, M. W., Zander, N. F., Kuhn, C. C., Crabb, J. W., Meyer, H. E. and Heilmeyer, L. M. G. The α and β subunits of phosphorylase kinase are homologues: cDNA cloning and primary structure of the β subunit. *Proc. Natl. Acad. Sci. USA* 85 (1988) 9381–9385

Lawrence, J. C., Chi, M. M. Y. and Lowry, O. H. Isozymes of phosphorylase kinase in rabbit skeletal muscle. Functional implications of differences in phosphorylase kinase and phosphorylase activities in individual muscle fibers. *J. Biol. Chem.* 261 (1986) 8556–8563

Lederer, B., van de Werve, G., de Barsy, T. and Hers, H. G. Glycogen phosphorylase and its converter enzymes in haemolysatis of normal human subjects and of patients with type VI glycogen storage disease. *Biochem. J.* 147 (1975) 23–35

Lederer, B., van de Werve, G., de Barsy, T. and Hers, H. G. The autosomal form of phosphorylase kinase deficiency in man: reduced activity of the muscle enzyme. *Biochem. Biophys. Res. Commun.* 92 (1980) 169–174

Lerner, A., Iancu, T. C., Bashan, W., Potashnik, R. and Moscs, S. A new variant of glycogen storage disease. *Am. J. Dis. Child.* 136 (1982) 406–410

Migion, B. R. and Huijing, F. Glycogen storage disease associated with phosphorylase kinase deficiency: evidence for X inactivation. *Am. J. Hum. Genet.* 26 (1974) 360–368

Mizuta, K., Hashimoto, E., Tsutou, A., Eishi, Y., Takemura, T., Narisawa, K. and Yamamura, H. A new type of glycogen storage disease caused by deficiency of cardiac phosphorylase kinase. *Biochem. Biophys. Res. Commun.* 119 (1984) 582–587

Morishita, Y., Nishiyama, K., Yamamura, H., Kodama, S., Negishi, H., Matsuo, M., Matsuo, T. and Nishizuka, Y. Glycogen phosphorylase kinase deficiency: a survey of enzymes in phosphorylase activating system. *Biochem. Biophys. Res. Commun.* 54 (1973) 833–841

Ohtani, Y., Matsuda, I., Iwamasa, T., Tamari, H., Origuchi, Y. and Miike, T. Infantile glycogen storage myopathy in a girl with phosphorylase kinase deficiency. *Neurology* (NY) 32 (1982) 833–838

Sakai, K., Matsumara, S., Okimura, Y., Yamamura, H. and Nishizuha, Y. Liver glycogen phosphorylase kinase. Partial purification and characterization. *J. Biol. Chem.* 254 (1979) 6631–6637

Schimke, R. N., Zakheim, R. M., Corder, R. C. and Hug, G. Glycogen storage disease type IX: Benign glycogenosis of liver and hepatic phosphorylase kinase deficiency. *J. Pediatr.* 83 (1973) 1031–1034

Servidei, S., Mitlay, L. A., Chodosh, J. and DiMauro, S. Fatal infantile cardiopathy caused by phosphorylase b kinase deficiency. *J. Pediatr.* 113 (1988) 82–85

Shuster, J. R., Chan, R. F. J. and Graves, D. J. Isolation and properties of the catalytically active γ-subunit of phosphorylase b kinase. *J. Biol. Chem.* 255 (1980) 2203–2210

Søvik, O., de Barsy, T. and Maehle, B. Phosphorylase kinase deficiency: severe glycogen storage disease with evidence of autosomal recessive mode of inheritance. *Eur. J. Pediatr.* 139 (1982) 210

Tuchman, M., Brown, B. I., Burke, B. A. and Ulstrom, R. A. Clinical and laboratory observations in a child with hepatic phosphorylase kinase deficiency. *Metabolism* 35 (1986) 627–633

Vandenheede, J. R., De Wulf, H. and Merlevede. Liver phosphorylase b kinase. Cyclic-AMP-mediated activation and properties of the partially purified rat-liver enzyme. *Eur. J. Biochem.* 101 (1979) 51–58

Willems, P. J., Gerver, W. J. M., Berger, R. and Fernandes, J. The natural history of liver glycogenosis due to phosphorylase b kinase deficiency. A longitudinal study of 41 patients. *Eur. J. Pediatr.* 149 (1990) 268–271

Zander, N. F., Meyer, H. E., Hoffmann-Posorske, E., Crabb, J. W., Heilmeyer, L. M. G. and Kilimann, M. W. cDNA cloning and complete primary structure of skeletal muscle phosphorylase kinase (α subunit). *Proc. Natl. Acad. Sci. USA* 85 (1988) 2929–2933

ANNOUNCEMENT

European Society for Pediatric Research

ANNUAL MEETING, Vienna 1990
September 23–27

Local Organizing Committee (Scientific Secretariat):
Prof. Dr K. WIDHALM
Dept. of Pediatrics, University of Vienna,
Währinger Gürtel 18–20, A-1097 Vienna, Austria
Tel: 0222/48 00/32 10, 0222/48 75 66
Telefax: 0222/43 34 84

PARTICIPATING WORKING GROUPS
Working Group on Mineral Metabolism
Working Groups on Neonatology
Working Group on Perinatal and Pediatric Microcirculation

SCIENTIFIC TOPICS (preliminary):
Inborn errors of metabolism
Allergology and immunodeficiency
Oncology
Pharmacology and antiviral agents
Preventive pediatrics
Pediatric surgery: liver transplantation
Scientific Contributions from all specialities of pediatrics are welcome
Poster Session
Workshops
Young Investigator Award

J. Inher. Metab. Dis. 13 (1990) 452–465

Muscle Glycogenosis

S. W. Moses
Department of Pediatrics, Faculty of Health Sciences, Ben Gurion University of the Negev, Beer-Sheva 84101, Israel

Summary: This review describes clinical, biochemical and genetic features of the four inborn errors affecting muscle glycogen breakdown, namely deficiencies of phosphorylase, phosphorylase kinase, amylo-1,6-glucosidase and acid α-glucosidase. They are characterized by a wide spectrum of clinical manifestation, affecting age of onset, clinical features, progress of disease and tissue involvement. Biochemically, variability of all four enzyme deficiencies is evident in terms of differences in residual enzyme present in tissues, and in the presence or absence of enzyme protein. Genetic heterogeneity, which has been documented in each of the enzyme deficiencies, manifests itself in terms of the presence, absence, quantity or size of mRNA. In phosphorylase deficiency heterogeneity has also been documented at the DNA level. In acid maltase deficiency nine mutant phenotypes have been described affecting various stages of lysosomal enzyme processing.

Since Claude Bernarde made his pioneering observation on glycogen metabolism over 130 years ago, it has become increasingly evident that the synthesis and breakdown of glycogen is a highly complex and tightly controlled process, involving substrates, intermediates, cofactors, activators, inhibitors, enzymic interconversions and hormonal interactions. Glycogen metabolism occurs in many tissues; however, its controls differ in each tissue and are adapted to the particular environment and metabolic requirements of each organ. Thus the regulation of glycogen synthesis and breakdown in the mammalian liver differs markedly from its regulation in muscle, each one serving a different function. In the liver glycogenolysis leads primarily to the production and liberation of glucose into the blood, whereas in muscle glycogenolysis provides substrates which enable ATP generation to be utilized during vigorous muscle contraction. While the resting muscle utilizes ATP, mainly derived from the breakdown of circulating glucose and free fatty acids, the amount of ATP available to support vigorous muscular contraction suffices only for about a second. Any extension of physical exercise requires short and long-term backup systems to provide the necessary high energy phosphate compounds. During contractile muscular activity, the levels of ADP and P_i rise rapidly, leading to an increased breakdown of creatine phosphate, by which ADP is rapidly phosphorylated to form ATP which can provide energy for an additional few seconds (Figure 1). Subsequently, through a cascadic activation of glycogenolytic enzymes initiated by epinephrine and an

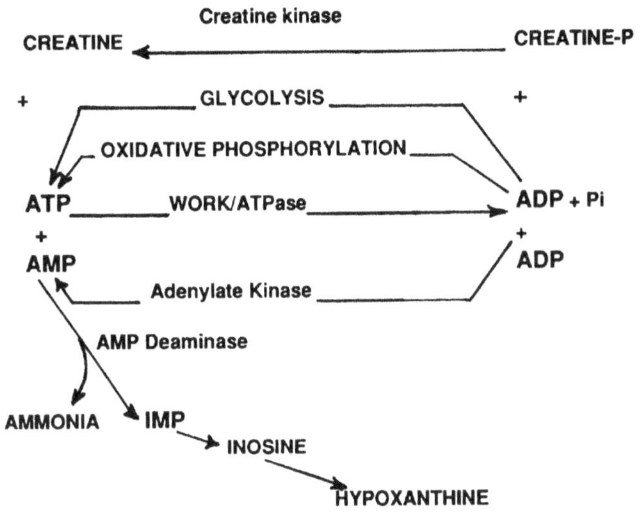

Figure 1 Alternative pathways of the production and breakdown of energy-rich compounds in muscle

increase in calcium ions in the cytosol, glycogen stores are broken down leading to an increase in the flux of glycolytic intermediates resulting in ATP formation and pyruvate and lactate accumulation. Pyruvate and acetyl CoA will, by fuelling the tricarboxylic acid cycle, provide reducing equivalents for further ATP production by oxidative phosphorylation. Adenylate kinase (also called myokinase) will be activated by the rise in ADP, providing an alternate reaction for ATP generation. As the adenylate kinase reaction is coupled to the adenylate deaminase reaction, AMP production leads to the formation of IMP, ammonia and subsequently inosine, adenosine and hypoxanthine. Since non-phosphorylated compounds can traverse the muscular membrane, ammonia and purine breakdown products can be detected in the efferent bloodstream of an exercising muscle (Mineo *et al.*, 1987). During prolonged submaximal exercise, the muscle switches to the utilization of other substrates such as circulating glucose and fatty acids which can subsequently also include amino acids.

In the present paper the four major muscular glycogenolytic enzyme deficiencies, affecting phosphorylase, phosphorylase *b* kinase, amylo-1,6-glucosidase and acid α-glucosidase will be discussed in terms of their clinical presentation, biochemical variations, molecular genetic heterogeneity and treatment.

GLYCOGEN PHOSPHORYLASE DEFICIENCY, GSD V, (McARDLE'S DISEASE)

Glycogen phosphorylase (EC 2.4.1.1) catalyses the initial step of glycogen breakdown by phosphorylytically removing 1,4 linked glucose residues in a stepwise fashion from the outer branches of the glycogen molecule, liberating glucose-1-phosphate. Skeletal muscle has a single isoenzyme which is separately coded from the liver isoenzyme. Consequently, patients with muscle phosphorylase deficiency will have normal liver phosphorylase and *vice versa*. The gene encoding human muscle phosphorylase has been mapped to the long arm of chromosome 11 (Lebo *et al*.,. 1984), cloned and sequenced (Burke *et al*., 1987).

Clinical variability

Since McArdle in 1951 described the cardinal features of this disease (McArdle, 1951), namely exercise intolerance, associated with myalgia and muscle stiffness relieved by rest, which in some cases is associated with myoglobinuria and even renal failure, a wide spectrum of clinical variants has been described. These include patients with excessive fatigue, poor stamina, muscle weakness without cramps, and muscle wasting (Engel *et al*., 1963). Age of onset has also been found to vary among patients: while most cases start in the form of a mild exercise intolerance in childhood which deteriorates with age, some develop clinical features at a later age. A 59-year-old patient with mild, painless, slowly progressive proximal muscle weakness and wasting which started in early childhood is on record (Abarbanel *et al*., 1987). On the other hand, patients with an early infantile fatal myopathy have been obseved (Di Mauro and Hartlage, 1978). The variability of this disease is well documented by DiMauro who summarized the clinical features and age of onset in 112 cases of myophosphorylase deficiency (DiMauro and Bresolin, 1986). In DiMauro's series 96% of patients suffered from the classical McArdle's syndrome, 50% of whom had myoglobinuria, while fixed weakness was found in 28% and wasting in 12% of cases. The clinical heterogeneity observed in this disease illustrates the importance of considering myophosphorylase deficiency in a wide variety of myopathies.

Muscle energy metabolism

It is expected that during vigorous exercise, myophosphorylase-deficient patients have a limited capacity to regenerate ATP through anaerobic and aerobic glycolysis. As a consequence no lactate accumulation will be observed during vigorous ischaemic exercise in such patients in contrast to normal muscle, and intracellular pH will not drop. The diminished pyruvate production will decrease the activity of the tricarboxylic acid cycle, and consequently effect oxidative phosphorylation, thus reducing oxygen consumption. It has been well documented by NMR techniques that in myophosphorylase-deficient patients vigorous muscular exercise is not associated with a decrease in intracellular pH or a depletion of ATP, while an increase in the P_i peak and a decrease in the phosphocreatine peak were found in the ^{31}P NMR spectra. Several investigators found during maximal tolerable muscle exertion a decrease in phosphocreatine and an increase in the P_i peaks (Lewis and Haller, 1985, Duboc *et al*., 1986). On the other hand, when patients were tested for their P_i/phosphocreatine ratios at different submaximal exercise rates, in myophosphorylase-deficient patients both exercise kinetics and post-exercise recovery were normal. This led Argov and colleagues (1987) to conclude that under submaximal exercising conditions, sufficient aerobic fuels are available and that mitochondrial activity was normal. These findings are in accord with the clinical observation of the 'second wind phenomenon' which relates to the capacity of myophosphorylase-deficient patients to continue, after an episode of exercise-induced myalgia and muscle stiffness, with submaximal activity for extended periods, utilizing circulating glucose and fatty acids for energy recovery. Vigorous exercise in such patients led to elevated levels of blood ammonia, inosine and hypoxanthine, suggesting an increased rate of breakdown of AMP. It is of interest to note that glucose infusions did not result in an elevation of blood lactate levels, but normalized both the NMR pattern and the blood ammonia levels, implying a shift of ATP synthesis from the creatine kinase and adenylate kinase reaction to aerobic glycolysis and oxidative phosphorylation (Lewis and Haller, 1986; Mineo *et al.*, 1987).

Family studies

Although pooled data from pedigree studies suggest an autosomal recessive mode of inheritance, unusual patterns have been found in isolated family pedigrees. A family with a symptom-manifesting heterozygote mother with 20% enzyme activity and a clinically unaffected father with 45% myophosphorylase activity has been described (Schmidt *et al.*, 1987).

An unusual family in which clinical manifestations of the disease could be traced in four generations, suggesting vertical transmission, was reported by Chui and Munsat (1976).

Biochemical variability of the enzyme protein

Different laboratories found biochemical heterogeneity in terms of detectable enzyme protein in myophosphorylase-deficient patients. In 85% of muscle biopsies from 48 patients with enzymatically proven myophosphorylase deficiency who represented different clinical variants of the disease, no cross-reacting material was found, while 12% had markedly reduced cross-reacting material and only one patient had a normal amount of protein (Servedei *et al.*, 1988a).

Molecular genetic heterogeneity

Daegelen and colleagues (1983) were the first to demonstrate in translation studies, using a rabbit reticulocyte cell-free system, the absence of a functional mRNA for myophosphorylase in two unrelated patients with McArdle's disease. Gautron and colleagues (1987) isolated muscle phosphorylase cDNA clones from a human cDNA library, and identified the clone by nucleotide sequencing. Northern blot analysis detected a 3.4 kilobase mRNA species which was specific for normal muscle phosphorylase. Presently Northern blotting has been performed in 12 patients. Pooled data (Gautron *et al.*, 1987, Servedei *et al.*, 1988a) show the following variability in amount and size of muscle phosphorylase mRNA: out of 11 patients examined, 10 were cross-reacting material negative. Of these 10, 6 patients had no detectable mRNA, 3 had normal size but decreased amounts of mRNA, one had truncated mRNA and one had mRNA of normal size. One patient with decreased amounts of cross-reacting material had normal sized mRNA. Pooled studies performed using Southern blot analysis of genomic DNA obtained from 15 patients, digested with different restriction enzymes, revealed identical restriction patterns in 14 patients, while in one Lebanese patient Rsa1 restriction length fragment polymorphism was detected (Anderson *et al.*, 1986; Gautron *et al.*, 1987; Servedei *et al.*, 1988).

The striking variability at the molecular genetic level is consistent with different mutations at the DNA or post-DNA level, possibly not unlike the molecular lesions demonstrated in thalassaemia.

PHOSPHORYLASE b KINASE DEFICIENCY

Phosphorylase *b* kinase (EC 2.7.1.38), the activating enzyme of glycogen phosphorylase, is composed of four subunits: α and β which have regulatory functions, γ which contains the catalytic site and δ which is identical to the calcium binding protein, calmodulin.

Clinical heterogeneity

Clinical variants appear with a wide spectrum (Table 1). A patient with hepatic phosphorylase kinase deficiency but normal muscle enzyme activity has been described (Hug *et al.*, 1969). Another autosomal recessively inherited variant in which both liver and muscle enzymes were affected was described separately in two families (Lederer *et al.*, 1980; Bashan *et al.*, 1981). Clinically these patients presented with hepatomegaly without muscle weakness. Among the myopathic forms, a severe muscular form which started in early infancy has been reported (Ohtani *et al.*, 1982),

Table 1 Variants of phosphorylase *b* kinase deficiency

Type	*Tissue involved*	*Mode of inheritance*	*Author*
IXa	Liver	Autosomal recessive	Hug (1969)
IXb	Leukocytes Liver?Muscle?	X-linked	Huijing (1969)
IXc	Liver,Muscle	Autosomal recessive	Lederer (1980) Bashan (1981
IX Infant	Muscle	?	Ohtani (1982)
IX Adult	Muscle	?	Abarbanel (1986
IX	Heart muscle	?	Mizuta (1984) Servidei (1988b)

while a late onset form with exercise intolerance and muscle cramps has been described (Abarbanel *et al.*, 1986). Two infants are on record who suffered from isolated myocardial phosphorylase kinase deficiency (Mizuta *et al.*, 1984; Servedei *et al.*, 1988b).

Isoenzymes

The marked clinical heterogeneity observed in this disease can be explained on the basis of the existence of tissue-specific isoenzymes which are under different genetic control. Different genetic defects of phosphorylase kinase involving different tissues have also been found in rodents. Evidence that the γ subunit of the liver differs from that of adult muscle and heart has been provided by Northern analysis of mRNA isolated from mouse tissue (Bender and Emerson, 1987), and by characterization of the human liver and muscle phosphorylase kinase. It is therefore conceivable that patients who present with tissue-specific phosphorylase kinase deficiency affecting either muscle or liver but not both have a mutation in their γ subunit, whereas if both tissues are involved an α or possibly a β subunit may be affected as they have been shown to be less tissue-specific (Van den Berg *et al.*, personal communication.)

DEBRANCHER ENZYME DEFICIENCY, GSD III

By removing branch points from the glycogen molecule the debranching enzyme amylo-1,6-glucosidase (EC 3.2.1.33) enables phosphorylase to extend glycogen breakdown to include inner layers of the glycogen molecule. The purified debrancher enzyme consists of a single polypeptide chain with two separate catalytic activities: an α-1,4-glucan transferase, and an α-glucosidase. In addition to the existence of several methods for assaying overall debrancher enzyme activity, the transfer and the hydrolytic activity can be separately assayed.

Distribution of enzyme activity in different tissues

A striking enzymic variability is found among patients regarding overall debrancher activity in tissue and the activities of the transfer and hydrolytic enzymes. On this basis, van Hoof and Hers (1967) subdivided glycogen storage disease type III patients into four groups according to the presence of residual activities of one or both enzymes in liver and muscle. They studied 45 patients with glycogen storage disease type III for the presence of the two activities both in liver and muscle, and found that 35 lacked the enzyme in both tissues while the remaining patients showed varying degrees of residual enzyme activities in muscle. In another study, out of 99 patients with glycogen storage disease type III reviewed, 65 were found to lack the enzyme in both liver and muscle. Of the remaining 33 patients, 12 in whom muscle enzyme activity was measured retained muscle enzyme activity (Illingworth-Brown, 1986). In predominantly North African Jewish cases studied in our laboratory in Israel, all 17 cases examined had both liver and muscle enzyme deficiencies.

Clinical features

Many patients present at an early age with liver involvement manifested by hepatomegaly and fasting hypoglycaemia, with no clinical evidence of myopathy. Some patients with muscle debrancher enzyme deficiencies show in addition to their hepatic involvement variable degrees of muscular weakness, and in a minority the muscle weakness, which may become manifest at different ages, predominates. In rare cases clinical, electromyographic and electron microscopic evidence of neuropathy can be found in addition to myopathy. The distribution of neuromuscular involvement in the Israeli case material is shown in Table 2 (Moses *et al.*, 1986). In addition to skeletal muscular involvement, evidence for cardiac muscular involvement has been found in the majority of patients studied: in most cases the involvement was based on electrocardiographic evidence of biventricular hypertrophy, which was frequently supported by abnormal echocardiographic findings. While 18 of the 19 patients had no cardiac symptoms, one patient had clinical evidence of cardiomyopathy (Table 3) (Moses *et al.*, 1989). On the basis of these findings it is advisable to evaluate the skeletal and cardiac muscular status in any patient who presents with glycogen storage disease type III.

Table 2 Neuromuscular evaluation of 17 GSD III patients

	No. of patients
Clinical:	
Little or no muscular weakness	11/17
Early onset weakness later improved	4/17
Late onset myopathy	2/17
Neuromyopathy	1/17
Laboratory:	
CPK elevation	17/17
EMG: Myopathic findings	9/10
Myo and neuropathic findings	2/10

Table 3 Cardiac involvement in 20 GSD III patients

	No. of patients
Clinical cardiomyopathy (gallop, atrial fibrillation, CHF)	1/20
X-ray (cardiomegaly)	2/20
Echocardiographic (left and right ventricular wall hypertrophy)	13/15
Electrocardiographic (left or biventricular hypertrophy)	19/20

Genetic heterogeneity

The marked tissue-dependent variation in the residual debrancher activity is consistent with the possibility that separate genetic controls affect liver and muscle. Similar conditions are explained in other diseases on the basis of different mutations occurring in tissue-specific isoenzymes. However, since the debrancher enzyme has been purified and found to exist in a single monomeric form which is apparently identical in liver and muscle, the genetic mechanism leading to the different expression of the enzyme in various tissues remains to be elucidated (Chen *et al.*, 1987).

mRNA of the debrancher enzyme was recently studied using cloned cDNA of the human debrancher enzyme. Northern blot analysis of lymphoid cells in four glycogen storage disease type III patients provided evidence for the following molecular heterogeneity: reduced mRNA was found in two cases, a smaller sized mRNA in one case, and no abnormality was detected in the fourth mRNA examined (Ding *et al.*, 1989)

ACID MALTASE DEFICIENCY , GSD II (POMPE'S DISEASE)

Acid maltase (EC 3.2.1.20), a lysosomal α-glucosidase optimally active at pH 4.0, releases glucose from maltose, oligosaccharides and glycogen. It hydrolyses both α-1,4 and α-1,6 linkages and can thus degrade glycogen. The gene coding for acid maltase has been mapped to the long arm of chromosome 17 and has been cloned (Konings *et al.*, 1984).

Clinical features

Acid maltase deficiency manifests a striking clinical heterogeneity. Three phenotypes have been recognized which differ from each other in age of onset, organ involvement and prognosis. The original Pompe's disease which was later called generalized glycogenosis is characterized by early infantile onset, hepatic, skeletal and cardiac muscle involvement, and a rapid downhill course leading to death in infancy. A late onset form which was subsequently described (Courtecouisse *et al.*, 1986) was later subdivided into a childhood and an adult form (Engel *et al.*, 1973). The childhood phenotype does not invariably present with cardiac involvement, and although clinical progress is slow, most patients do not usually survive the second decade of their life. Adult onset acid maltase deficiency presents typically in the form of a limb-girdle type myopathy which is frequently associated with respiratory failure.

Isolated cases have been reported who presented with characteristic features of acid maltase deficiency including lysosomal glycogen accumulation, but in whom no enzyme defect could be detected (Tachi *et al.*, 1988). An unusual family was described in which the index case suffered from infantile acid maltase deficiency with markedly increased muscle glycogen while his grandfather suffered from adult onset acid maltase deficiency with no abnormal glycogen deposition in his muscles (Busch *et al.*, 1979).

Prevalence

While this disease is relatively rare in the Western European countries, it is the most common type of glycogen storage disease found in Taiwan (Lin *et al.*, 1987). Clustering of cases has also been described among Israeli Arabs; 18 out of 20 cases diagnosed in Israel during the last 15 years occurred among unrelated Arabs, 16 of whom had the infantile form of acid maltase deficiency. A marked heterogeneity was found in pH profiles of muscle and leukocyte enzyme activities among patients (Bashan *et al.*, 1988).

Molecular genetics

α-Glucosidase formation was studied in fibroblasts of an adult acid maltase deficiency patient. Northern blot analysis using a cloned α-glucosidase cDNA showed a markedly reduced quantity of the 3.4 kb α-glucosidase mRNA indicating that either synthesis or stability of mRNA is affected (Van der Horst *et al.*, 1987) In another study of mRNA in cell lines from two infantile onset acid maltase deficiency patients, diversity was found at the molecular level: the 3.4 kb mRNA was not detected in one of the cell lines, while the mRNA was present in the other. Examination of DNA with restriction enzymes did not show any major deletion in either of these patients (Martiniuk *et al.*, 1986). On the other hand, restriction length fragment polymorphism was detected in an Indian acid maltase deficient family (Van der Ploeg *et al.*, 1988).

Molecular heterogeneity

The biosynthesis, processing, targeting, packaging and trimming of lysosomal enzymes proceeds through several well-defined intracellular steps, which will be described in brief detail: the high molecular weight precursor synthesized by ribosomes is glycosylated in the endoplasmic reticulum by transfer of a high mannose oligosaccharide from a lipid-linked intermediate to the nascent polypeptide. After additional side chain modifications, the protein reaches the *cis* compartment of the golgi apparatus where mannose residues are phosphorylated to mannose-6-phosphate, which constitutes a recognition marker for the mannose-6-phosphate receptor situated in the *trans* golgi network.

A receptor dependent transport vesicle forms and buds off the golgi network to enter the endolysosome. Within the endolysosome the receptor dissociates and the phosphate moiety is cleaved off, whereupon a limited proteolysis reduces the 110 kDa precursor to the final 70–76 kDa form. The molecular diversity present in acid maltase deficiency was presented in an elegant study by Reuser and colleagues (1987) who investigated the biosynthesis and *in situ* localization of acid α-glucosidase and its precursors in cultured fibroblasts from 30 acid maltase deficiency patients. Biosynthetic forms of α-glucosidase were electrophoretically separated and identified by immunoblotting. The intracellular location of the mutant enzyme was determined by immunoelectron microscopy. By these methods the presence and location of the

110 kDa precursor, the rate of phosphorylation and the presence and location of the mature (70–76 kDa) forms were identified and their enzymic activity measured. It was found that while the endoplasmic reticulum and the golgi complex were normally labelled, lysosomes were deficient in α-glucosidase. The 110 kDa was the only molecular form detectable in all but one of the various mutants, while the intermediate 95 and the mature 76 and 70 kDa forms were partially or completely lacking.

Recently Van der Ploeg and colleagues (1988) found an acid glucosidase precursor of reduced size which was not processed to the mature enzyme. In fibroblasts of some patients, α-glucosidase tended to disappear from the vesicular elements of the *trans* golgi reticulum, and only a fraction of the mutant enzyme seemed to reach the lysosome. A phosphorylation defect could be demonstrated in some cell lines. Reuser and colleagues raised the possibility that in such mutants acid α-glucosidase is secreted rather than sequestered in lysosomes. Lysosomal content of mature catalytically active α-glucosidase was relatively higher in the adult than in the infantile form of acid maltase deficiency but exceptions were noted. Nine different mutant phenotypes were identified by these methods (Reuser *et al.*, 1987; Van der Ploeg *et al.*, 1988)

Enzyme replacement

Hug and Schubert (1967) were the first to try to replace the missing enzyme in a patient with the infantile form of acid maltase deficiency by parenteral administration of purified enzyme extracted from *Aspergillus niger*. Although liver glycogen concentrations decreased to normal levels, the patient succumbed to the disease. Similar experiments performed with human placental enzyme (Hers and De Barsy, 1973) as well as with bone marrow transplantation (Watson *et al.*, 1986) were unsuccessful. Recently successful enzyme replacement in lysosomes of cultured skeletal muscle cells of a patient with the infantile form of acid maltase deficiency has been reported. While using the mannose phosphate receptor on the membrane as a target for a high mannose-containing enzyme precursor purified from human urine, efficient uptake of α-glucosidase into lysosomes and reversal of glycogen storage was demonstrated in tissue culture. (Van der Ploeg *et al.*, 1988)

DIETARY THERAPY

As no primary therapy of the enzyme defect is presently available in any of the muscle glycogenoses, the main therapeutic efforts are dietary in nature. Patients with debrancher enzyme deficiencies have in their early years limited fasting tolerances with hypoglycaemia which are being addressed with frequent feedings, nocturnal gastric infusions of glucose and uncooked cornstarches from two to three years of age.

High protein diets have been advocated in patients with acid maltase deficiency, debrancher enzyme deficiency and muscle phosphorylase deficiency. The rationale behind this therapeutic approach was that an abnormal muscle protein metabolism exists in these myopathies. This has been shown in exercising muscle in phosphorylase-deficient patients where in contrast to normal muscle, in which alanine is released, a net uptake of alanine occurs (Wahren *et al.*, 1973). Debrancher enzyme-deficient patients were found to have low serum branched chain amino acids which are known to be taken up by muscle (Slonim *et al.*, 1983a). In acid maltase deficiency an accelerated protein turnover was found in muscle (Umpleby *et al.*, 1987). It has been suggested that a high protein diet can be beneficial in various ways: it can provide amino acids for muscle protein synthesis, it can be utilized as an alternative fuel for muscle energy metabolism, and it can replace muscle-derived amino acids for gluconeogenesis in the liver. While this treatment resulted in some clinical improvement in a patient with McArdle's disease (Slonim and Goans, 1985), protein administration did not effect the NMR spectrum of an exercising myophosphorylase-deficient patient (Argov *et al.*, 1987). Clinical benefit was more striking but not invariably effective in the myopathic form of debrancher enzyme deficiency (Slonim *et al.*, 1984).

A high protein diet did not prevent the downhill course in the infantile form of acid maltase deficiency whereas some functional improvement was noted in the childhood form of the disease (Slonim *et al.*, 1983b). On the basis of the data presently available it seems warranted to try an innocuous regime of a high protein diet in muscle glycogenosis with functional deficits, except in the infantile form of AMD; however, clinical benefit is not always to be expected.

CONCLUSION

It becomes evident from this review that each of the inborn errors of muscle glycogen metabolism occurs with a wide range of phenotypic variability, in some cases differing markedly from the original clinical description of the disease. Variability can affect age of onset, clinical features, progress of disease, tissue involvement, mode of inheritance and molecular heterogeneity. In some diseases the severity of the clinical features can be correlated with the degree of enzyme deficiency or the involvement of a specific isoenzymic subunit; in other cases some basic questions remain to be elucidated: for example, how in each of the enzyme deficiencies can the frequently observed phenotypic heterogeneity be explained on a molecular basis? What causes some patients with phosphorylase or phosphorylase kinase deficiency to suffer from exercise induced muscle cramps while other patients present with exercise unrelated muscle weakness? What is the basis for the wide spectrum of clinical manifestation in muscle debrancher enzyme deficiency which cannot be explained on the basis of residual enzyme activity? What causes the differences between the hypotonic and the asymptomatic forms of phosphorylase kinase deficiency, or the variability in the age of onset and clinical manifestations in the various forms of acid maltase deficiency? Is there a correlation between this recently found genetic heterogeneity and the striking clinical variability observed in muscle glycogenosis, and if so what is it?

Recent developments have broadened our knowledge and deepened our understanding as to the metabolic derangements, biochemical variations and molecular genetic heterogeneity found in this group of diseases. The information gained, which has had limited application in terms of patient handling, has proved useful for prenatal diagnoses while the present knowledge has been successfully applied in preliminary trials of treatment in the form of enzyme replacement, albeit still as mentioned before, at the tissue culture level.

REFERENCES

Abarbanel, J. M., Bashan, N., Potashnik, R., Moses, S. W. and Herishanu, Y. Adult muscle phosphorylase kinase deficiency. *Neurology* 36 (1986) 560–562

Abarbanel, J. M., Potashnik, R., Frisher, S., Moses, S. W., Osimani, A. and Herishanu, Y. Myophosphorylase deficiency: the course of an unusual congenital myopathy. *Neurology* 37 (1987) 316–318

Anderson, L., Fletterick, R., DiMauro, S., Hwang, P., Gorin, F. and Lebo, R. V. Restriction enzyme analysis of McArdle's syndrome gene locus. *Muscle and Nerve* 9 (1986) 231 (abstract)

Argov, Z., Bank, W. J., Maris, J. and Chance, B. Muscle energy metabolism in McArdle's syndrome by *in vivo* phosphorus magnetic resonance spectroscopy. *Neurology* 37 (1987) 1720–1724

Bashan, N., Iancu, T. C., Lerner, A., Frazer, D., Potashnik, R. and Moses, S. W. Glycogenosis due to liver and muscle phosphorylase kinase deficiency. *Pediatr. Res.* 15 (1981) 299–303

Bashan, N., Potashnik, R., Barash, V., Gutman, A. and Moses, S. W. Glycogen storage disease type II in Israel. *Isr. J. Med. Sci.* 24 (1988) 224–227

Bender, P. K. and Emerson, C. P. Skeletal muscle phosphorylase kinase catalytic subunit mRNA are expressed in heart tissue but not in liver. *J. Biol. Chem.* 262 (1987) 8799–8805

Burke, J., Hwang, P., Anderson, L., Lebo, R., Gorin, F. and Fletterick, R. Intron/Exon structure of the human gene for the muscle isozyme of glycogen phosphorylase. *Proteins* 2 (1987) 177–187

Busch, H. F. M., Koster, J. F. and van Weerden, T. W. Infantile and adult-onset acid maltase deficiency occurring in the same family. *Neurology* 29 (1979) 415–416

Chen, Y. T., He, J. K., Ding, J. H. and Brown, B. I. Glycogen debranching enzyme: Purification, antibody characterisation, and immunoblot analysis of type III glycogen storage disease. *Am. J. Hum. Genet.* 41 (1987) 1002–1015

Chui, L. A. and Munsat, T. L. Dominant inheritance of McArdle's syndrome. *Arch. Neurol.* 33 (1976) 636–641

Courtecuisse, V., Royer, P., Habib, R., Monniere, C. and Demos, J. Glycogenose musculaire pare deficit d'alpha-1,4-glucosidase simulant une dystrophy musculaire progressive. *Arch. Franc. Pediatr.* 22 (1965) 1153–1164

Daegelen, D., Munnich, A., Levin, M. J., Girault, A., Goasguen, J., Kahn, A. and Dreyfus, J. C. Absence of functional messenger RNA for glycogen phosphorylase in the muscle of two patients with McArdle's disease. *Ann. Hum. Genet.* 47 (1983) 107–115

DiMauro, S. and Hartlage, P. L. Fatal infantile form of muscle phosphorylase deficiency. *Neurology* 28 (1978) 1124–1129

DiMauro, S. and Bresolin, N. Phosphorylase deficiency. In Engel, A. G. and Banker, B. Q. (eds.), *Myology*, McGraw-Hill, New York, 1986, pp. 1585–1601

Ding, J. H., Harris, D. A., Bing-Zi, Y. and Chen, Y. T. Cloning of cDNA for human muscle glycogen debrancher, the enzyme deficient in type III glycogen storage disease. *Pediatr. Res.* 25 (1989) 140 A

Duboc, D., Jehenson, P., Tran Dinh, S., Marsac, C., Syrota, A. and Fardeau, M. Phosphorus NMR spectroscopy study of muscular enzyme deficiencies involving glycogenolysis and glycolysis. *Neurology* 37 (1978) 663–671

Engel, A. G., Gomez, M. R., Seybold, M. E. and Lambert, E. H. The spectrum and diagnosis of acid maltase deficiency. *Neurology* 23 (1973) 95–106

Engel, W. K., Eyerman, E. L. and Williams, H. E. Late onset type of skeletal muscle phosphorylase deficiency. A new familial variety with completely and partially affected subjects. *N. Engl. J. Med.* 268 (1963) 135–137

Gautron, S., Daegelen, D., Mennecier, F., Dubocq, D., Kahn, A. and Dreyfus, J. C. Molecular mechanisms of McArdle's disease (muscle glycogen phosphorylase deficiency). *J. Clin. Invest.* 79 (1987) 275–281

Hers, H. G. and De Barsy, T. Type II glycogenosis (acid maltase deficiency). In Hers, H. G. and Van Hoof, F. (eds.) *Lysosomes and Storage Diseases*, Academic Press, New York, 1973, pp. 197–216.

Hug, E., Schubert, W. K. and Chuck, G. Deficient activity of phosphorylase and accumulation of glycogen in the liver. *J. Clin. Invest.* 48 (1969) 704–715

Hug, G. and Schubert, W. K. Lysosomes in type II glycogenosis. Changes during administration of extract from *Aspergillus niger*. *J. Cell. Biol.* 35 (1967) C1–C6

Illingworth-Brown, B. Debranching and branching enzyme deficiencies. In Engel, A. G. and Banker, B. Q. (eds.), *Myology*, McGraw-Hill, New York, 1986, pp. 1653–1662

Lebo, R. V., Gorin, F., Fletterick, R. J., Lao, F. T., Cheung, M. C., Bruce, B. D. and Kan, Y. W. High resolution chromosome sorting and DNA spot-blot analysis assign McArdle's syndrome to chromosome 11. *Science* 225 (1984) 57–59

Lederer, B., Van de Werve, G., De Barsy, T. and Hers, H. G. The autosomal form of phosphorylase kinase deficiency in man: reduced activity of the muscle enzyme. *Biochem. Biophys. Res. Commun.* 92 (1980) 169–174

Lewis, S. F. and Haller, R. G. The pathophysiology of McArdle's disease: clues to regulation in exercise and fatigue. *J. Appl. Physiol.* 61 (1986) 391–401

Lin, C. Y., Hwang, B., Hsiao, K. J. and Jin, Y. R. Pompe's disease in China and prenatal diagnosis by determination of α-glucosidase activity. *J. Inher. Metab. Dis.* 10 (1987) 11–17

Martiniuk, F., Mehler, M., Pellicer, A., Tzall, S., La Badie, G., Hobart, C., Ellenbogen, A. and Hirschhorn, R. Isolation of a cDNA for human acid α-glucosidase and detection of genetic heterogeneity for mRNA in three α-glucosidase-deficient patients. *Proc. Natl. Acad. Sci. USA* 83 (1986) 9641–9644

McArdle, B. Myopathy due to a defect of muscle glycogen breakdown. *Clin. Sci.* 24 (1951) 13–33

Mineo, I., Kono, N., Hara, N., Shimizu, T., Yamada, Y., Kawachi, M., Kiyokawa, H., Wang, Y. L. and Tarui, S. Myogenic hyperuricemia: a common pathophysiologic feature of glycogenosis types III, V, and VII. *N. Engl. J. Med.* 317 (1987) 75–80

Mizuta, K., Kashimoto, E. and Tsutou, A. A new type of glycogen storage disease caused by deficiency of cardiac phosphorylase kinase. *Biochem. Biophys. Res. Commun.* 119 (1984) 582–587

Moses, S. W., Gadoth, N., Bashan, N., Ben-David, E., Slonim, A. and Wanderman, K. L. Neuromuscular involvement in glycogen storage disease type III. *Acta Paediatr. Scand.* 75 (1986) 289–296

Moses, S. W., Wanderman, K. L., Myroz, A. and Friedman, M. Cardiac involvement in glycogen storage disease type III. *Eur. J. Pediatr.* 431 (1989) 1–3

Ohtani, I., Matzuda, I., Iwasama, T., Tamari, H., Origuchi, Y. and Miike, T. Infantile glycogen storage myopathy in a girl with phosphorylase kinase deficiency. *Neurology* 32 (1982) 833–838

Reuser, A. J. J., Kroos, M., Willemsen, R., Swallow, D., Tager, J. M. and Galjaard, H. Clinical diversity in glycogenosis type II. *J. Clin. Invest.* 79 (1987) 1689–1699

Schmidt, B., Servidei, S., Gabbai, A. A., Silva, A. C., de Sousa Bulle de Oliveira, A. and DiMauro, S. McArdle's disease in two generations: autosomal recessive transmission with manifesting heterozygote. *Neurology* 37 (1987) 1558–1561

Servedei, S., Shanske, S., Zeviani, M., Lebo, R., Fletterick, R. and DiMauro, S. McArdle's disease: biochemical and molecular genetic studies. *Ann. Neurol.* 24 (1988a) 774–781

Servidei, S., Metlay, L. A., Chodosh, J. and DiMauro, S. Fatal cardiopathy caused by phosphorylase *b* kinase deficiency. *J. Pediatr.* 113 (1988b) 82–85

Slonim, A. E. and Goans, P. J. Myopathy in McArdle's syndrome. Improvement with a high protein diet. *N. Engl. J. Med.* 312 (1985) 355–359

Slonim, A. E., Coleman, R. A., Moses, S., Bashan, N., Shipp, E. and Mushlin, P. Amino acid disturbance in type III glycogenosis: differences from type I glycogenosis. *Metabolism* 32 (1983a) 70–74

Slonim, A. E., Coleman, R. A., McElligot, M. A., Najjar, J., Hirschhorn, K., Labadie, G. U., Mrak, R., Evans, O. B., Shipps, E. and Presson, R. Improvement of muscle function in acid maltase deficiency by high protein therapy. *Neurology* 33 (1983b) 34–38

Slonim, A. E., Coleman, R. A. and Moses, S. W. Myopathy and growth failure in debrancher enzyme deficiency: Improvement with high-protein nocturnal enteral therapy. *J. Pediatr.* 105 (1984) 906–911

Tachi, N., Tachi, M., Sasaki, K., Tomita, H., Wakai, S., Annaka, S., Minami, R., Tsurui, S. and Sugie, S. Glycogen storage disease with normal acid maltase: skeletal and cardiac muscle. *Pediatr. Neurol.* 5 (1989) 60–63

Umpleby, M., Wiles, C. M., Trend, P., Scobie, I. N., Macleod, A. F., Spencer, G. T. and Sonsken, P. H. Protein turnover in acid maltase deficiency before and after treatment with high protein diet. *J. Neurol. Neurosurg.* and *Psychiatry* 50 (1987) 587–592

Van der Horst, G. T. J., Hoefsloot, E. H., Kroos, M. A. and Reuser, A. J. J. Cell free translation of human lysosomal α-glucosidase: evidence for reduced precursor synthesis in an adult patient with glycogenosis type II. *Biochim. Biophys. Acta* 910 (1987) 123–129

Van der Ploeg, A. T., Loonen, M. C. B., Bolhuis, P. A., Busch, H. M. F., Reuser, A. J. J. and Galjaard, H. Receptor mediated uptake of acid α-glucosidase corrects lysosomal storage in cultured skeletal muscle. *Pediatr. Res.* 24 (1988) 90–94

Van Hoof, F. and Hers, H. G. The subgroups of type III glycogenosis. *Eur. J. Biochem.* 2 (1967) 265–270

Wahren, J., Felig, P., Havel, R. J., Jorfeldt, L., Pernow, B. and Saltin, B. Amino acid metabolism in McArdle's syndrome. *N. Engl. J. Med.* 288 (1973) 774–777

Watson, G. J., Gardner-Medwin, D., Goldfinch, M. E. and Pearson, A. D. J. Bone marrow transplantation for glycogen storage disease type II (Pompe's disease). *N. Engl. J. Med.* 314 (1986) 385

J. Inher. Metab. Dis. 13 (1990) 466–475

Inherited Disorders of Carbohydrate Metabolism in Children Studied by ^{13}C-Labelled Precursors, NMR and GC–MS

A. LAPIDOT
Department of Isotope Research, Weizmann Institute of Science, 76100 Rehovot, Israel

Summary: Glucose carbon recycling, glucose production and glucose turnover in glycogen storage disease type I and type II patients and control subjects were determined by a novel approach – mass isotopomer analysis of plasma ^{13}C glucose. Changes in the isotopomer distribution of plasma ^{13}C glucose were found only in glycogen storage disease type III patients and control subjects. Glucose carbon recyling parameters were also derived from ^{13}C NMR spectra of plasma glucose C-1 splitting pattern. Our results eliminate a mechanism for glucose production in glycogen storage disease type I children involving gluconeogenesis. However, glucose release by amylo-1,6-glucosidase activity is in agreement with our results.

A quantitative determination of the metabolic pathways of fructose conversion to glucose in normal children, and in children with disorders of fructose metabolism was derived from ^{13}C NMR measurement of plasma ^{13}C glucose isotopomer populations following [U-^{13}C]fructose administration. A direct pathway from fructose, bypassing fructose-1-phosphate aldolase, to fructose-1,6-diphosphate in controls and hereditary fructose intolerant children (47% and 27%, respectively) was identified. In children with fructose-1,6-diphosphatase deficiency, only the gluconeogenic substrates were ^{13}C labelled but no synthesis of glucose from [U-^{13}C]fructose occurred. The significantly lower (by 68%) conversion of fructose to glucose in hereditary fructose intolerance, as compared to control subjects, and non-conversion in fructose-1,6-diphosphatase deficient subjects after [U-^{13}C]fructose ($\sim$ 20 mg/kg) administration can serve as the basis of a safe diagnostic test for patients suspected of inborn errors of fructose metabolism and other defects involving gluconeogenesis.

The release of glucose from the cell produced either by glycogenolysis or gluconeogenesis involves the hydrolysis of glucose-6-phosphate by glucose-6-phosphatase (EC 3.1.3.9). As a result of impairment of glucose-6-phosphatase activity, children with glycogen storage disease type I are susceptible to hypoglycaemia during short periods of fasting (Howell and Williams, 1982). However, a limited amount of endogenous glucose production was found in these children (Tsalikian *et al.*,, 1984; Schwenk *et al.*, 1986; Kalderon *et al.*, 1988). A novel method based on mass isotopomer distribution in glycogen glucose from infused [U-^{13}C]glucose has been introduced by us (Kalderon *et al.*, 1986) and was recently used to determine glucose recycling in glycogen storage disease and control subjects (Kalderon *et al.*, 1988; 1989a). We have recently shown that the source of endogenous glucose production is not gluconeogenesis, in contrast to patients with amylo-1,6-glucosidase (debrancher enzyme; EC 3.2.1.33) deficiency (glycogen storage disease type III), whose endogenous glucose is mainly derived from gluconeogenic precursors (Kalderon *et al.*, 1989a).

A non-invasive and non-radioactive approach was recently undertaken to assess the mechanism by which glucose is produced in children with glycogen storage disease type I (Lapidot *et al.*, 1988; Kalderon *et al.*, 1989b). D-[U-^{13}C]glucose was administered to patients with glycogen storage disease type I and glycogen storage disease type III and compared with control subjects. Glucose carbon recycling was determined by monitoring ^{13}C NMR resonances of plasma glucose at position C-1 coupled to C-2. Endogenous dilution by non-labelled glucose molecules in comparison to dilution by recycled glucose molecules enabled us to suggest mechanisms for glucose production in two types of glycogen storage disease patients, type I and type III. Other enzymatic defects in glucose production are currently being investigated using a similar methodological approach.

An inborn deficiency in the ability of aldolase B (EC 2.1.2.13) to split fructose-1-phosphate is found in humans with hereditary fructose intolerance. An inborn deficiency of fructose-1,6-diphosphatase (fructose-1,6-biphosphatase, hexose diphosphatase, EC 3.1.3.11) is a severe disorder of gluconeogenesis, threatening life in the first few years (Gitzelmann *et al.*, 1985). D-[U-^{13}C]fructose was given to these patients and control children and ^{13}C NMR measurements of plasma glucose isotopomer populations were performed. Our results reveal that splitting of fructose-1-phosphate (F-1-P) by aldolase, the well-known pathway in the conversion of fructose to glucose, accounts for only approximately 50% of the total amount of fructose conversion to glucose; phosphorylation of F-1-P to F-1,6-diP accounts for the other part. Thus, an understanding of inherited disorders of carbohydrate metabolism should clarify our knowledge of normal metabolism and define biochemical adaptations available to the human organism.

EXPERIMENTAL PROCEDURES

Subject and study design: The studies included control infants and patients with glycogen storage disease types I and III, hereditary fructose intolerance or fructose-1,6-diphosphatase deficiency. A total of 13 studies were performed in glycogen storage disease and control subjects, each of whom received a primed dose-constant nasogastric infusion of D-[U^{13}C]glucose (99% ^{13}C enriched) (or an infusion diluted with non-labelled glucose solution) at a rate of 0.4–6.0 mg kg^{-1} min^{-1}; blood samples were taken at intervals up to 100 min to determine steady state conditions as previously described (Kalderon *et al.*, 1989a, 1989b). The hereditary fructose intolerance and fructose-1,6-diphosphatase deficient patients were on strict low fructose diets and were in good health when [U^{13}C]fructose measurements were carried out. A total of 18 studies were performed in these patients and control subjects after fasting (7–9 h), each of whom received a primed dose-constant nasogastric infusion of D-(U-^{13}C]fructose (99% ^{13}C enriched) at a rate of 0.3–0.5 mg kg^{-1} min^{-1} (Gopher *et al.*, 1989).

This study received the approval of the Human Studies Commitee of Hadassah Medical Centre, Jerusalem, the Kaplan Hospital, Rehovot, and the Rambam Hospital, Haifa. Informed consent was obtained from the parents of the children.

Materials: D-[U-^{13}C]glucose was prepared in our laboratory from algae grown on $^{13}CO_2$ < 99% enriched (Lapidot and Kahana, 1986) and D-[U-^{13}C]fructose was obtained from D-[U-^{13}C]glucose (99% enriched) by glucose isomerase conversion.

NMR spectroscopy: High resolution ^{13}C NMR spectra were obtained with a Bruker AM 500 MHz spectrometer operating at 125.76 MHz.

Determination of isotopic enrichments of ^{13}C glucose at position C-1: Plasma glucose recycling was determined either by comparing the ^{13}C isotopomer populations of the infused D-[U-^{13}C]glucose to plasma ^{13}C glucose, by mass spectrometry techniques (Kalderon *et al.*, 1989a), or by measuring ^{13}C resonance of glucose at position C-1 coupled to glucose C-2 with ^{13}C NMR (Kalderon *et al.*, 1989b), thereby measuring intramolecular dilution of glucose at position C-2 in comparison to C-1.

Mass isotopomer analysis of plasma glucose: This was determined by selective ion monitoring by gas chromatography–mass spectrometry as previously described (Kalderon *et al.*, 1989a).

RESULTS AND DISCUSSION

The mechanisms of glucose production and recycling in glycogen storage disease type I and glycogen storage disease type III

The primary enzymatic defect in glycogen storage disease type I prevents the generation of free glucose from glucose-6-phosphate derived from either glycogenolysis or gluconeogenesis. It has therefore been assumed that the hypoglycaemia observed in patients with glycogen storage disease type I results from a defect in glucose production. A progressive increase in endogenous glucose production (1.1 to 3.5 mg kg^{-1} min^{-1}) in glycogen storage disease type I patients, found in our study and by others (Tsalikian *et al.*, 1984), indicates that glucose is released in glycogen storage disease type I children lacking glucose-6-phosphatase activity. The mechanism(s) by which glycogen storage disease type I subjects produce glucose is not clear. The aim of our studies is to evaluate the contribution of alternative pathways for glucose production in glycogen storage disease types I and III patients. Under normal conditions D[U-^{13}C]glucose is converted into D[U-^{13}C]lactate and D[U-^{13}C]alanine, as a result of glycolysis in the peripheral tissues (and in the liver), and newly synthesized glucose can be produced in the liver by gluconeogenesis. Thus, the recycling of glucose carbons back to glucose through the three carbon molecule pool provides an estimate of gluconeogenic activity. The ratio of plasma glucose molecules having less than six ^{13}C atoms per molecule to molecules of six ^{13}C per molecule has been used to calculate the extent of glucose carbon recycling (Kalderon *et al.*, 1988, 1989a) (see equations 1 and 2).

$$NR = P_6 / \sum_{n=1}^{6} 6(P_n) \qquad \text{(equation 1)}$$

NR in equation 1 is the ratio of the number of molecules of glucose having six ^{13}C atoms (P_6) to the total number of molecules of glucose having one to six ^{13}C atoms (P_n).

The NR value of the infused glucose is 0.93 ± 0.01, due to some contribution of P_5 and P_4 to the main isotopomer P_6. Correction for 'isotopic impurities' is included in equation 2, where GR is the calculated glucose recycling:

$$GR = \left[1 - \frac{\text{NR (plasma glucose)}}{\text{NR (infused glucose)}}\right] \times 100 \qquad \text{(equation 2)}$$

Although endogenous glucose production in glycogen storage disease type I patients varied as a function of glucose infusion rates, no indication of plasma glucose recyling was found in any of the glycogen storage disease type I patients, whereas a significant change in isotopomer distribution was found in glycogen storage disease type III patients, corresponding to 50% glucose carbon recycling (Kalderon *et al.*, 1989a).

To assess the mechanism by which glucose is produced in glycogen storage disease type I, a new approach was developed (Lapidot *et al.*, 1988; Kalderon *et al.*, 1989b) for measuring hepatic glucose recycling, by monitoring ^{13}C NMR resonances of plasma glucose at position C-1 coupled to C-2. Linear regression analysis of β-glucose C-1 doublet to singlet (d/s) peak areas as a function of ^{13}C enrichment of glucose C-1 is presented in Figure 1. It represents a dilution curve of D[U-^{13}C]glucose by unlabelled glucose molecules. The d/s peak area values derived from the ^{13}C NMR plasma glucose C-1 splitting pattern of glycogen storage disease type I patients (as a function of their ^{13}C enrichments) coincided with the dilution curve. These results indicate that the plasma glucose of glycogen storage disease type I subjects comprises only a mixture of [99%-U-^{13}C]D-glucose and unlabelled glucose and lacks any recycled glucose. Significantly different glucose carbon recyling values were obtained for glycogen storage disease type III patients in comparison to glycogen storage disease type I patients (Figure 1), as a result of a greatly reduced degree of C-1, C-2 coupling. Only residual hepatic activity of glucose-6-phosphatase in glycogen storage disease type I would result in newly synthesized recycled glucose; since our findings reveal that glucose production in these patients is non-recycled, the proposed mechanism based on residual glucose-6-phosphatase activity (Tsalikian *et al.*, 1984) can be eliminated. However, glucose release by amylo-1,6-glucosidase activity would result in endogenous production of non-^{13}C-labelled and non-recycled glucose carbon, as was found in our study. In contrast, in glycogen storage disease type III

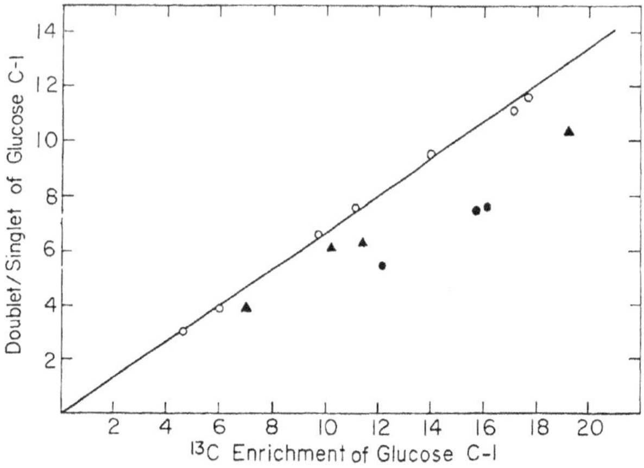

Figure 1 Glycogen storage disease type I plasma glucose C-1 d/s as a function of glucose C-1 ^{13}C enrichment (○), values coincide with the standard dilution curve (———). Glycogen storage disease type III patients (●) and control subjects (▲) deviate from the standard dilution curve.

patients gluconeogenesis is suggested as the major route for endogenous glucose synthesis. The significant difference between the glucose C-1 splitting pattern of glycogen storage disease type III plasma and control subjects in comparison to glycogen storage disease type I plasma can be used as a parameter for estimating glucose recycling.

Our recent findings (unpublished results) that glycogen storage disease type I patients could not release ^{13}C glucose following ^{13}C fructose administration, support the mechanism suggested for glucose production in glycogen storage disease type I patients (Kalderon *et al.*, 1989a). In contrast, gluconeogenesis is the main route for glucose production in glycogen storage disease type III, thus the conversion of ^{13}C fructose to ^{13}C glucose in these patients was found to be similar to that in normal controls (unpublished results).

Either the ^{13}C NMR or the mass isotopomer analysis procedures using ^{13}C labelled tracers can be developed as a non-invasive diagnostic test for inborn enzymatic defects involving gluconeogenesis.

Fructose metabolism in man, a suggested mechanism

An inborn deficiency in the ability of aldolase B to split fructose-1-phosphate is found in humans with hereditary fructose intolerance (Gitzelmann *et al.*, 1985). Since aldolase B is a key enzyme in fructose metabolism, elucidation of fructose metabolic pathways in hereditary fructose intolerance should throw light on the contribution of different pathways of fructose conversion in the normal subject and define the range of metabolic adaptation available. In most cases of hereditary fructose intolerance, final diagnosis of aldolase B deficiency is usually performed on liver biopsy specimens. Although the advantages of using stable isotope-labelled fructose for *in vivo* diagnosis of hereditary fructose intolerance in infants and young children are evident, such a technique has not yet been developed.

The main site of fructose metabolism is the liver. Cleavage of fructose-1-phosphate to triose phosphate and subsequent condensation to fructose-1,6-diphosphate is accepted to be the primary pathway of fructose conversion to glucose (Hers, 1957). Since fructose once it reaches the bloodstream is utilized rapidly, plasma ^{13}C NMR spectra taken after [U-^{13}C]fructose infusion for approximately 70 min, (at the rate of 0.3–0.5 mg/kg per min) do not contain ^{13}C resonances corresponding to [U-^{13}C] fructose (preliminary results, Lapidot *et al.*, 1989). The ^{13}C enrichment of plasma glucose derived from the infused [U-^{13}C]fructose is in the range of 0.5–3.9% (atom % excess), thus the ^{13}C NMR glucose C-1 centre peak arises mainly from the non-enriched glucose carbon (1.1%) while the doublet resonances of ^{13}C glucose arise from glucose C-1 coupled to C-2 (Figure 2). Thus the doublet to singlet (d/s) ratio of glucose C-1 is a reflection of its enrichment as observed when compared to GC–MS results (Gopher *et al.*, 1990a; Lapidot *et al.*, 1989).

Linear regression analysis of β-glucose C-1 d/s peak areas as a function of [U-^{13}C] fructose infusion rates is shown in Figure 3 for hereditary fructose intolerance and control subjects. The significant difference between the slopes of the curves derived from hereditary fructose intolerance patient data and from control subject measure-

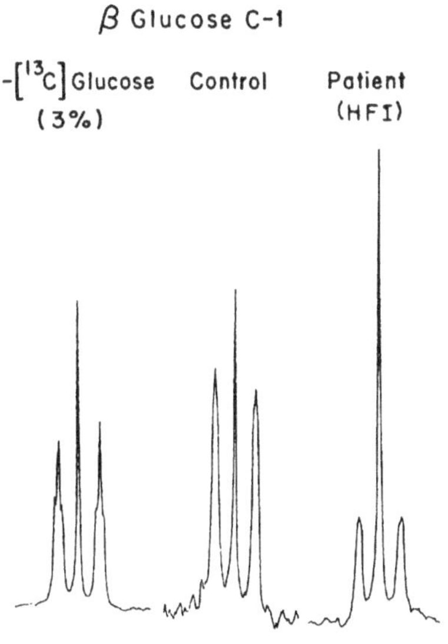

Figure 2 Expanded ^{13}C NMR views of a β-glucose C-1 of control and hereditary fructose intolerance subjects, and [U-^{13}C]glucose (3%, in a mixture with non-labelled glucose).

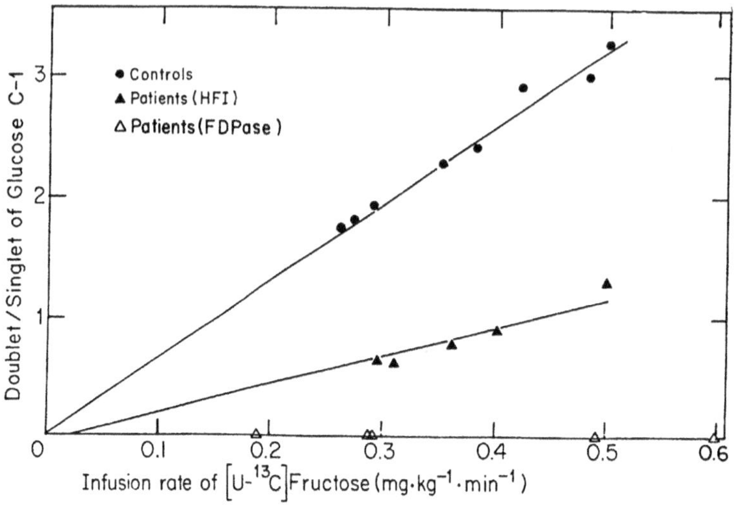

Figure 3 Linear regression analysis of proton-decoupled ^{13}C NMR of the β-glucose C-1 fraction d/s ratio as a function of [U-^{13}C]fructose (99%) infusion rates, in control subjects (●) and hereditary fructose intolerance patients (▲) ($r = 0.990$; $y = 0.034 + 6.465x$ and $r = 0.980$; $y = -0.074 \pm 2.480x$ respectively), in comparison to fructose-1,6-diphosphatase patients (△).

ments indicates that the conversion of fructose to glucose declined by 68% in hereditary fructose intolerance patients.

Quantitation of fructose metabolic steps in normal and hereditary fructose intolerance children was based on ^{13}C NMR measurements of plasma glucose isotopomer populations. The isotopomer populations at position C-4 of two (C_3-$^*C_4$-$^*C_5$) or three ($^*C_3$-$^*C_4$-$^*C_5$) adjacent ^{13}C atoms permitted us to quantitate the metabolic pathways of fructose conversion to glucose in the human liver. For example, Figure 4 illustrates that the 5-line multiplet observed for α and β C-4 is the consequence of the presence of a mixture of isotopomers. The apparent triplet resonances are due to glucose *C-4 coupled to *C-3 and *C-5, and the doublet resonances are those of glucose *C-4 coupled to *C-5. The singlet resonance of C-4 is mainly from the natural abundance of ^{13}C (1.1%). The relative areas of the individual components of the multiplet were measured. The results lead us to suggest that two main pathways are responsible for conversion of fructose to glucose in humans, a direct and an indirect phosphorylation pathway of fructose-1-phosphate to fructose-1,6-diphosphate; each one accounts for approximately 50% (in control subjects) of the total conversion (Figure 5).

In our recent studies on children with fructose-1,6-diphosphatase deficiency (Gopher *et al.*, 1990), the occurrence of an initial phosphorylation of fructose to fructose-6-phosphate is not in agreement with the non-labelled glucose values observed after [U-^{13}C]fructose admininstration to five fructose-1,6-diphosphatase deficient patients

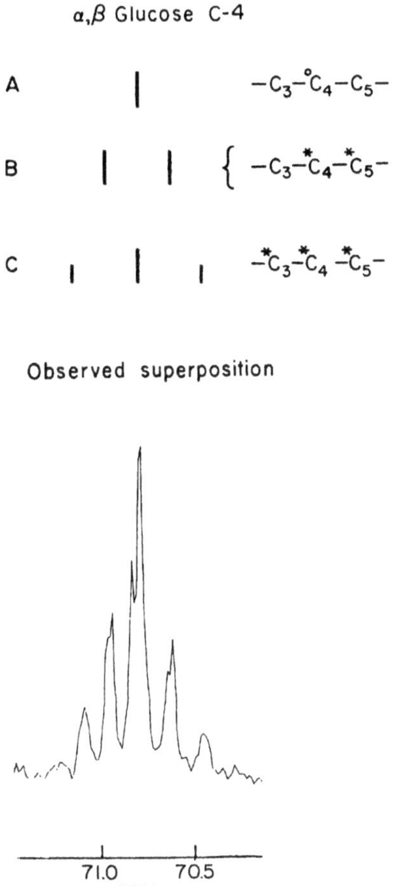

Figure 4 Schematic presentation of isotopomer population of α,β-glucose *C-4 coupled to one or two adjacent ^{13}C atoms. The corresponding observed superpositions are extended views of the spectra obtained from a control subject. C_3-$^0C_4$-C_5 is the natural abundance peak of glucose C-4. Since the centre peak of the triplet resonances coincided with the natural abundance peaks, triplet resonances were calculated by multiplying by 2 the outer peak areas.

(Figure 3). Since in these patients the deficiency is in the fructose-1,6-diphosphatase activity but not in the hexokinase activity, phosphorylation of fructose to fructose-6-phosphate might be expected. However, our findings show that after [U-^{13}C]fructose administration to fructose-1,6-diphosphatase deficient children, only the gluconeogenic precursors, lactate, alanine and glycerol are ^{13}C enriched and not the glucose itself. This indicates that there is a direct pathway from fructose, bypassing fructose-

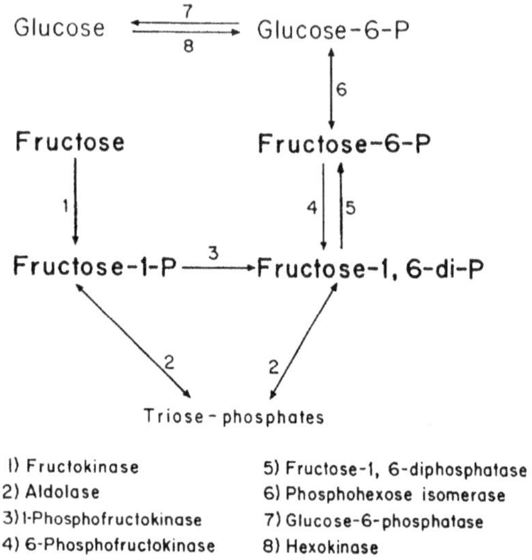

Figure 5 Schematic presentation of fructose conversion to glucose in human liver; a suggested mechanism for fructose-1-phosphate bypassing fructose-1-phosphate aldolase to fructose-1,6-diphosphate by 1-phosphofructokinase.

1-phosphate aldolase, to fructose-1,6-diphosphate in these patients but since their fructose-1,6-diphosphatase activity is impaired, glucose is not formed via this pathway.

The significantly different degree of conversion of fructose to glucose obtained in hereditary fructose intolerance in comparison to fructose-1,6-diphosphatase deficient children can be used as a diagnostic criterion. The procedure described can serve as the basis of a safe diagnostic test for patients suspected of having inborn errors of fructose metabolism.

ACKNOWLEDGEMENTS

To my coworkers listed in the references: Drs Kalderon, Gopher, Gutman, Korman, Mandel and Vaisman; and to the Israel Academy of Science and Ministry of Health for supporting this research.

REFERENCES

Gitzelmann, R., Steinmann, B. and Van de Berghe, G. Essential fructosuria, hereditary fructose intolerance, and fructose-1,6-diphosphatase deficiency. In: *The Metabolic Basis of Inherited Disease* (5th edn.), New York, McGraw-Hill, 1985, pp. 118–139

Gopher, A., Vaismann, N., Mandel, H. and Lapidot, A. Determination of fructose metabolic pathways in normal and fructose-intolerant children: A ^{13}C NMR study using [U-^{13}C] fructose. *Proc. Natl. Acad. Sci. USA* (1990a) in press

Gopher, A., Gutman, A. and Lapidot, A. Metabolic studies in patients with fructose-1,6-diphosphatase deficiency by [U-^{13}C]fructose with ^{13}C NMR, development of a diagnostic test. (1990b) (submitted for publication)

Hers, H. G. *Le Metabolism du Fructose*, Edition Arscia, Brussels, 1957

Howell, R. R. and Williams, J. C. The glycogen storage disease. In: *The Metabolic Basis of Inherited Disease* (5th edn.), McGraw-Hill, New York, 1982, pp. 141–166

Kalderon, B., Gopher, A. and Lapidot, A. Metabolic pathways leading to liver glycogen repletion *in vivo*, studied by GC–MS and NMR. *FEBS Lett.* 204 (1986) 29–32

Kalderon, B., Lapidot, A., Korman, S. H. and Gutman, A. Glucose recycling and production in children with glycogen storage disease type I, studied by gas chromatography/mass spectrometry and [U-^{13}C]glucose. *Biomed. Environ. Mass Spectrom.* 16 (1988) 305–308

Kalderon, B., Korman, S. H., Gutman, A. and Lapidot, A. Glucose recyling and production in glycogenosis type I and III: stable isotope technique study. *Am. J. Physiol.* 257 *Endocrinol. Metabol.* 20 (1989a) (E346–353)

Kalderon, B., Korman, S. H., Gutman, A. and Lapidot, A. Estimation of glucose carbon recycling in children with glycogen storage disease. A ^{13}C NMR study using [U-^{13}C]glucose. *Proc. Natl. Acad. Sci. USA* 89 (1989b) 4990–4994

Lapidot, A. and Kahan, Z. Biological process for preparing compounds labelled with stable isotopes. *Trends in Biotechnol.* 4 (1986) 2–4

Lapidot, A., Kalderon, B., Korman, S. H. and Gutman, A. *In vivo* diagnosis of glycogen storage diseases by [U-^{13}C]glucose and ^{13}C NMR. *Society of Magnetic Resonance in Medicine* (1988) p. 249

Lapidot, A., Gopher, B. and Vaisman, N. Fructose metabolism in hereditary fructose intolerance and control children. *Society of Magnetic Resonance in Medicine* (1989) p. 571

Schwenk, W. F. and Haymond, M. W. Optimal rate of external glucose administration in children with glycogen storage disease type I. *N. Engl. J. Med.* 314 (1986) 682–685

Tsalikian, E., Simmons, P., Gerich, J. E., Howared, C. and Haymond, N. W. Glucose production and utilization in children with glycogen storage disease type I. *Am. J. Physiol.* 247 *Endocrinol. Metabol.* 10 (1984) E513–E519

J. Inher. Metab. Dis. 13 (1990) 476–486

Galactose Disorders: an Overview

J. B. HOLTON
Department of Clinical Chemistry, Southmead Hospital, Bristol BS10 5NB, UK

Summary: There are three separate disorders of galactose metabolism of clinical importance. Galactokinase deficiency mainly causes cataracts which regress without complications providing a galactose-free diet is started early enough. UDPgalactose-4-epimerase deficiency seems extremely rare. A common feature of the two reported cases is nerve deafness. Galactose-1-phosphate uridyl transferase deficiency poses the greatest problems because of the poor long-term outcome in spite of a galactose-restricted diet, and with no clear indications of how and when the underlying damage occurs. Recent evidence of low erythrocyte and tissue UDPgal levels, associated with ovarian dysfunction, may indicate impaired galactoside synthesis. Administration of uridine corrects the UDPgal depletion and trials in which it is added to the galactose-restricted diet have begun.

There are three clinically significant disorders of galactose metabolism (Segal, 1989) which are due to deficiencies of galactokinase (EC 2.7.1.6), galactose-1-phosphate uridyl transferase (transferase, EC 2.7.7.10) and uridine diphosphate galactose-4-epimerase (epimerase, EC 5.1.3.2). There is a variant of epimerase deficiency in which the enzyme abnormality is confined mainly to erythrocytes, and there are no obvious clinical sequelae (Gitzelmann, 1972). This variant will not be discussed any further in this paper.

BIOCHEMISTRY

Galactose metabolism

The pathways of galactose metabolism, and associated enzyme reactions, are shown in Figure 1. The principal object of the main pathway, through gal-1-P and UDPgal, has been considered to be the conversion of large amounts of galactose to glc-1-P, which is particularly important in the infant whose carbohydrate source is lactose. The overall conversion of the galactose moiety to glucose is carried out by epimerase, in which inversion of the H and OH groups on C-4 occurs.

The critical requirement for epimerase in the metabolism of a galactose load was demonstrated by observations in an epimerase-deficient patient (Henderson *et al.*, 1983). On a small daily intake of galactose of about 1 g, the main metabolite which accumulated in erythrocytes was the substrate for epimerase, UDPgal. On larger

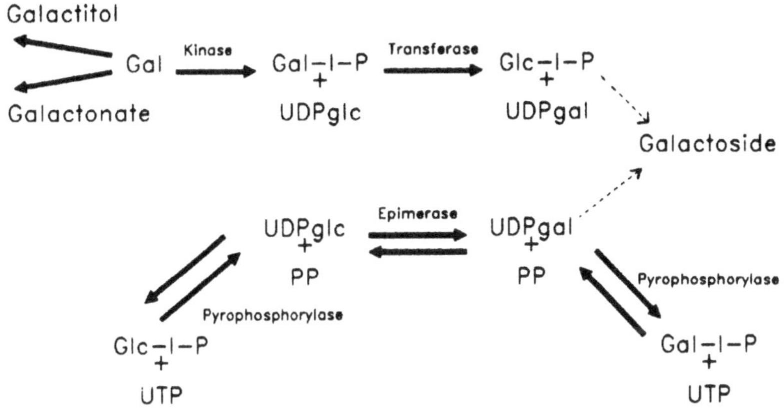

Figure 1 Pathways of galactose metabolism. The main route for galactose metabolism is via galactokinase (kinase), galactose-1-phosphate uridyl transferase (transferase), uridine diphosphate galactose-4-epimerase and UDP-glucose pyrophosphorylase. A second pathway allowing interconversion of glucose and galactose metabolites involves UDPglc and UDPgal pyrophosphorylase, and epimerase.

supplements of galactose, 2–4 g/day, the concentration of UDPgal reached a plateau, but gal-1-P concentrations increased progressively and became greater than those of UDPgal. This apparent inability to metabolize gal-1-P could be due to a depletion of UDPglc and/or the competitive inhibition of UDPglc by UTP in the transferase reaction.

Synthesis of galactosides

The other important aspect of galactose metabolism is the requirement to incorporate it into complex oligosaccharides, glycoproteins and glycolipids (galactosides) which use UDPgal as the necessary galactosyl donor. UDPgal is a product of the transferase reaction but may also be made from glc-1-P, involving pyrophosphorylase and epimerase. In transferase deficiency it has been assumed that adequate UDPgal synthesis would be maintained by the latter pathway. However, Shin and colleagues (1985) reported that UDPgal concentrations were low in erythrocytes of treated transferase-deficient patients. This finding has been confirmed and extended by Ng and colleagues (1987) and their results are shown in Table 1. Patients with complete transferase deficiency had erythrocyte UDPgal concentrations of about 40% of normal, but those with a variant form of the disorder, with less than 1–2.5% of normal transferase, had normal concentrations of the cofactor. Both groups of patients had normal concentrations of erythrocyte UDPglc and similarly increased concentrations of gal-1-P. A depletion of UDPgal in transferase deficiency was also found in liver and skin fibroblasts.

The implication of the above observation is that some transferase activity is

Table 1 Erythrocyte gal-1-P, UDPglc and UDPgal levels in transferase-deficient subjects and low activity variants[a]

	Patients *Classical*[b] ($n = 26$)	*Variants*[b] ($n = 3$)	*Controls*
Gal-1-P (mg/100 ml RBC)	2.66 ± 0.53	2.25 ± 0.47	0
UDPglc (μmol/100 g Hb)	38.9 ± 14.6	44.1 ± 10.2	38.1 ± 7.1
UDPgal (μmol/100 g Hb)	3.88 ± 1.79	9.40 ± 3.53	10.3 ± 3.5

[a] From Ng *et al.*, (1987)
[b] Classical patients had no measurable transferase activity, variant patients had 1–2% of normal transferase levels

essential to maintain normal UDPgal concentrations. This is interesting in the context of the recent cloning of the transferase gene (Reichardt and Berg, 1988) and its location on the short arm of chromosome 9, next to the gene for galactosyl transferase (Reichardt, personal communication). This is supportive of a rôle for transferase in maintaining UDPgal concentrations, at least in evolutionary terms.

The depletion of UDPgal in transferase deficiency does not necessarily indicate reduced availability of cofactor for transfer of galactose into complexes, but abnormal galactoside synthesis is being considered as a pathogenetic mechanism in the disorder. Experimental evidence for an effect on galactose incorporation into glycoproteins of transferase deficient cultured skin fibroblasts grown on a galactose-free medium has been obtained (Dobbie *et al.*, 1990). Transferase-deficient fibroblasts had a significant lowering of the galactose/mannose and the galactose + sialic acid/mannose ratios compared to control cells (Table 2).

On the first discovery of an epimerase-deficient child (Holton *et al.*, 1981) there

Table 2 Carbohydrate composition of transferase deficient and control cell lines grown on a galactose-depleted medium

Cell type	*μg mannose/ mg protein*	*μg galactose/ mg protein*	*μg (sialic acid + galactose)/ μg mannose*	*μg galactose/ μg mannose*
Controls ($n = 8$)	0.85 ± 0.25	0.83 ± 0.21	1.46 ± 0.37	1.00 ± 0.22
Transferase deficient ($n = 6$)	0.78 ± 0.37	0.60 ± 0.32	1.08[a] ± 0.13	0.77[a] ± 0.08

[a] Difference control and transferase deficient cell lines, $p < 0.05$
Skin biopsies were cultured and stored by standard techniques. In the experiments, cells were grown for at least three passages in TC 199 culture medium supplemented with 10% v/v fetal calf serum which had been dialysed against three changes of 50 volumes of isotonic saline to remove uncombined galactose. The cells were then washed in three changes of phosphate buffer saline and harvested with trypsin/EDTA solution. The cell suspension was centrifuged and the supernatant discarded. The cells were re-suspended in water, an aliquot removed for protein estimation and the remainder was lyophilized after freezing in liquid nitrogen. The carbohydrate composition of the lyophilized cells was determined by gas liquid chromatography.

was concern that galactose restriction would lead to UDPgal depletion, since synthesis through transferase would be reduced and a lack of epimerase would prevent endogenous production from glc-1-P. However, Creiger and colleagues (1986) demonstrated that the human epimerase-deficient fibroblasts could synthesize a galactose-rich glycoprotein, LDL receptor, quite normally when grown on a galactose depleted medium. On the other hand, Chinese hamster ovary mutant cell lines which were epimerase deficient could not make normal LDL receptor grown under the same conditions. The key to this difference seemed to be that hamster cell lines were completely deficient in epimerase, but the human cells had a low level of enzyme activity. Gillett (1985) has found that liver epimerase activity in the same patient was about 10% of normal and the K_m of this enzyme was identical to that of two controls.

These observations suggest that the abnormal enzyme is structurally altered and unstable. The presence of significant amounts of epimerase would confirm that galactose supplements should be unnecessary in this condition.

Metabolite abnormalities in the galactose disorders

In uncontrolled galactokinase deficiency the principal metabolite of the accumulated galactose is galactitol (Gitzelmann, 1967). It is probable that galactonic acid is also a product of galactose metabolism in this disorder, as in transferase deficiency (see later). As UDPgal depletion appears to be a consequence of transferase deficiency, it might be anticipated that it will also be a feature of galactokinase deficiency because of a reduction in the flux of gal-1-P through the transferase reaction. However, galactokinase deficiency is incomplete (Gitzelmann *et al.*, 1974) and the residual enzyme activity may be sufficient to maintain normal UDPgal levels.

In transferase-deficient galactosaemic patients prior to galactose restriction there are large accumulations of gal-1-P, galactitol and galactonic acid. It is recognized that the first and second of these compounds persist in low, but abnormal, amounts on the galactosaemia diet (Donnell *et al.*, 1963). Previously mentioned reductions in UDPgal concentrations were recorded in patients on galactose-restricted diets and it should be questioned whether this abnormality is present prior to treatment. It could be postulated that UDPgal synthesis is increased from gal-1-P in these circumstances, although this might be achieved at the expense of UTP depletion (Figure 1).

In untreated epimerase deficiency it may be presumed that the pattern of galactose metabolites is similar to that in transferase deficiency except that an increased erythrocyte UDPgal concentration has been demonstrated (Henderson *et al.*, 1983). This appears to be the only situation in which increased UDPgal occurs, and clinical features unique to this condition could therefore be due to this particular biochemical aberration.

The origin of galactose-1-phosphate in galactose-restricted transferase-deficient patients

It was mentioned in the preceding section that gal-1-P levels remain slightly increased in erythrocytes of galactose-restricted transferase-deficient patients. The origin of this gal-1-P has usually been considered to be endogenous synthesis from glc-1-P via UDPglc and UDPgal. The evidence for this was discussed by Gitzelmann and Hansen (1980). Pourci and colleagues (1985) questioned this explanation and have proposed an alternative hypothesis, which supposes that small amounts of free galactose are available in the diet and from the catabolism of galactosides for conversion to gal-1-P. The latter hypothesis would be more consistent with the recent finding of low UDPgal concentrations and the persistent galactitol levels which presumably arise from free galactose. It could be important to clarify this question if it was thought necessary to reduce gal-1-P levels below those achieved by current dietary practice.

CLINICAL EFFECTS

Galactokinase deficiency (McKusick 23020)

The predominant feature of galactokinase deficiency is bilateral cataracts, and fortunately with early diagnosis and dietary restriction of galactose these will resolve without surgical intervention. The question of cataracts and galactose metabolism is discussed more fully in a separate paper (Endres and Shin, 1990). The other notable complication is Pseudotumour cerebri, but this occurs very rarely and has been described more often in transferase deficiency (Huttenlocher *et al.*, 1970). It is tempting to document this as a true complication of the galactose disorders because of a known high brain concentration of galactitol before treatment and the accepted osmotic effect of the hexitol. However, since the problem is so rare it might suggest that a second causative event is needed for the complication to occur.

Transferase deficiency (McKusick 23040)

The well-known natural history of transferase deficiency is usually modified at an early stage by the introduction of a galactose-restricted diet which is very effective in reversing the acute toxic effects of the disease. The diagnosis, which precedes dietary intervention, relies on clinical suspicion, newborn population screening or early testing in families known to be at high risk. There has been much debate on whether newborn screening should be introduced generally (Ng, 1987).

In order to examine the need for screening in the UK, Green, Holton, Leonard and Honeyman (personal communication) have studied the presenting features of all patients diagnosed clinically during 1988 (Table 3). This data is compared with that from an early series from Los Angeles (Donnell *et al.*, 1980). It appears that in the UK diagnosis was achieved generally at an earlier stage of the disease and prior to the development of the more severe signs. The pattern of clinical features was not dissimilar to that found in screened populations (Buist *et al.*, 1988), although in this group of infants some are completely asymptomatic at the time of discovery. Unfortunately, the UK survey is not designed to ascertain all neonatal deaths from transferase deficiency, which is another consideration in the case for neonatal screening. A controlled study of screening and non-screening in the same population

Table 3 Clinical features in transferase deficiency patients diagnosed clinically

Clinical feature	*UK survey* (1988) No. (% of total cases = 16)	*Los Angeles survey* (1949–78) No. (% of total cases = 43)
Jaundice	13 (81)	34 (79)
Failure to thrive	5 (31)	23 (53)
Septicaemia	1 (6)	5 (12)
Urinary tract infection	1 (6)	
Hepatomegaly	3 (18)	39 (90)
Splenomegaly	1 (6)	
'Hepatitis'	3 (18)	
Vomiting	2 (12)	17 (39)
Cataracts	2 (12)	19 (44)

would be necessary to investigate this factor.

Most concern is directed towards the long-term complications of the disease. A recent collaborative study of 340 patients (Table 4) has emphasized the basic problems and Buist and colleagues (1989) have analysed the results further. Typically, mental development appears normal in the early years of life but there is a progressive deterioration in performance, particularly of certain tests, during school years (Sardharwalla and Wraith, 1987). It is not clear whether this is a real change in brain function or whether it is due to a changing emphasis of developmental tests with age. There is a significant correlation between low IQ and the speech disorder. In respect to the question of newborn screening, the collaborative study confirmed previous conclusions (Donnell *et al.*, 1980) that long-term outcome is not affected by time of diagnosis and commencement of treatment. A small number of patients with progressive, severe neurological disorders, notably tremor, hypotonia and ataxia,

Table 4 A survey of long-term outcome in 340 cases of diet treated galactosaemia (Buist *et al.*, 1988)

	Clinical symptoms	*Newborn screening*	*Known relative*
Total number in group	149	147	44
Median age and range (years)	10 (0–38)	3.5 (0–21)	13 (0–32)
Median age on starting diet and range (days)	25 (3–550)	9 (2–45)	1 (1–7)
Late onset complications (age at assessment)	*Percentage showing complications*[a] (total no. assessed)		
Developmental delay ($\geqslant$ 6 years)	45 (95)	36 (36)	32 (25)
Speech abnormality ($\geqslant$ 4 years)	53 (105)	57 (63)	70 (27)
Ovarian dysfunction ($\geqslant$ 12 years)	87 (38)	80 (5)	80 (15)
Growth retardation ($\geqslant$ 1.5 years)	21 (126)	14 (106)	12 (28)

[a] None of the differences between diagnostic groups reach significance

have been reported (Lo *et al.*, 1984). These cases may be due to a completely separate pathological mechanism or may be extreme examples of a much larger problem.

Epimerase deficiency

Only two cases of generalized epimerase deficiency have been reported in the literature (Holton *et al.*, 1981; Sardharwalla *et al.*, 1987). Table 5 summarizes the presenting features of the patients, which display the same range of signs and symptoms as those of transferase deficiency, except that hypotonia is specifically mentioned as a feature of epimerase deficiency. The older patient has been maintained on a completely galactose-restricted diet for much of her life, whereas the second patient has been given galactose supplements. The long-term outcome of the children is not dissimilar (MacFaul and Sardharwalla, personal communications). The most interesting common problem is nerve deafness which is not a feature of transferase deficiency, and they both have mild mental retardation but no evidence of ovarian dysfunction.

PATHOGENESIS

A knowledge of the mechanisms involved in the pathology of the galactose disorders is required, amongst other reasons, to plan a logical approach to treatment. Current information on pathogenesis is quite inadequate in this respect. The hypotheses which exist can all be categorized by the abnormalities which occur in the concentration of three metabolites; galactitol, galactose-1-phosphate and UDPgal.

Traditionally, cataract formation, which occurs in all three disorders, has been explained by the accumulation of galactitol in the lens. This is partly because increased galactitol is the principal biochemical abhormality in galactokinase deficiency and cataracts are the only confirmed clinical sign in the disorder.

In experimental animals galactitol accumulation is associated with osmotic swelling of the lens and this may be the primary event in cataract formation, although there are many other biochemical changes occurring.

Another hypothesis explaining cataract formation depends on myo-inositol depletion as a key link in the process. A depletion of lens myo-inositol is established

Table 5 Early features of epimerase deficiency

Patient 1 (Holton *et al.*, 1981)	*Patient* 2 (Sardharwalla *et al.*, 1987)
Jaundice	Jaundice
Poor feeding/weight loss	Poor feeding/weight loss
Vomiting	–
Hypotonia	Hypotonia
Galactosuria	Galactosuria
Amino aciduria	Amino aciduria
–	Septicaemia
–	Cataracts

(Stewart *et al.*, 1968) and it has an importance in phospholipid metabolism and many aspects of cell function. Polyol accumulation and myo-inositol depletion have been implicated in both diabetic and galactosaemic cataract formation (Broekhuyse, 1968). In addition, myo-inositol depletion and deranged phospholipid metabolism have been proposed as the mechanism of diabetic neuropathy, through an effect on nerve conduction (Finegold *et al.*, 1983), and of mental retardation in galactosaemia (Berry *et al.*, 1981). In the galactosaemic work, synaptosomes prepared from the cerebra of galatose-intoxicated rats showed an impairment of phosphatidyl inositol turnover when stimulated by acetyl choline. Attractive though this last hypothesis is, it is difficult to explain why mental retardation is not also a feature of galactokinase deficiency.

Gal-1-P has been suggested as the cause of acute toxic signs in transferase deficiency and has also been linked to most of the long-term abnormalities occurring in this disorder. However, direct evidence for this hypothesis is lacking. Gal-1-P has been considered to cause a reduction in energy availability through inhibition of several enzymes involved in glucose metabolism (Sidbury, 1960). Although inhibition has been found *in vitro*, it cannot be demonstrated *in vivo* in the experimental animal. Alternatively, energy depletion could arise because of the trapping of ATP in gal-1-P and the futile metabolism of this compound in transferase deficiency. Animal model experiments inducing liver necrosis by galactose analogues would appear to support this hypothesis (Starling and Keppler, 1977). Reduced liver ATP and erythrocyte UTP concentrations have been found in transferase deficient patients.

The possibility that reduced UDPgal concentrations are a cause of the pathology of transferase deficiency has been discussed earlier. The only evidence for any clinical link is an apparent correlation between erythrocyte UDPgal concentrations and the occurrence of ovarian dysfunction (Kaufman *et al.*, 1988). The ovary has a particularly high content of complexed galactose and therefore might be particularly sensitive to UDPgal depletion. The important rôle of galactoproteins and galactolipids in cellular function would suggest that this pathogenetic mechanism could be of wider significance.

When does the damage causing long-term complications of transferase deficiency arise?

The biggest current problems in the galactose disorders are the long-term complications in transferase deficiency. More successful treatment almost certainly requires a knowledge of not only how damage resulting in long-term complications is caused, but also when it originates. High concentrations of galactose, galactitol and gal-1-P have been found in fetal liver and blood at least from the middle of the second trimester (Allen *et al.*, 1980). There is no information on UDPgal concentrations in the fetus. Evidence that damage might occur prenatally depends on animal studies in which high levels of galactose were fed during pregnancy. The closest similarity between the abnormalities seen in the offspring and the human is in the ovarian changes. However, it is also considered that there is a postnatal component in the ovarian dysfunction (Kaufman *et al.*, 1986). It should be noted that there is no evidence that maternal galactose restriction in pregnancy reduces the accumulation of metabolites in the transferase-deficient fetus (Irons *et al.*, 1985), or that it improves the long-term outcome.

It is surprising that according to evidence mentioned earlier (Buist *et al.*, 1988), the period between birth and commencement of dietary treatment is not critical in determining long-term outcome, particularly since the concentrations of galactose metabolites are usually highest at this time. Concentrations of UDPgal have not been recorded during this uncontrolled time.

The possibility that damage occurs whilst the child is on treatment has to be considered. It has been mentioned that gal-1-P and galactitol concentrations remain slightly elevated in spite of galactose restriction. On the other hand, no correlation between erythrocyte gal-1-P concentrations when a galactose-restricted diet was established and long-term outcome has been found (Buist *et al.*, 1989). Reduced UDPgal levels, with the possible implications, have been found during dietary galactose restriction.

TREATMENT

The rationale of changes to treatment regimes for transferase deficiency are not firmly based at the present time. It is probable that most effort will be directed towards correction of UDPgal concentrations. It has been demonstrated that oral administration of uridine restores erythrocyte UDPgal concentration to normal. This appears to have no immediate adverse effects and was continued for nine months in two patients with some possible benefit (Kaufman, 1989). It is obvious that these claims should be tested with large scale and long-term controlled studies. The same effect on UDPgal concentrations might be achieved by giving smaller amounts of orotic acid and it is interesting that this compound was used therapeutically in transferase deficiency many years ago (Tada *et al.*, 1962). It has also been shown to prevent liver necrosis induced in rats by galactosamine. A correction of UDPgal concentration and possibly other metabolic abnormalities might be achieved by inducing small increases in transferase activity (Segal, 1989) and administration of inositol could be considered in order to correct its possible depletion. Although the last approach is empirical, just as the others described, it has the advantage that it is not likely to be harmful.

PRENATAL DIAGNOSIS

Prenatal diagnosis of transferase deficiency by enzyme estimation in chorionic villus biopsies, or in cultured amniotic fluid cells, and by amniotic fluid galactitol assays, is simple and accurate (Holton *et al.*, 1989). Unfortunately, the gene probe has not been found to be useful in prenatal diagnosis. At present, prenatal diagnosis is undertaken rarely but should perhaps be considered more seriously until alternative and better methods of treatment are established.

REFERENCES

Allen, J. T., Gillett, M., Holton, J. B., King, G. S. and Pettit, B. R. Evidence of galactosaemia *in utero*. *Lancet* 1 (1980) 603

Berry, G., Yandrasitz, J. R. and Segal, S. Experimental galactose toxicity: effects on synaptosomal phosphatidylinositol metabolism. *J. Neurochem* 37 (1981) 888–891

Broekhuyse, R. Changes in myo-inositol permeability in the lens due to cataractacous condition. *Biochim. Biophys. Acta* 163 (1968) 269–272

Buist, N. R. M., Waggoner, D., Donnell, G. N., Levy, H. The effect of newborn screening in galactosaemia: results of the international survey. *Abstracts of the 26th Annual Symposium of the Society for the Study of Inborn Errors of Metabolism*, SSIEM, 1988, p. 53

Buist, N. R. M., Waggoner, D. and Donnell, G. N. The international galactosaemia survey: final results. *Abstracts of the 27th Annual Symposium of the Society for the Study of Inborn Errors of Metabolism*, SSIEM, 1989, 0–7

Creiger, M., Kingsley, D. M. and Holton, J. B. Structure and function of low density lipoprotein in epimerase deficiency galactosaemia. *N. Engl. J. Med.* 314 (1986) 1257–1258

Dobbie, J. A., Holton, J. B. and Clamp, J. R. Defective galactosylation of proteins in cultured skin fibroblasts from galactosaemic patients. *Ann. Clin. Biochem.* (1990) (In press)

Donnell, G. N., Bergren, W. R., Perry, G. and Koch, R. Galactose-1-phosphate in galactosaemia. *Paediatrics* 31 (1963) 802–810

Donnell, G. N., Koch, R., Fischer, K., Ng, W. G. Clinical aspects of galactosaemia. In Burman, D., Holton, J. B. and Pennock, C. A. (eds.), *Inherited Disorders of Carbohydrate Metabolism*, MTP Press, Lancaster, 1980, pp. 103–115

Endres, W. and Shin, Y. S. Cataract and metabolic disease. *J. Inher. Metab. Dis.* 13 (1990) 509–576

Finegold, D., Lattimer, S. A., Nolle, S., Bernstein, M. and Greene, D. A. Polyol pathway activity and myo-inositol metabolism: a suggested relationship in the pathogenesis of diabetic neuropathy. *Diabetes* 32 (1983) 988–922

Gillett, M. G. Investigation of human uridine 5′-phosphate-4-epimerase. MSc Thesis, University of Bath, 1985.

Gitzelmann, R. Hereditary galactokinase deficiency, a newly recognised cause of juvenile cataracts. *Pediatr. Res.* 1 (1967) 14–23

Gitzelmann, R. Deficiency of uridine diphosphate galactose-4-epimerase in blood cells of an apparently healthy infant. *Helv. Paediatr. Acta* 27 (1972) 125–130

Gitzelmann, R. and Hansen, R. G. Galactose metabolism, hereditary defects and their clinical significance. In Burman, D., Holton, J. B. and Pennock, C. A. (eds.), *Inherited Disorders of Carbohydrate Metabolism*, MTP Press, Lancaster, 1980, pp. 61–101

Gitzelman, R., Wells, H. J. and Segal, S. Galactose metabolism in a patient with hereditary galactokinase deficiency. *Eur. J. Clin. Invest.* 4 (1974) 79–84

Henderson, M. J., Holton, J. B. and McFaul, R. Further observations in a case of uridine diphosphate galactose-4-epimerase deficiency with a severe clinical presentation. *J. Inher. Metab. Dis.* 6 (1983) 17–20

Holton, J. B., Gillett, M. G., McFaul, R. and Young, R. Galactosaemia: a new severe variant due to uridine diphosphate galactose-4-epimerase deficiency. *Arch. Dis. Child.* 56 (1981) 885–887

Holton, J. B., Allen, J. T. and Gillett, M. G. Prenatal diagnosis of disorders of galactose metabolism. *J. Inher. Metab. Dis.* 12 Suppl. 1 (1989) 202–206

Huttenlocher, R. R., Hillman, R. E. and Hsia, Y. E. Pseudotumour cerebri in galactosaemia. *J. Pediatr.* 76 (1970) 902–905

Irons, M., Levy, H. L., Pueschel, S. and Castree, K. Accumulation of galactose-1-phosphate in the galactosaemic fetus despite maternal milk avoidance. *J. Pediatr.* 107 (1985) 261–263

Kaufman, F. R., Donnell, G. N., Roe, T. F. and Kogut, M. D. Gonadal function in patients with galactosaemia. *J. Inher. Metab. Dis.* 9 (1986) 140–146

Kaufman, F. R., Xu, Y.. K., Ng, W. G., Donnell, G. N. Correlation of ovarian function with galactose-1-phosphate uridyl transferase level in galactosaemia. *J. Pediatr.* 112 (1988) 754–756

Kaufman, F., Ng., W. G., Xu, Y. K., Giudici, T., Donnell, G. N. Treatment of patients with classical galactosaemia with oral uridine. *Abstracts of the 27th Annual Symposium of the Society for the Study of Inborn Errors of Metabolism*, SSIEM 1989, 0–8

Lo, W., Packman, S., Nash, S., Schmidt, R. N., Ireland, S., Diamond, I., Ng, W. G., Donnell, G. N. Curious neurologic sequelae in galactosaemia. *Pediatrics* 73 (1984) 309–312

Ng, W. G. Summary of the galactosaemia workshop. In Therrell, B. L. (ed.) *Advances in Neonatal Screening*, Excerpta Medica, Amsterdam, 1987, pp. 221–222

Ng, W. G., Xu, Y. K., Kaufman, F. and Donnell, G. N. Deficit of uridine diphosphate galactose (UDPgal) in galactosaemia. *Am. J. Human. Genet.* 41 Suppl. (1987) A12

Pourci, M. L., Mangeot, M. and Lemmonier, A. Origin of the galactose-1-phosphate present in erythrocytes and fibroblasts of treated galactosaemic patients. *IRCS Med. Sci.* 13 (1985) 1232–1233

Reichardt, J. K. V. and Berg, P. Cloning and characterization of a cDNA encoding human galactose-1-phosphate uridyl transferase. *Mol. Biol. Med.* 5 (1988) 107–122

Sardharwalla, I. B. .and Wraith, J. E. Galactosaemia. *Nutrition and Health* 5 (1987) 175–188

Sardharwalla, I. B., Wraith, J. E., Bridge, C., Fowler, B. and Roberts, S. A. A patient with a severe type of epimerase deficiency galactosaemia. *Abstracts of the 25th Annual Symposium of the Society for the Study of Inborn Errors of Metabolism*, SSIEM, 1987, 91

Segal, S. Disorders of galactose metabolism. In Scriver, C. R., Beaudet, A. L., Sly, W. S. and Valle, D. (eds.), *The Metabolic Basis of Inherited Disease*, McGraw-Hill, New York, 1989, pp. 453–480

Segal, S. and Rogers, S. Regulation of galactose metabolism: implications for therapy. *J. Inher. Metab. Dis.* 13 (1990) 487–500

Shin, Y. S., Rieth, M., Hoyer, S. and Endres, W. Uridine diphosphogalactose, galactose-1-phosphate and galactitol concentrations in patients with classical galactosaemia. *Abstracts of the 23rd Annual Symposium of the Society for the Study of Inborn Errors of Metabolism*, SSIEM, 1985, p. 35.

Sidbury, J. B. The role of galactose-1-phosphate in the pathogenesis of galactosaemia. In Gardner, L. I. (ed.), *Molecular Genetics and Human Disease*, Charles, C. Thomas, Springfield, Illinois, 1960, pp. 61–82

Starling, J. J. and Kepler, D. O. R. Metabolism of 2-deoxy-D-galactose in liver induces phosphate and uridylate trapping. *Eur. J. Biochem.* 80 (1977) 373–379

Stewart, M. A., Kurien, M. M., Sherman, W. R. and Cotlier, E. V. Inositol changes in nerve and lens of galactose fed rats. *J. Neurochem.* 15 (1968) 941–946

Tada, K., Kudo, Z., Ohno, T., Akabane, J. and Chica, R. Congenital galactosaemia and orotic acid therapy with promising results. *Tohoku J. Exp. Med.* 77 (1962) 340–342

J. Inher. Metab. Dis. 13 (1990) 487–500

Regulation of Galactose Metabolism: Implications for Therapy

S. SEGAL and S. ROGERS
Division of Biochemical Development and Molecular Diseases, Children's Hospital of Philadelphia and the Department of Pediatrics and Medicine, University of Pennsylvania School of Medicine, Philadelphia, Pennsylvania, USA

Summary: In view of evidence that dietary therapy of galactose-1-phosphate uridyltransferase deficiency has failed to prevent complications of the disorder, there is a need for new strategies in treatment. The enhancement of residual enzyme activity in tissues of galactosaemic patients should provide such an approach. This possibility is derived from knowledge of the regulation of transferase activity in normal animal tissues. The pertinent observations summarized herein are: (1) that hepatic transferase activity is modulated by various cellular metabolites, uridine nucleotides being of particular significance; (2) that transferase activity in the young rat liver is subject to developmental programming with a several-fold increase after birth; (3) that transferase activity in pregnant rat liver is significantly increased which may be related to hormonal effects of progesterone; and (4) that pharmacological doses of folic acid may increase transferase activity. The basis of such regulation can give insight into sufficient augmentation of the residual activity to increase galactose utilization and thereby better the long-term outcome.

Galactose restriction has been considered a satisfactory basis for therapy ever since Mason and Turner (1935) described how removing galactose from the diet eliminated the acute galactose toxicity syndrome in a patient with galactose-1-phosphate uridyltransferase deficient galactosaemia. Recent evidence, however, has indicated that there are 'clouds over galactosaemia' (Lancet, Editorial, 1982). Despite early diagnosis and the institution of a galactose-free diet there appears to be an inability to prevent some degree of mental retardation (Fishler *et al.*, 1980; Komrower, 1982) or ovarian failure (Kaufman *et al.*, 1981; Steinmann *et al.*, 1981), and there have been reports of neurological ataxia syndromes appearing in well-treated older patients (Lo *et al.*, 1984; Friedman *et al.*, 1989). A recent survey of over 300 patients indicates that there is developmental delay, speech abnormality, ovarian dysfunction and growth retardation in a large number of patients, independent of the time after birth of the institution of dietary restriction (Buist *et al.*, 1988). The reason for the inefficacy of galactose restriction is at present obscure.

There are two prevalent theories for the poor outcome in this disease. The first of these, espoused by Gitzelmann (Gitzelmann, 1969; Gitzelmann and Hansen, 1974; Gitzelmann *et al.*, 1975) is that there is continuous self-intoxication due to the endogenous production of galactose-1-phosphate from uridine diphosphate galactose. The second one, recently proposed by Ng and colleagues (1987), is based on the observation (Shin *et al.*, 1985) that there is a depletion of cellular UDPgalactose and postulates a resulting impairment of the synthesis of critical complex substances containing galactose. Figure 1 shows the Leloir pathway where ordinarily exogenous galactose is phosphorylated by ATP, the resulting galactose-1-phosphate (gal-1-P) interacting with UDPglucose by the activity of transferase to form UDPgalactose, which undergoes epimerization to UDPglucose. The sugar in the latter then enters the glucose pathway by a cleavage to glucose-1-phosphate. With a block in transferase, ingestion of galactose is associated with accumulation of gal-1-P and, via alternate paths, galactitol and galactonate. With elimination of dietary galactose one would expect no gal-1-P accumulation but this is not the case, with high cellular levels being observed in the best treated patients. Gitzelmann (1969) proposed that gal-1-P is formed via pyrophosphorylitic cleavage of UDPgalactose (indicated by PP in Figure 1) which is derived by epimerization of ever present UDPglucose readily formed from UTP and glucose-1-phosphate. The gal-1-P is thought to be related to the continuing toxicity (Komrower, 1982; Gitzelmann and Steinmann, 1984). The low level of UDPgalactose in galactose-1-phosphate uridyltransferase deficient tissues has led Ng and colleagues (Kaufman *et al.*, 1989) to believe that UDPgalactose depletion results in decreased glycoprotein and galactolipid synthesis, which is the basis for long-term complications. Why cell UDPgalactose is low is not clear since it can be formed from UDPglucose.

With failure of dietary therapy it appears there is a need for new strategies in the treatment of the galactose-1-phosphate uridyltransferase deficient disorder. One approach is possible enhancement of residual enzyme activity. This would result in

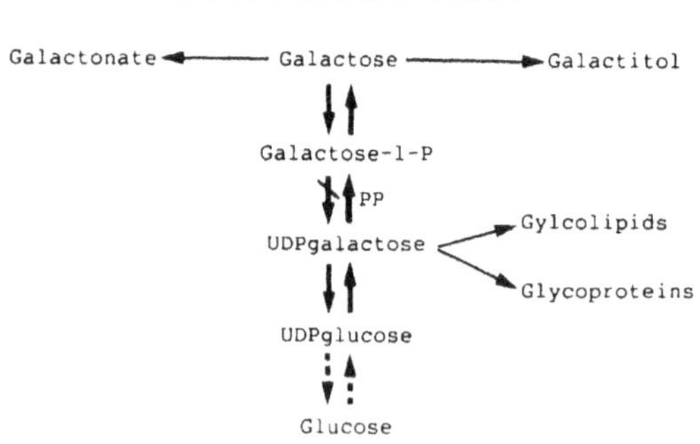

Figure 1 Reactions of the pathway of galactose metabolism responsible for the galactose–glucose interconversion

an increased flux through the pathway with a decrease in gal-1-P and an increase in UDPgalactose, thus satisfying the basis of toxicity of both prevalent theories. From our own studies of ^{14}C-galactose oxidation by galactosaemic patients, we know that there is residual metabolic capacity (Segal *et al.*, 1965; Segal and Cuatrecasas, 1968). Most patients produce galactose-1-phosphate uridyltransferase protein (Tedesco and Mellman, 1971) and some have small amounts of red cell galactose-1-phosphate uridyltransferase activity (Kaufman *et al.*, 1988). Recent studies in our laboratory have shown detectable galactose-1-phosphate uridyltransferase in Percoll-fractionated reticulocytes when whole blood has no assayable activity (Kelley *et al.*, 1989). Galactosaemic fibroblasts possess considerable galactose-1-phosphate uridyltransferase activity soon after subculture which diminishes with confluency (Russell and DeMars, 1967).

REGULATION OF GALACTOSE-1-PHOSPHATE URIDYLTRANSFERASE

Described below are our studies on the regulation of normal transferase activity in rat liver with the idea that knowledge of how transferase is regulated can give us an insight into the possible augmentation of the residual enzyme activity in the deficient patient. There are four aspects of the regulation of galactose metabolism which should be emphasized: the metabolic regulation of enzyme activity; developmental programming; pregnancy and progesterone effects; and pharmacological effects, notably with folic acid.

The metabolic regulation of enzyme activity

That there is metabolic regulation of transferase activity became evident when we observed that normal suckling rat liver perfused with galactose resulted in an increase in the specific activity of transferase within 30 min (Rogers and Segal, 1981). This and the previous findings that diet could regulate galactose metabolizing enzymes in intestine (Stifel *et al.*, 1968) led us to study the effect of a high galactose diet on the Leloir pathway enzymes in young adult rat livers (Rogers *et al.*, 1989a). As shown in Figure 2, there is a marked and persistent increase in transferase, a transient increase in epimerase and little alteration in galactokinase after six days of feeding a 40% galactose diet. A physiological counterpart to this study is shown in Table 1. In hepatocytes isolated from livers of rats on the experimental diet there is an increased uptake of galactose, a higher conversion to glucose and an enhanced conversion to lactate. This suggests that transferase is indeed capable of manipulation by metabolic influence.

Table 2 summarizes the regulation of galactose-metabolizing enzymes. Galactokinase is inhibited by both its substrate and its product (Cuatrecasas and Segal, 1965), which would indicate that there is a decrease in galactose phosphorylation when a block exists in transferase or epimerase activity. More importantly, transferase is also inhibited by high levels of its substrates, gal-1-P and UDPglucose (Bertoli and Segal, 1966). Glucose-1-phosphate, a product, is perhaps one of the most potent metabolic inhibitors. Of particular significance is the fact that uridine nucleotides,

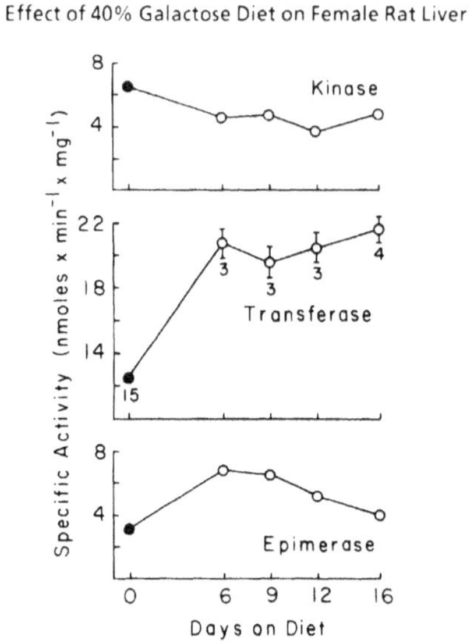

Figure 2 Effect of an isocaloric 40% galactose diet on the specific activities of the galactose-metabolizing enzymes. The solid symbol refers to activities found prior to initiating the diet. Data shown (Rogers *et al.*, 1989a) are the average ± SEM for *n* animals as indicated in the middle panel. Standard errors for galactokinase and epimerase are within the size of the symbols. Levels of each enzyme shown during the diet are statistically different ($p < 0.001-0.05$) from that found at day 0 with the exception of that found for epimerase at day 16.

Table 1 The metabolism of [1-^{14}C] galactose by hepatocytes from galactose-fed adult rats

	Control (n/mg/30 min)	*Galactose*	*p*
Galactose uptake	19.86 ± 1.03(7)	27.75 ± 3.29(9)	< 0.05
Conversion to glucose	3.97 ± 0.81(7)	12.67 ± 3.02(9)	< 0.02
Conversion to lactate	4.85 ± 0.51(8)	10.53 ± 1.38(9)	< 0.01

Hepatocytes isolated from rats fed 40% galactose for 7 days were incubated with 4 mmol/L [1-^{14}C]galactose for 30 min. Data is taken from Rogers *et al.*, 1989a

Table 2 Regulation of galactose metabolizing enzymes

Enzyme	*Regulation*
Galactokinase	Galactose, Gal-1-P
Uridyltransferase	Gal-1-P, UDPGlu, Glu-1-P, UDP, UTP
UDPGal-4-epimerase	NAD, NADH, pH, UMP, UDP

UTP and UDP, are competitive inhibitors of UDPglucose for the enzyme (Segal and Rogers, 1971). As a matter of fact, from the steady-state concentrations of UDPglucose and UTP we know to exist in cells, it would appear that the transferase is normally operating in a restrained or inhibited manner (Cohn and Segal, 1973). Epimerase is also regulated, especially by NAD which stimulates it and NADH which inhibits it (Isselbacher and Crane, 1961). The ingestion of ethanol can make any of us temporarily galactosaemic by increasing NADH. It is also inhibited by uridine nucleotides, especially uridine monophosphate (Cohn and Segal, 1970).

The inhibition of uridine-containing nucleotides is of great consequence, since the administration of uridine has been advocated as a therapeutic modality to increase tissue UDPgalactose levels (Kaufman *et al.*, 1989), and thereby enhance glycoprotein and galactolipid synthesis. In fact, many parents in the US are trying to obtain uridine for their affected children. However, the administration of uridine may be a two-edged sword. Table 3 shows the results obtained when suckling rat liver homogenates were assayed for transferase activity in the presence of various levels of uridine. There is a significant inhibition of the enzyme as the amount of uridine in the homogenate is increased. Uridine is a non-linear competitive inhibitor of UDPglucose and a non-competitive inhibitor of gal-1-P (Rogers and Segal, 1989). In addition, there is a significant inhibition of transferase when UTP levels are increased (Rogers and Segal, 1971) and there is an additive effect of uridine and UTP. This translates into inhibition of galactose metabolism. Table 4 shows data obtained when the intact suckling rat liver was perfused with 4 mmol/L galactose plus 1 mmol/L uridine and various metabolites were measured. Uridine causes a three-fold increase in UTP to a level where inhibition of the transferase would occur. This, together with the circulating uridine, results in more than a doubling of galactose-1-phosphate (Rogers and Segal, 1989).

Galactose-1-phosphate uridyltransferase can be responsive to change in its cellular environment. The implication of this is that residual flux through the Leloir pathway might be manipulated by metabolic means. A corollary is that the regulation by uridine nucleotides has to be taken into account in any attempt to change cellular UDPgalactose levels by the administration of uridine. If Gitzelmann and colleagues

Table 3 Inhibition of rat liver transferase by uridine and UTP

Concentration (mmol/L)	*Uridine* (% inhibition)	*UTP* (% inhibition)
0.10	20	—
0.20	41	—
0.25	—	47
0.4	66	—
0.5	—	56
1.0	59	99

Uridine and UTP were added to the soluble fraction of tissue homogenates. Data was taken from Segal and Rogers, 1971 and Rogers and Segal, 1989

Table 4 **Effect of uridine on metabolites in isolated perfused liver of suckling rats**

Metabolite	*Control*	*Uridine*	*p*
	(μmol per g wet weight)		
Galactose-1-phosphate	0.15 ± 0.02(11)	0.33 ± 0.03(8)	< 0.001
Glucose-1-phosphate	0.14 ± 0.02(18)	0.08 ± 0.02(8)	< 0.01
UDPglucose	0.20 ± 0.01(18)	0.22 ± 0.03(6)	NS
UTP	0.06 ± 0.01(16)	0.19 ± 0.02(5)	< 0.001

Livers were perfused for 30 min with 4 mmol/L galactose with and without uridine. Data is taken from Rogers *et al.*, 1989b

(1975) are correct that endogenous gal-1-P production is associated with long-term toxicity, the inhibition of any residual transferase as a result of uridine administration would indeed, be detrimental rather than therapeutic.

Developmental programming

The second aspect of regulation is that of developmental programming. Figure 3 shows the pattern of enzyme-specific activities in rat liver during fetal and postnatal development. The significant finding is that after a rise in late gestation there is a marked increase in galactose-1-phosphate uridyltransferase activity in the postpartum period, peaking at around 8–10 days (Bertoli and Segal, 1966; Rogers *et al.*, 1989b).

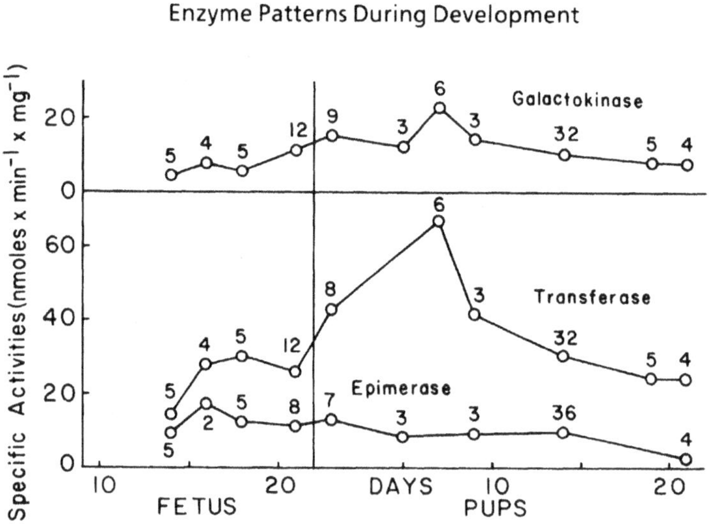

Figure 3 Changes in levels of the galactose-metabolizing enzymes of rat fetal and pup liver. The number of animals used for each data point is indicated above the symbol. Data is from Rogers *et al.*, 1989b.

There is then a precipitous fall-off with a subsequent gradual decrease to adult levels which occurs by about 40 days of life. The mechanisms for this programming are not understood and are not explained by the galactose-containing diet. Figure 4 shows the physiological consequences of the high transferase in the postpartum period. Galactose disposition when measured in hepatocytes isolated from animals of various ages shows a marked increase in the first two weeks of life in the ability to take up galactose, to convert it to glucose and lactate, and to oxidize the sugar to CO_2 (Rogers *et al.*, 1983). The implication is that understanding the mechanism of this age-related increase in galactose-1-phosphate uridyltransferase could provide information used to enhance residual activity in the galactosaemic patient.

Pregnancy and progesterone

The third aspect of regulation involves pregnancy and progesterone. We and others have shown that when a high galactose diet is fed to pregnant rats cataracts are not induced as they would be when virgin females are placed on the same diet for the

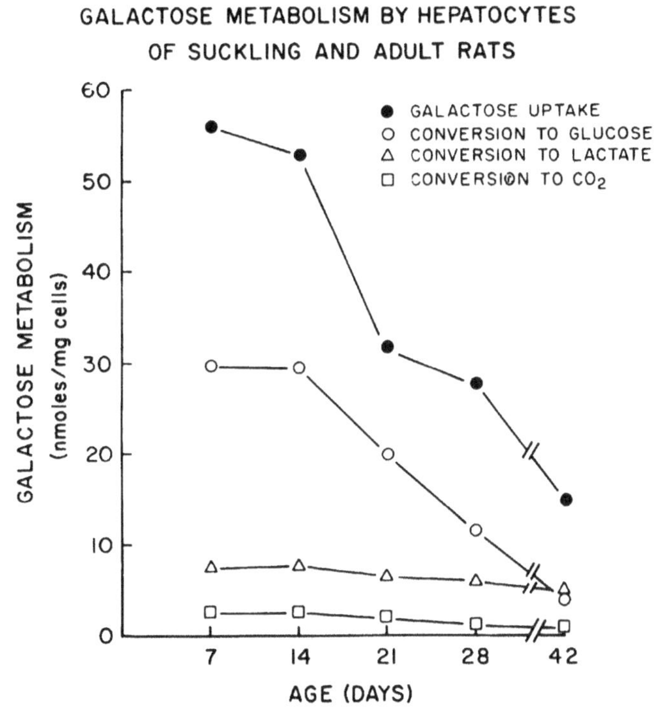

Figure 4 Comparison of 4 mmol/L [1-^{14}C]galactose metabolism during postnatal development. Data is from Rogers *et al.*, 1983.

same period of time (Segal and Bernstein, 1963; Unakar, 1979). This finding may be related to the observation that progesterone administered (2 mg/day) to normal weanling rats fed a 30% galactose diet has a protective effect in delaying the onset of cataracts (Pesch *et al.*, 1960). These results led us to undertake a study of the specific activity of the galactose metabolizing enzymes in the pregnant rat since little is known about galactose metabolism in this condition (Rogers *et al.*, 1989b). Figure 5 shows that during pregnancy, while hepatic galactokinase specific activity is slightly altered, that of transferase activity almost doubles by the 10th day. Figure 6 reveals the distribution of enzyme activity at term in the pregnant rat liver, clearly demonstrating that, of the enzymes measured, transferase is elevated in the liver of most pregnant rats. This has led us to speculate that the protection of the pregnant rat from the effects of a high galactose diet may be related to the increase in hepatic transferase activity. Obviously, the pregnant state, which is characterized by high levels of oestrogen and progesterone, has focused attention on the effect of the hormones on transferase. Our preliminary data suggest that transferase activity in the liver of virgin females given high doses of progesterone is, indeed, increased. The implication of these studies is that the ability to enhance galactose-1-phosphate uridyltransferase offers protection from galactose toxicity which may be achieved by hormonal mimicry of pregnancy. Indeed, the early administration of hormones and ovarian cycling of galactosaemic females could have long-term beneficial effects.

Pharmacological effects of folic acid

A number of years ago Hermann and colleagues (Rosenberg *et al.*, 1969a, b, 1970) showed that the administration of large doses of folate to humans could enhance the

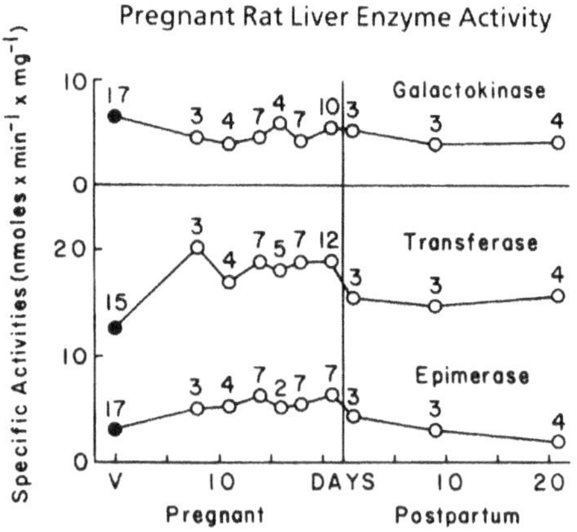

Figure 5 Changes in the levels of the galactose-metabolizing enzymes during pregnancy and lactation. Data (Rogers *et al.*, 1989b) represent averages $\pm$ SEM for *n* animals shown above each point. Some SEM are within the size of the symbol. All of the data shown during pregnancy are significantly different to that shown for the virgin (V), $p \leq 0.05$, except for galactokinase at day 14 and term.

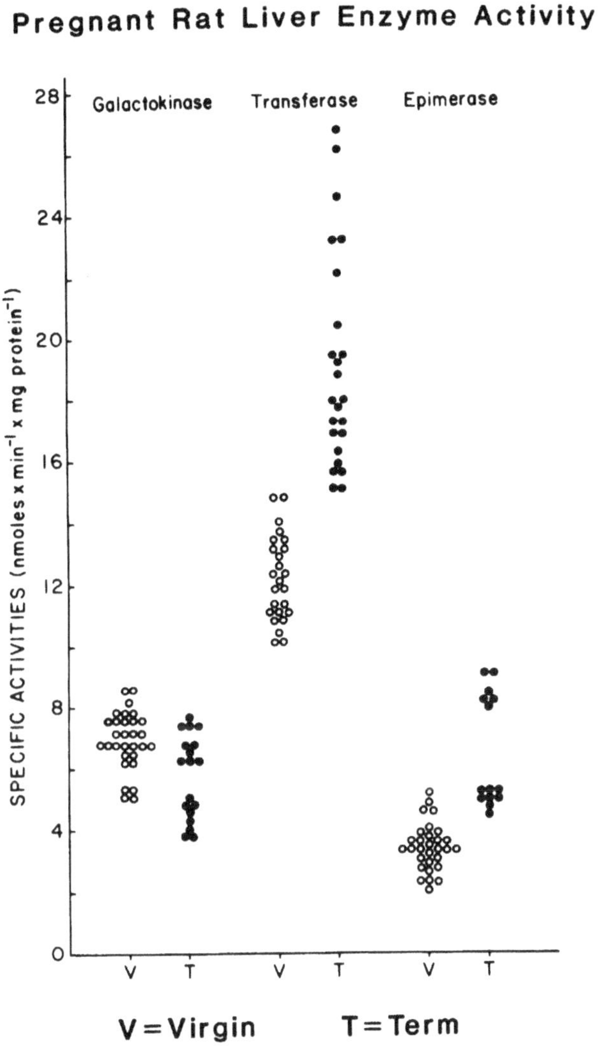

Figure 6 Comparison of the ranges of enzyme-specific activities for virgin and term maternal rat livers (Rogers *et al.*, 1989b).

activity of glycolytic and gluconeogenic enzymes in the intestinal mucosa (Rosensweig *et al.*, 1969a, 1969b, 1970). They also showed that folate given to humans with fructose 1,6-diphosphatase deficiency could enhance the residual activity of this enzyme in the intestinal mucosa and relieve the hypoglycaemia symptoms which were found in the patient (Taunton *et al.*, 1978). We have studied the effects of folate on normal galactose metabolism and have observed: (1) that in the perfused suckling rat liver there is an increase in galactose utilization and in transferase (Rogers and Segal, 1984); (2) that the intact suckling rat shows an increase in galactose oxidation after seven days of treatment with folate (Rogers and Segal, unpublished observation); and (3) that explants of fetal rat liver cultured with folate result in an increase in transferase activity (Rogers and Segal, unpublished observation). Figure 7 shows that the specific activity of transferase during perfusion of suckling rat liver with galactose is significantly higher in folate-treated rats. The increase is most apparent at the end of the study when the activity of the enzyme appears to fall. At the same time, if the

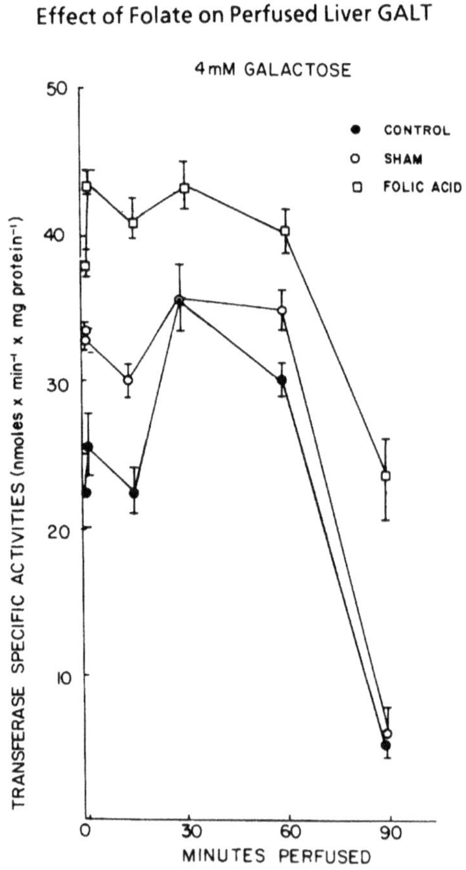

Figure 7 Effect of folic acid treatment on the specific activity of transferase during perfusion of suckling rat livers (Rogers *et al.*, 1984). Initial concentration of the recirculating media was 4 mmol/L galactose.

effect of folate on galactose uptake of these perfused suckling livers is measured, there is a marked increase and change in the kinetics of uptake of galactose (Figure 8). When the oxidation of ^{14}C-galactose was measured for 5 h in suckling rats who had been treated from day 7 to day 14 with 1 mg of folate, there was a significant increase in the ability of these animals to oxidize galactose to $^{14}CO_2$ to the extent of about 50%. The implication is that galactose metabolism in the normal can be enhanced by compounds known to increase galactose-1-phosphate uridyltransferase.

CONCLUSIONS

It appears that normal transferase enzyme can be manipulated, programmed in the newborn, and altered by changes in hormonal state and by pharmacological agents. Whether these various factors can enhance the residual transferase activity found in galactosaemic patients remains to be determined. We are in the process of carrying out small pilot studies to determine if, indeed, progesterone and folate can influence the galactosaemic patient's ability to metabolize ^{13}C-galactose. At the present time, in the absence of genetic manipulation to increase transferase activity, alteration of the metabolic state to enhance residual transferase activity appears to be a viable alternative. It should be pointed out that the levels of transferase activity do not have to be greatly increased in order to effect a change in the ability to metabolize galactose. We have demonstrated in the black galactosaemic who can metabolize

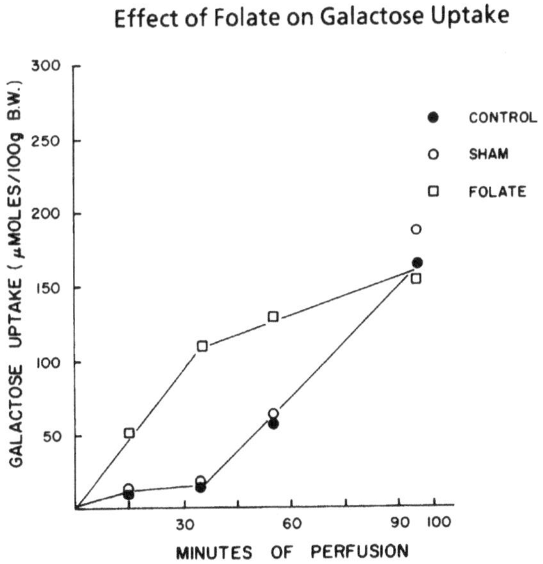

Figure 8 Effect of folic acid administration on galactose uptake by livers of suckling rats perfused with 4 mmol/L galactose (Rogers *et al.*, 1984).

considerable amounts of galactose (Segal *et al.*, 1965) that the residual galactose-1-phosphate uridyltransferase activity is only 10% of normal (Rogers *et al.*, 1970; Segal *et al.*, 1971). The Los Angeles group has reported that galactosaemic females with detectable red cell transferase have normal UDPgalactose levels and no ovarian functional abnormality (Kaufman *et al.*, 1988). In other metabolic disorders such as homocystinuria, when pyridoxine added to affected cultured cells increases the deficient enzyme activity from 4 to 8%, the vitamin can reverse the patient's abnormal metabolic pattern (Mudd *et al.*, 1989).

Although there appears to be a 'cloud over galactosaemia' at the present time, our increasing knowledge leads us to believe that there may be a break in the clouds before long as a result of our search for alternative strategies in the therapy of this disorder.

REFERENCES

Bertoli, D. and Segal, S. Developmental aspects and some characteristics of mammalian galactose-1-phosphate uridyltransferase. *J. Biol. Chem.* 241 (1966) 4023-4029

Buist, N., Waggoner, D., Donnell, G. and Levy, H. The effects of newborn screening on prognosis in galactosemia: results of the international survey. Abs. 26th SSIEM Annual Symposium, Glasgow, 6–9 September 1988, p. 53

Cohn, R. M. and Segal, S. Regulation of mammalian liver uridine diphosphogalactose-4-epimerase by pyrimidine nucleotides. *Biochim. Biophys. Acta* 222 (1970) 533–536

Cohn, R. M. and Segal, S. Galactose metabolism and its regulation. *Metabolism* 22 (1973) 627–642

Cuatrecasas, P. and Segal, S. Mammalian galactokinase: developmental and adaptive characteristics in rat liver. *J. Biol. Chem.* 240 (1965) 2382–2388

Fishler, K., Koch, R., Donnell, G.N. and Wenz, E. Developmental aspects of galactosemia from infancy to childhood. *Clin. Pediatr.* 19 (1980) 38–44

Friedman, J. H., Levy, H. L. and Boustany, R. M. Late onset neurologic syndromes in galactosemic siblings. *Neurology* 39 (1989) 741–742

Gitzelmann, R. Formation of galactose-1-phosphate from uridine diphosphate galactose in erythrocytes from patients with galactosemia. *Pediatr. Res.* 3 (1969) 279–286

Gitzelmann, R. and Hansen, R. G. Galactose biogenesis and disposal in galactosemics. *Biochim. Biophys. Acta* 372 (1974) 374–378

Gitzelmann, R. and Steinmann, B. Galactosemia: How does long-term treatment change the outcome? *Enzyme* 32 (1984) 37–46

Gitzelmann, R., Hansen, R. G. and Steinmann, B. Biogenesis of galactose, a possible mechanism of self-intoxification in galactosemia; in Hommes and Van den Berg (eds.), *Normal and Pathological Development of Energy Metabolism*, Academic Press, London, 1975, pp. 25–37

Isselbacher, K. J. and Crane, S. M. Studies on the inhibition of galactose oxidation by ethanol. *J. Biol. Chem.* 236 (1961) 2394–2398

Kaufman, F. R., Kogut, M. D., Donnell, G. N., Goebelsmann, U., March, C. and Koch, R. Hypergonadotropic hypogonadism in female patients with galactosemia. *N. Engl. J. Med.* 304 (1981) 994–998

Kaufman, F. R., Xu, Y. K., Ng, W. G. and Donnell, G. N. Correlation of ovarian function with galactose-1-phosphate uridyltransferase levels in galactosemia. *J. Pediatr.* 112 (1988) 754–756

Kaufman, F. R., Ng, W. G., Xu, Y. K., Cridici, T., Kaleito, T. A. and Donnell, G. N. Treatment of patients (PTS) with classical galactosemia (G) with oral uridine. *Abs. Am. Soc. Pediatr. Res.*, April 1989

Kelley, R. I., Feinberg, D. M. and Segal, S. Galactose-1-phosphate uridyltransferase in density-fractionated erythrocytes: Studies of normal and mutant enzymes. *Hum. Genet.* 82 (1989) 99–103

Komrower, G. M. Galactosemia – thirty years on. The experience of a generation. *J. Inher. Metab. Dis.* 5 (1982) 96–104

Lancet editorial. 'Clouds over galactosaemia'. *Lancet* 1 (1982) 1379–1380

Lo, W., Packman, S., Nash, S., Schmidt, K., Ireland, S., Diamond, I., Ng, W. and Donnell, G. Curious neurologic sequelae in galactosemia. *Pediatrics* 73 (1984) 309–312

Mason, H. H. and Turner, M. E. Chronic galactosemia. *Am. J. Dis. Child.* 50 (1935) 359

Mudd, S. H., Levy, H. L. and Skovby, F. Disorders transsulfuration. In Scriver, C.R., Beaudet, A. L., Sly, W. S. and Valley, D. (eds.), *The Metabolic Basis of Inherited Disease*, McGraw-Hill, New York, (1989), pp. 693–734

Ng, W. G., Xu, Y. K., Kaufman, F. and Donnell, G. N. Uridine nucleotide sugar deficiency in galactosemia: implications. *Clin. Res.* 35 (1987) 212A

Pesch, L., Segal, S. and Topper, Y. J. Progesterone effects on galactose metabolism in prepubertal patients with congenital galactosemia and in rats maintained on high galactose diets. *J. Clin. Invest.* 39 (1960) 178–184

Rogers, S. R. and Segal, S. Changing activities of galactose-metabolizing enzymes during perfusion of suckling rat liver. *Am. J. Physiol.* 240 (1981) E333–E339

Rogers, S. and Segal, S. Enhanced galactose metabolism in isolated perfused livers of folate-treated suckling rats. *Metabolism* 33 (1984) 634–640

Rogers, S. and Segal, S. Effects of uridine on hepatic galactose-1-phosphate uridyltransferase. *Enzyme* 42 (1989) 53–60

Rogers, S., Holtzapple, P. G., Mellman, W. J. *et al.* Characteristics of galactose-1-phosphate uridyltransferase in intestinal mucosa of normal and galactosemic humans. *Metabolism* 19 (1970) 701–708

Rogers, S., Guerra, M. and Segal, S. Galactose metabolism in suckling and adult isolated rat hepatocytes. *Pediatr. Res.* 17 (1983) 609–616

Rogers, S. R., Bovee, B. W., Saunders, S. L. and Segal, S. Galactose as a regulatory factor of its own metabolism by rat liver. *Metabolism* 38 (1989a) 810–815

Rogers, S., Bovee, B. W., Saunders, S. L. and Segal, S. Activity of hepatic galactose-metabolizing enzymes in pregnant rat and fetus. *Pediatr. Res.* 25 (1989b) 161–166

Rosensweig, N. S., Herman, R. H. and Stifel, F. B. Dietary regulation of glycolytic enzymes. VI. Effect of dietary sugars and oral folic acid on human jejunal pyruvate kinase, phosphofructokinase and fructosediphosphatase activities. *Biochim. Biophys. Acta* 208 (1970) 373–380

Rosensweig, N. S., Herman, R. H., Stifel, F. B. *et al.* Regulation of human jejunal gycolytic enzymes by oral folic acid. *J. Clin. Invest.* 48 (1969a) 2038–2045

Rosensweig, N. S., Stifel, F. B., Herman, Y. F. *et al.* Regulation of human jejunal glycolytic enzymes by oral folic acid: time and dose response. *Am. J. Clin. Nutr.* 22 (1969b) 677–678

Russell, J. D. and DeMars, R. UDPglucose: D-galactose-1-phosphate uridyltransferase in cultured human fibroblasts. *Biochem. Genet.* 1 (1967) 11–14

Segal, S. and Bernstein, H. Observations on cataract formation in the newborn offspring of rats fed a high galactose diet. *J. Pediatr.* 62 (1963) 363–370

Segal, S. and Cuatrecasas, P. The oxidation of ^{14}C-galactose by patients with congenital galactosemia. Evidence for a direct oxidative pathway. *Am. J. Med.* 44 (1968) 340–347

Segal, S. and Rogers, S. Nucleotide inhibition of mammalian liver galactose-1-phosphate uridyltransferase. *Biochim. Biophys. Acta* 250 (1971) 351–360

Segal, S., Blair, A. and Roth, H. The metabolism of galactose by patients with congenital galactosemia. *Am. J. Med.* 38 (1965) 62–70

Segal, S., Rogers, S. and Holtzapple, P.G. Liver galactose-1-phosphate uridyltransferase: Activity in normal and galactosemic subjects. *J. Clin. Invest.* 50 (1971) 500–506

Shin, Y. S., Rieth, M., Hoyer, S. and Endres, W. Uridine diphosphogalactose, galactose-1-phosphate and galactitol concentration in patients with classical galactosemia. Abs. 23rd SSIEM Annual Symposium Proceedings *Inborn Errors of Metabolism*, Liverpool, 1985

Steinmann, B., Gitzelmann, R. and Zachmann, M. Hypogonadism and galactosaemia. *N. Engl. J. Med.* 305 (1981) 464–465

Stifel, F. B., Herman, R. H. and Rosensweig, N. S. Dietary regulation of galactose-metabolizing enzymes: Adaptive changes in rat jejunum. *Science* 162 (1968) 692–693

Taunton, O. D., Green, H., Stifel, F. B. *et al.* Fructose-1, 6-diphosphate deficiency hypoglycemia and response to folate therapy in a mother and her daughter. *Biochem. Med.* 19 (1978) 260–276

Tedesco, T. A. and Mellman, W. J. Galactosemia: Evidence of a structural gene mutation. *Science* 172 (1971) 727–728

Unakar, N. J., Smart, T., Reddan, J. R. and Devlin, I. Regression of cataracts in the offspring of galactose fed rats. *Ophthalmic Res.* 11 (1979) 52–64

J. Inher. Metab. Dis. 13 (1990) 501–508

The Mechanisms of Cataract Formation

C. Schmitt and O. Hockwin
Medizinische Einrichtungen der Rheinischen Friedrich Wilhelms Universität Bonn, Abteilung für Experimentelle Ophthalmologie, Sigmund Freud Straße 25, D-5300 Bonn, FRG

Summary: This review summarizes current knowledge concerning cataract formation. Metabolically induced forms of cataract are discussed, but mainly aspects of cataract formation in older patients are described, especially with respect to lens protein modifications and epidemiological results. In most cases, cataract in older people is a multifactorial process and therefore cataracts appear in a multitude of different morphological types. Only accurate documentation of lens disturbances and the use of reproducible methods can provide more detailed information about the complexity of the disease cataract.

Attempts to explain the disease 'cataract' are as old as the disease itself. One of the first ideas concerning the pathological mechanisms led to the term cataract because of the assumption that humour flowing down from the brain (κατὰφεῖν) would close the pupillary region. In the meantime, considerable progress has been made in the field of cataract research. This is especially the case where the cataract is assoociated with diseases in which the pathogenic mechanisms could be found. Moreover, there exist countless biochemical, histological and epidemiological results which have made contributions to a better understanding of this extraordinarily complex disease. Nevertheless, the mechanisms leading to the most frequent lens opacifications, namely opacifications with increasing age, are nearly unknown. Hypotheses and model systems have been developed which in combination with experimental results and epidemiological surveys have become the essential basis for further research in cataract development.

METABOLIC CATARACTS

Metabolically induced cataracts mostly appear in early childhood since the underlying inborn disorders of metabolism often cause damage to the very susceptible developing pre- or postnatal lens. One of these cataracts is the diabetic cataract, which thanks to optimized insulin substitution hardly develops to its full extent. The following mechanism is believed to cause the development of cataracts in untreated diabetes. Lack of insulin causes glucose accumulation not only in blood but also in the aqueous humour and in the lens. Within the lens reduction of glucose to sorbitol takes place via the aldose reductase pathway. Further sorbitol metabolism proceeds very slowly; the resulting accumulation of sorbitol is followed by an osmotic swelling of the lens fibres. Typical findings of a fully developed diabetic cataract are snowflake-like opacifications of the anterior and posterior lens cortex. This kind of lens disturbance is fairly seldom seen in older diabetic patients, whose lens changes do not really vary from those of other 'normal' people. However, diabetic patients have an earlier onset of cataracts (Anthonisen, 1936; Kinoshita, 1964).

Also osmotically induced are the cataracts of galactosaemia which is caused by a lack of galactose-1-P-uridyltransferase in its classical form, or a lack of galactokinase. By reducing the C-1-aldehyde group the osmotically effective sugar polyol galactitol is formed from the excess galactose. Its accumulation within the lens leads to opacifications of the embryonic nucleus (Kinoshita, 1965). In the case of α-mannosidosis the accumulation of mannose-enriched oligosaccharides gives rise to opacifications of the posterior lens capsule.

Besides these inborn errors of sugar metabolism disorders of amino acid metabolism can play an important role in cataract development. In Lowe's syndrome, for example, we find different kinds of opacifications probably as the result of synthesis of abnormal lens proteins. As a consequence of disturbed lens growth, the lenses moreover remain smaller and thinner than usual. Of interest in disorders of amino acid metabolism is the observation of cataract development in phenylketonuric animals after feeding with 4-chlorphenylalanine. In man, however, there is no evident relationship between phenylketonuria and cataract development (Wegener *et al.*, 1984). Also well known is cataract formation in rats after feeding with a tryptophan-free diet (Ohrloff *et al.*, 1978).

In addition to the diseases already mentioned, there are many cataract associated syndromes. Last but not least are the cataracts which develop following intrauterine viral infections such as rubella, toxoplasmosis and cytomegalic virus as well as cataracts secondary to other eye diseases or cataracts resulting from traumatic injuries to the eye.

CATARACTS OF OLD AGE

All types of metabolic cataract together only constitute a very small number compared to the most common cataract, the cataract of old age, unfortunately often called 'senile cataract'. Biochemical investigations of age-related changes in lens metabolism as well as studies of experimentally induced cataracts have made essential contributions to the elucidation of the mechanisms involved in cataract formation with increasing age. Different cataract models give proof of the fact that quite different pathological actions produce morphologically widely varying kinds of cataracts. This, together with the findings following combined treatment of animals with different cataractogenic factors, emphasizes the complexity of cataract formation (Hockwin *et al.*, 1969). Cataract formation in old age depends on many damaging influences and must be considered as a multifactorial process in most cases. One major factor which has hindered the research on cataract formation in older people and sometimes still hinders further progress today is the uncritical and undifferentiated grouping of a great variety of morphologically different cataract types under the term 'senile cataract'.

But is the ageing process itself the cause of cataract, and is cataract really an unavoidable disease for all people reaching a certain age? This question can clearly be answered in the negative: there are many 80-year-olds with acceptable visual acuity whereas some 50-year-olds have to undergo cataract surgery because of advanced lens opacifications. Nevertheless, it is evident that with increasing age the incidence of cataract also increases markedly. This gives rise to the question as to which physical and biochemical lens properties, and especially which changes during the ageing process are responsible for the formation of cataract.

One of the best known phenomena to occur with increasing age is an increased yellow to brown coloration of the lens nucleus (Klang, 1948). This is accompanied by a decrease in lens transmission in the wavelengths between 300 and 400 nm (Lerman and Borkman, 1976). This change is supposed to be due to a photochemically induced degradation of intrinsic lens tryptophan to N-formylkynurenine by means of oxygen radicals. This assumption coincides with epidemiological results revealing significantly higher cataract extraction rates in areas of the USA where sunlight is present for the longest time compared to areas with moderate climates and shorter sunlight duration (Hiller *et al.*, 1977). Moreover, within a given geographical region the prevalence of the brownish nuclear cataract is higher amongst people who are living and working mostly outdoors compared to people spending most of their time indoors (Zigman *et al.*, 1979).

These observations emphasize the importance of lens biochemistry, especially of the lens proteins, since in the end modifications of lens proteins are responsible for changes in physical properties of the lens. The lens transparency is mainly ensured by a special arrangement of its constituent proteins as well as an equilibrium between these proteins and the lens water content (Trokel, 1962). Impairment of this balance can be caused by either osmotically-induced swelling or by a defect in a metabolic step. Moreover, modification of the protein structure itself can produce lens opacification. These changes can occur during the biosynthesis of lens proteins which only lasts until the lens fibre formation is finished. Fibre formation starts from the epithelial cells of the lens equator – the so-called germinative zone. The mature lens fibres stop protein synthesis at the time when they lose their nuclei. The fibres then surround already existing lens fibres, therefore all lens fibres remain within the lens for the whole lifespan of the individual (Spencer, 1985). There is no loss of cells as there is in the skin by means of shedding of the superficial cells. Thus a second possibility for protein changes is by means of post-translational modifications, affecting both structural proteins and enzyme molecules. With increasing age, for example, a progressive reduction in the essential energy providing anaerobic glycolysis takes place as a consequence of modifications of the key enzymes of the carbohydrate metabolism (Hockwin and Ohrloff, 1981). The subsequent impairment of crucial energy-dependent metabolic steps renders the lens more susceptible to additional endo- and/or exogenous damaging influences, thus increasing the disposition to the formation of lens opacifications. Some of these postsynthetic protein alterations are deamidation, glycolysation, phosphorylation, formation of disulphide bonds and mixed disulphides, racemization of optical active parts, proteolysis, formation of aggregates, and oxidation of methionine (Hockwin, 1985). As a result of the modifications of the structural proteins, increased light scattering caused by protein conversion and the formation of high molecular weight aggregates occurs (Benedek, 1971).

The post-translational modifications would be expected mainly to affect the oldest lens fibres, situated in the lens nucleus. However, about 75% of all cataracts in old age reveal a surprisingly transparent lens nucleus, but at the same time they show markedly advanced opacities in the cortical region, which reflect a hazard to the younger lens fibre cells. This phenomenon might be due to alterations concerning the general state of health with increasing age on the one hand, or to drug treatment of certain age related diseases, which might affect the lens metabolism. Starting from this assumption a working hypothesis on cataract formation has been developed in our department, not concentrating just on a simple cause and effect relationship, but keeping very much in mind the susceptibility of the lens to a multitude of influences (Hockwin *et al.*, 1969).

Two terms need to be mentioned: co- and syncataractogenesis (Figure 1). Cocataractogenesis means the intensification of a direct cataractogenic influence by a second subliminal factor. When a cataract appears only after a combined application of two subliminal factors, this is termed syncataractogenesis. Appreciable research in the last few years has been based on this working hypothesis. This model also proved to be very worthwhile in preclinical drug safety studies, since it offers the possibility of detecting subliminal cataractogenic potential in combining the drug in question with other lens-damaging factors in animal experiments. The aim of the drug safety studies thereby is the specific search for the cataractogenicity of one well-defined exogenous influence.

Statistical analyses of epidemiological surveys in contrast mostly supply first indications of a possible cataractogenic potential of certain risk factors. For example, there exists a higher prevalence of cataract in people with hypertension, but whether

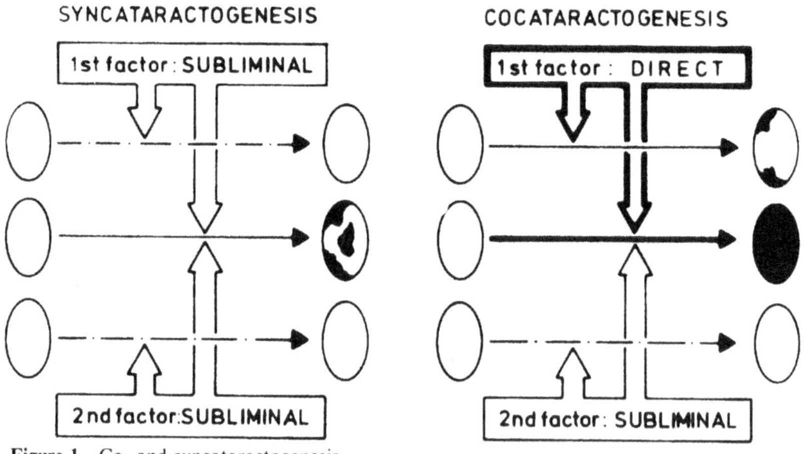

Figure 1 Co- and syncataractogenesis.

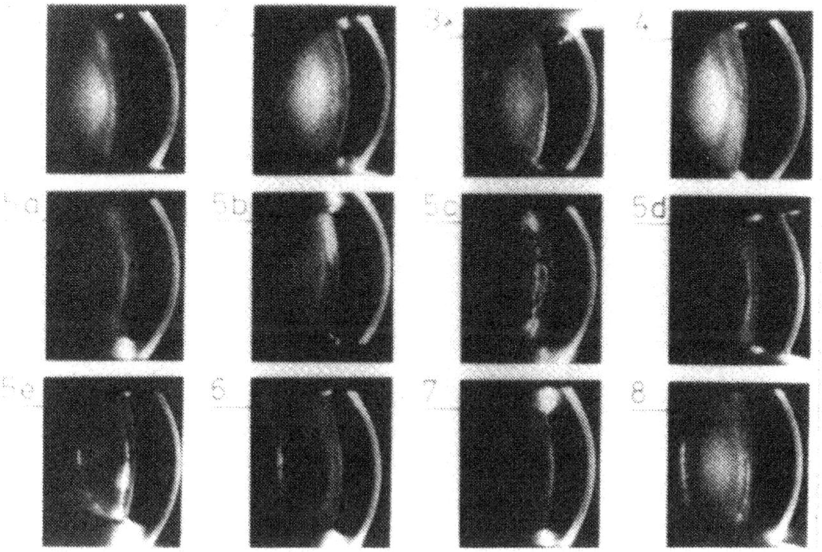

1 nuclear opacity	2 nucleus and posterior capsule	3 nucleus, anterior and posterior capsule	4 nucleus and anterior cortex
5a water clefts and spokes	5b wedge-shaped cataract	5c cataracta coronaria	5d deeper anterior cortex
5e anterior and posterior cortex	6 posterior subcapsular opacity	7 anterior and posterior capsule	8 total lens opacity

Figure 2 Cataract classification system.

there is a causal relationship between hypertension and the development of lens opacifications is unproven. Possible influences of antihypertensive drugs have also to be taken into account (Kahn *et al.*, 1977). There exists also a hypothesis that heavy smoking and drinking, and working on military bases are risk factors in cataract development (Harding and van Heyningen, 1989). Such epidemiological results mainly depend on the formulation of a question and on the availability of important information concerning the general state of health.

Potential risk factors discovered by means of epidemiological studies need to be critically tested in animal experiments. It is of the utmost importance, not only to prove or exclude a relation between risk and cataract, but also to describe the cataract morphology as accurately as possible according to a comprehensive classification system (see Figure 2), and to document the findings using an objective documentation system. Only in this way is there a possibility of evaluating the multifactorial cause and effect chain, thereby possibly interfering with the process of cataract development one day by drug treatment. For documentation, the system of Scheimpflug photography of the anterior eye segment has been available for about 10 years (Hockwin *et al.*, 1978). By providing reproducible lens photographs with sufficient depth of field this method allows an exact morphological localization of lens opacifications to be

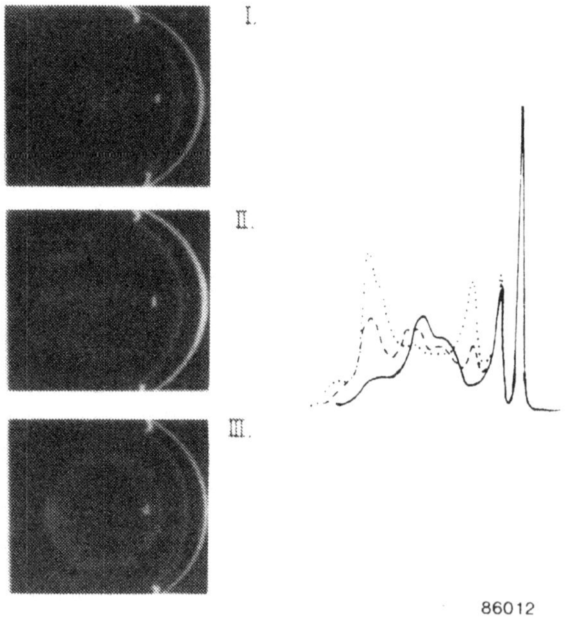

Figure 3 Development of a supranuclear cataract in rats after naphthalene feeding and presentation of the corresponding densitograms of the lens photographs from investigation I (———) II (----) and III (·······)

made. Additionally, follow-up studies of any given lens disturbance are possible by comparing the first photograph with later ones of the same lens (see Figure 3).

CONCLUSION

To conclude, the following crucial aspects of cataractogenesis ought to be emphasized:
1. Ageing itself is certainly a factor not to be underestimated in cataractogenesis, but age alone as the simple cause of cataract can be excluded.
2. A variety of metabolic disorders can cause changes in the composition of the supporting aqueous humour, leading to lens impairment.
3. Protein modifications, as a consequence of disturbed protein biosynthesis or as a consequence of post-translational changes, can give rise to opacifications of the lens by disorganizing the protein structure and thereby inducing a protein–water imbalance. One post-translational alteration, the sunlight-induced coloration of the lens nucleus, should be particularly emphasized with special respect to the discussion about the reduction in the ozone layer.
4. A multitude of environmental and nutritional factors as well as diseases and the drugs taken to treat them are thought to be involved in the process of cataract formation. Further efforts in epidemiological research and in ocular drug safety studies are needed to evaluate them.
5. Only an objective and reproducible documentation of lens irregularities can hope to provide objective and clinically relevant data.

REFERENCES

Anthonisen, H. The frequency of diabetic cataract and diabetic glaucoma as compared to the frequency of diabetes in the general population of Denmark. *Acta Ophthalmol.* (*Kbh.*) 14 (1936) 150–158

Benedek, G. Theory of transparency of the eye. *Appl. Opt.* 10 (1971) 459–472

Harding, J.J. and van Heyningen, R. Beer, cigarettes and military work as risk factors for cataract. In Hockwin, O., Sasaki, K. and Leske, M.C. (eds.), Risk factors for cataract development. *Dev. Ophthalmol.*, Karger, Basel, 1989, pp. 13–16

Hiller, R., Giacometti, L. and Yuen, K. Sunlight and cataract: an epidemiological investigation. *Am. J. Epidemiol.* 105 (1977) 450–459

Hockwin, O., Biochemie des Auges. *Klinische Monatsblätter für Augenheilkunde, Beiheft* 107, Enke, Stuttgart, 1985

Hockwin, O., Okamoto, T., Bergeder, H.D., Klein, W., Ferrari, L. and Streit, W. Genesis of cataracts. Cumulative effects of subliminal noxious influences. *Ann. Ophthalmol.* 1 (1969) 321–325

Hockwin, O., Dragomirescu, V. and Koch, H.R. Spezialkamera für die Augenphotographie. *DFG-Mitteilungen* 3 (1978) 17–20

Hockwin, O. and Ohrloff, C. Enzymes in normal, ageing, and cataractous lenses. In Bloemendal (ed.), *Molecular and Cellular Biology of the Eye Lens*, Wiley, New York, 1981, pp. 367–413

Kahn, H.A., Leibowitz, H., Ganley, J. *et al.* The Framingham eye study. I. Outline and major prevalence findings. *Am. J. Epidemiol.* 106 (1977) 17

Kinoshita, J.H. Selected topics in ophthalmic biochemistry. *Arch. Ophthalmol.* 72 (1964) 554–572

Kinoshita, J.H. Cataracts in galactosemia. *Invest. Ophthalmol.* 4 (1965) 786–799

Klang, G. Measurements and studies of the fluorescence of the human lens *in vivo*. *Acta*

Ophthalmol. Suppl. 31 (1948) 1–152

Lerman, S. and Borkman, R.F. Spectroscopic evaluation and classification of the normal, ageing, and cataractous lens. *Ophthalmic Res.* 8 (1976) 335–353

Ohrloff, C., Stoffel, C., Koch, H.R. *et al.* Experimental cataracts in rat due to tryptophan-free diet. *Graefes Arch. Ophthalmol.* 205 (1978) 73

Spencer, W.H. *Ophthalmic Pathology*, Saunders, Philadelphia, 1985

Trokel, S. The physical basis for the transparency of the lens. *Invest. Opthalmol.* 1 (1962) 493-502

Wegener, A., Münch, C., Byrd, D.J., Jaeger, W., Hockwin, O. and Bours, J. Die Morphologie von Linsenveränderungen bei experimentell phenylketonurischen Ratten mit ohne Tryptophanmangeldiät. *Fortschr. Ophthalmol.* 81 (1984) 626–628

Zigman, S., Datiles, M. and Torczynski, E. Sunlight and human cataracts. *Invest. Ophthalmol.* 18 (1979) 462–467

J. Inher. Metab. Dis. 13 (1990) 509–516

Cataract and Metabolic Disease

W. Endres and Y. S. Shin
Universitäts-Kinderklinik, Lindwurmstrasse 4, D-8000 München 2, FRG

Summary: In addition to the already recognized metabolic diseases which have been associated with cataract formation, e.g. galactosaemia, galactokinase deficiency, Lowe's syndrome and diabetes, several other disorders can also lead to the development of cataracts. They are sorbitol dehydrogenase deficiency, uridine diphosphate galactose-4-epimerase deficiency, marginal maternal transferase and galactokinase deficiency, galactitol and sorbitol accumulation of unknown origin, heterozygosity for galactosaemia and galactokinase deficiency as well as the carrier state for Lowe's syndrome. In this review these metabolic disorders have been divided into five groups according to the age at the first appearance of lens clouding and the possible means of treatment have been discussed.

In more than 90% of congenital cataract the aetiology remains unknown. Most of these cataracts are inherited as a dominant trait. Only a small number of congenital cataracts are known to be due to metabolic disorders. Since some of these diseases have been detected quite recently and, at least in some cases, lens clouding can be prevented by dietary means, it is worthwhile drawing the attention of paediatricians and ophthalmologists to the possibility of early diagnosis and treatment.

An additional aim of this review is to differentiate the metabolic disorders leading to cataract formation into various groups according to the age at onset of lens clouding. This may also be helpful in the differential diagnosis of inborn errors of metabolism presenting with cataracts.

DISEASE-RELATED FIRST APPEARANCE OF CATARACT

As shown in Table 1, the disorders have been divided into five groups according to the age at onset of cataract: at birth, during the further newborn period, in infancy, in childhood and in adulthood.

At birth

The prenatal development of lens clouding is a universal finding in patients with Lowe's oculo–cerebro–renal syndrome (McKusick 30900) (Lowe *et al.*, 1952; Abbassi *et al.*, 1968). We also demonstrated cataractous changes with lenticonus opacification

Table 1 Cataract in metabolic disorders

Time when first visible	*Disorder*
At birth	Lowe's syndrome Zellweger syndrome Rhizomelic chondrodysplasia punctata Sorbitol dehydrogenase deficiency
In the newborn (after 5 days)	Galactosaemia (Gal-1-P uridyl transferase deficiency) UDP galactose-4-epimerase deficiency Marginal maternal galactokinase deficiency Hyperglycinuria
	Single observation: Metachromatic leukodystrophy
In the infant (after 4 weeks)	Galactokinase deficiency Partial galactokinase deficiency Marginal maternal galactokinase deficiency Galactitol or sorbitol accumulation of unknown origin α-Mannosidosis Sialidosis Hypoglycaemia
	Single observations: Hypobetalipoproteinaemia and vitamin E deficiency Mitochondrial myopathy and lactic acidosis Vitamin D deficiency rickets Lactose intolerance
In the child	Diabetes mellitus Wilson's disease Hypoparathyroidism Pseudohypoparathyroidism
	Single observations: Cerebellar atrophy, mental retardation and myopathy Menkes' disease Alport's syndrome
In the adult	Heterozygosity for Gal-1-P uridyl transferase deficiency Heterozygosity for galactokinase deficiency Carriers for Lowe's syndrome Lactose absorbers Riboflavin deficiency Gyrate atrophy with hyperornithinaemia Glucose-6-phosphate dehydrogenase deficiency Cerebrotendinous xanthomatosis Myotonic dystrophy

in a fetus at risk for Lowe's syndrome as early as the 24th week of gestation (Endres *et al.*, 1977).

In disorders of peroxisome biogenesis, e.g. in Zellweger syndrome (Heymans, 1984; McKusick 21410) and rhizomelic chondrodysplasia punctata (Lazarow and Moser, 1989; McKusick 21510), cataracts are a frequent observation at birth.

In 1982 Vaca and colleagues described several predominantly male members of a Mexican family with cataracts and reduced sorbitol dehydrogenase (EC 1.1.1.14) activity (McKusick 18250) in red blood cells. Shin and colleagues (1984) described a German family where a father and his son had cataracts and reduced sorbitol dehydrogenase activity in red blood cells. However, the grandfather of the family described by Vaca and colleagues (1982), who also had reduced sorbitol dehydrogenase activity in red blood cells, was completely normal without any signs of lens clouding. A further study concerning the pathogenetic relationship between sorbitol dehydrogenase deficiency and the development of cataracts is therefore necessary. Possible additional factors should be considered, such as an increased aldose reductase (EC 1.1.1.21) activity as observed in diabetic rats (Varma and Kinoshita, 1974), which can contribute to a sorbitol accumulation in lenses or sorbitol dehydrogenase isozymes in tissues other than in red blood cells. The determination of sorbitol in plasma (Shin *et al.*, 1985b) may be an excellent means of proving the cause of cataract as well as controlling a potential therapy.

Cataract in the newborn

In some patients with galactosaemia due to galactose-1-phosphate uridyl transferase (EC 2.7.7.12) deficiency (Mason and Turner, 1935; Holton, 1990; McKusick 23040) lens opacities can be detected within the first week of life (Segal, 1989). In these patients aldose reductase catalyses the conversion of accumulated galactose to its polyol, galactitol, which leads to swelling of the lens fibres. If dietary galactose restriction is initiated early, the cataract can regress fully. The incidence of cataract in galactosaemic patients detected by clinical symptoms is about 50% (Buist *et al.*, 1988). However, 13% of 147 patients found by newborn screening already had cataracts in the neonatal period (Buist *et al.*, 1988).

Holton and colleagues (1981) and Sardharwalla and colleagues (1988) each reported a patient with a generalized uridine diphosphate galactose-4-epimerase (EC 5.1.3.2) deficiency (McKusick 23035) whose clinical symptoms were similar to those usually found in patients with classical galactosaemia. In one of these patients cataracts were present on slit lamp examination (Sardharwalla *et al.*, 1988). However, cataracts have also been observed in some patients with peripheral epimerase deficiency who were otherwise healthy (Shin *et al.*, 1985a). Cataracts have even been found in heterozygotes for peripheral epimerase deficiency (Jakobs *et al.*, 1990). In all three genetic constellations (generalized epimerase deficiency, peripheral epimerase deficiency and the heterozygous state for peripheral epimerase deficiency) elevated plasma galactitol levels have been demonstrated (Jakobs *et al.*, 1990). It can therefore be postulated that galactitol accumulation in the lens could be a main cause of the cataract development.

Harley and colleagues (1974) demonstrated that 75 mothers of children with cataracts had somewhat reduced galactokinase activities in red blood cells but these were not compatible with the heterozygous state of galactokinase deficiency. They made a similar observation in 36 mothers whose galactose-1-phosphate uridyl transferase activities were reduced but not significantly different from those of controls and concluded that 'these results are interpreted as strong evidence that marginal maternal deficiency of either or both enzymes, in the face of substantial lactose intake during pregnancy, may contribute to the formation of cataracts during developmental life.' This interpretation, however, has been questioned by Winder and colleagues (1985) on the basis of observations on a small number of families with established enzyme deficiencies and/or cataracts. Further investigations concerning the lactose intake in mothers of such families during pregnancy are also necessary in order to elucidate this point.

The association of cataract with hyperglycinuria in six members of a Finnish kindred with autosomal dominantly inherited cataract (Similä and Käär, 1974) may be an incidental observation. The same may be true for the single observation of cataract in a newborn infant with metachromatic leukodystrophy (Endres, 1986). Nevertheless, these findings indicate a complexity in cataract formation.

Cataract in infancy

Galactokinase (EC 2.7.1.6) deficiency (McKusick 23020), first described by Gitzelmann (1965; 1967), leads to cataract formation during the first months of life and is the sole clinical manifestation of the disease. In one patient lens opacities have been observed as early as the age of three weeks (Thalhammer *et al.*, 1968).

Beutler and colleagues (1973) and Beutler and Matsumoto (1978) reported a statistical correlation of the partial reduction in the galactokinase activity with cataract development during the first year of life. Similar observations have been made by Kaloud and colleagues (1975). Marginal maternal galactokinase deficiency as mentioned previously may lead to lens clouding beyond the newborn period (Harley *et al.*, 1974).

Some infants with cataract and normal galactose metabolizing enzymes in red blood cells have been found to have elevated plasma concentrations of galactitol (Jakobs *et al.*, 1988). Jakobs and colleagues (1990) recently reported that an increased sorbitol concentration was also observed in some cataract patients with a normal sorbitol dehydrogenase activity in red blood cells. Currently no comprehensible explanations for this polyol accumulation in plasma have been found and the cause remains speculative.

In addition cataracts have been observed in disorders of glycoprotein degradation including α-mannosidosis (Öckerman, 1967; Kjellman *et al.*, 1969; McKusick 24850) and sialidosis (Durand *et al.*, 1977; Beaudet and Thomas, 1989; McKusick 25655). It has also been well established that hypoglycaemia from different causes during infancy can result in cataract formation (Merin and Crawford, 1971; Koivisto *et al.*, 1972).

Isolated cases of infantile cataract have been described in metabolic disorders such as hypobetalipoproteinaemia and vitamin E deficiency (Griffiths *et al.*, 1988), mitochondrial myopathy of skeletal and heart muscle associated with lactic acidosis after exercise (Sengers *et al.*, 1975), vitamin D deficiency rickets (Hochman and Mejlszenkier, 1977) and lactose intolerance (Hirashima *et al.*, 1979).

Cataract in childhood

Cataracts developed during childhood (mainly during adolescence) may be due to diabetes mellitus, Wilson's disease (McKusick 27790), hypoparathyroidism and pseudohypoparathyroidism. According to Danks (1989) lenticular opacities have been observed in 15–20% of all patients with Wilson's disease. Cataracts have been seen occasionally in patients suffering from cerebellar atrophy, mental retardation and myopathy (Herva *et al.*, 1987), Menkes' kinky hair disease (Sakano *et al.*, 1982) and children with Alport's syndrome (Schatz, 1971).

Cataract in adults

Cataracts have been observed among adult subjects who were heterozygous for galactose-1-phosphate uridyl transferase deficiency (Prchal *et al.*, 1978; Burke *et al.*, 1988; Brivet *et al.*, 1989) or for galactokinase deficiency (Monteleone *et al.*, 1971; Prchal *et al.*, 1978). The cataract formation among the respective heterozygotes, however, may depend upon the galactose intake. Lenticular opacities have also been seen in carriers of the gene for Lowe's syndrome (Gardner and Brown, 1976; Hittner *et al.*, 1982).

Rinaldi and colleagues (1984) observed a prevalence of persistent high lactase activity in adult Neapolitans with cataracts. The authors interpreted this finding as an increased susceptibility to cataracts in adults absorbing a higher amount of galactose from a lactose-containing diet.

Riboflavin deficiency in red blood cells has been demonstrated in eight adult patients with cataracts (Prchal *et al.*, 1978). Since riboflavin deficiency has also been associated with the development of cataracts in animals, it can be assumed that it was directly responsible for the cataract formation in humans.

Finally, rare disorders such as gyrate atrophy with hyperornithinaemia (Valle and Simell, 1989; McKusick 25887), glucose-6-phosphate dehydrogenase deficiency (Luzzatto and Mehta, 1989; McKusick 30590), cerebrotendinous xanthomatosis (Björkhem and Skrede, 1989; McKusick 21370) and myotonic dystrophy (Harper, 1989; McKusick 16090) can be associated with the development of cataract.

CONCLUSIONS

The age-related classification of cataract formation presented here may be helpful in the differential diagnosis of a certain group of metabolic diseases. The causes of cataract formation are indeed diverse and the time of onset is also variable. We need further investigations in order to estimate the validity of the correlations reported between disease and cataract. In particular, this might be true for sorbitol dehydrogenase deficiency, partial galactokinase defiency, heterozygosity for galactose-1-phosphate uridyl transferase deficiency or for galactokinase deficiency, marginal maternal galactokinase deficiency, and galactitol or sorbitol accumulation of unknown origin.

The early and accurate detection of possible causes for the cataract may be helpful in preventing its formation by appropriate measures. In most diseases no specific treatment is available. In patients with a defect in galactose metabolism dietary galactose restriction is the main objective. An important question lies, however, in the therapy for pregnant mothers homozygous or heterozygous for one of the disorders in galactose metabolism. The extremely high levels of galactose-1-phosphate in red blood cells during the newborn period in galactosaemic patients suggests that the galactose metabolism is very active during the prenatal as well as the neonatal period. Galactose toxicity may therefore occur in infants with such mothers even though they are completely healthy otherwise. Further studies are needed for a definite regime for treatment.

REFERENCES

Abbassi, V., Lowe, C. U. and Calcagno, P. L. Oculo–cerebro–renal syndrome. *Am. J. Dis. Child.* 115 (1968) 145–168

Beaudet, A. L. and Thomas, G. H. Disorders of glycoprotein degradation: mannosidosis, fucosidosis, sialidosis, and aspartylglycosaminuria. In Scriver, C. R., Beaudet, A. L., Sly, W. S. and Valle, D. (eds.), *The Metabolic Basis of Inherited Disease*, McGraw-Hill, New York, 1989, pp. 1603–1621

Beutler, E. and Matsumoto, F. Galactokinase and cataracts. *Lancet* 1 (1978) 1161

Beutler, E., Matsumoto, F., Kuhl, W., Krill, A., Levy, N., Sparkes, R. and Degnan, M. Galactokinase deficiency as a cause of cataracts. *N. Engl. J. Med.* 228 (1973) 1203–1206

Björkhem, I. and Skrede, S. Familial diseases with storage of sterols other than cholesterol: Cerebrotendinous xanthomatosis and phytosterolemia. In Scriver, C. R., Beaudet, A. L., Sly, W. S. and Valle, D. (eds.), *The Metabolic Basis of Inherited Disease*, McGraw-Hill, New York, 1989, pp. 1283–1302

Brivet, M., Migayron, F., Roger, J., Cheron, G. and Lemonnier, A. Lens hexitols and cataract formation during lactation in a woman heterozygote for galactosaemia. *J. Inher. Metab. Dis.* 12, Suppl. 2 (1989) 343–345

Buist, N., Waggoner, D., Donnell, G. and Levy, H. The effects of newborn screening on prognosis in galactosemia: results of the international survey. *Proceedings of the 26th SSIEM Symposium (1988)* p. 53, ISBN 1-870617-01-0

Burke, J. P., O'Keefe, M., Bowell, R. and Naughton, E. R. Cataracts in children with classical galactosaemia and in their parents. *J. Inher. Metab. Dis.* 11, Suppl. 2 (1988) 246–248

Danks, D. M. Disorders of copper transport. In Scriver, C. R., Beaudet, A. L., Sly, W. S. and Valle, D. (eds.), *The Metabolic Basis of Inherited Disease*, McGraw-Hill, New York, 1989, pp. 1411–1431

Durand, P., Gatti, R., Cavalieri, S., Borrone, C., Tondeur, M., Michalski, J.-C. and Strecker, G. Sialidosis (mucolipidosis I). *Helv. Paediatr. Acta* 32 (1977) 391–400

Endres, W. Unpublished observation (1986)

Endres, W., Schaub, J., Stefani, F. H., Wirtz, A. and Zahn, V. Cataract in a fetus at risk for oculo–cerebro–renal syndrome (Lowe). *Klin. Wochenschr.* 55 (1977) 141–144

Gardner, R. J. M. and Brown, N. Lowe's syndrome: Identification of carriers by lens examination. *J. Med. Genet.* 13 (1976) 449–454
Gitzelmann, R. Deficiency of erythrocyte galactokinase in a patient with galactose diabetes. *Lancet* 2 (1965) 670–671
Gitzelmann, R. Hereditary galactokinase deficiency, a newly recognized cause of juvenile cataracts. *Pediatr. Res.* 1 (1967) 14–23
Griffiths, R. D., Taylor, C. J., Isherwood, D. M. and Jackson, M. J. Fat malabsorption, vitamin E deficiency, scoliosis and cataracts. *J. Inher. Metab. Dis.* 11, Suppl. 2 (1988) 153–154
Harley, J. D., Irvine, S., Mutton, P. and Gupta, J. D. Maternal enzymes of galactose metabolism and the 'inexplicable' infantile cataract. *Lancet* 2 (1974) 259–261
Harper, P. S. The muscular dystrophies. In Scriver, C. R., Beaudet, A. L., Sly, W. S. and Valle, D. (eds.), *The Metabolic Basis of Inherited Disease*, McGraw-Hill, New York, 1989, pp. 2869–2902
Herva, R., von Wendt, L., von Wendt, G., Saukkonen, A.-L., Leisti, J. and Dubowitz, J. A syndrome with juvenile cataract, cerebellar atrophy, mental retardation and myopathy. *Neuropediatrics* 18 (1987) 164–169
Heymans, H. S. A. Cerebro–hepato–renal (Zellweger) syndrome. Clinical and biochemical consequences of peroxisomal dysfunction. Thesis, University of Amsterdam, 1984
Hirashima, Y., Shinozuka, S., Ieiri, T., Matsuda, I., Ono, Y. and Murata, T. Lactose intolerance associated with cataracts. *Eur. J. Pediatr.* 130 (1979) 41–45
Hittner, H. M., Carroll, A. J. and Prchal, J. T. Linkage studies in carriers of Lowe oculo–cerebro–renal syndrome. *Am. J. Hum. Genet.* 34 (1982) 966–971
Hochman, H. I. and Mejlszenkier, J. D. Cataracts and pseudotumor cerebri in an infant with vitamin D-deficiency rickets. *J. Pediatr.* 90 (1977) 252–254
Holton, J. B. Galactose disorders: an overview. *J. Inher. Metab. Dis.* 13 (1990) 476–486
Holton, J. B., Gillett, M. G., MacFaul, R. and Young, R. Galactosaemia: a new variant due to uridine diphosphate galactose-4-epimerase deficiency. *Arch. Dis. Child.* 56 (1981) 885–887
Jakobs, C., Douwes, A. C., Kok, R. M., De Jong, A., Endres, W. and Shin, Y. S. Elevated plasma galactitol levels in patients with congenital cataracts without enzyme defects. *Eur. J. Pediatr.* 147 (1988) 446
Jakobs, C., Douwes, A. C., Brockstedt, M., Stellaard, F., Endres, W. and Shin, Y. S. Plasma polyol levels in patients with cataract. *J. Inher. Metab. Dis.* 13 (1990) 517–522
Kaloud, H., Sitzmann, F. C., Schenker, H. and Prestele, H. Enzymaktivitätswerte des Galaktosestoffwechsels bei der sogenannten Cataracta congenita. *Dtsch. Med. Wochenschr.* 100 (1975) 873–876
Kjellman, B., Gamstrop, I., Brun, A., Öckerman, P.-A. and Palmgren, B. Mannosidosis: a clinical and histopathologic study. *J. Pediatr.* 75 (1969) 366–373
Koivisto, M., Blanco-Sequeiros, M. and Krause, U. Neonatal symptomatic and asymptomatic hypoglycaemia: a follow-up study of 151 children. *Dev. Med. Child. Neurol.* 14 (1972) 603–614
Lazarow, P. B. and Moser, H. W. Disorders of peroxisome biogenesis. In Scriver, C. R., Beaudet, A. L., Sly, W. S. and Valle, D. (eds.), *The Metabolic Basis of Inherited Disease*, McGraw-Hill, New York, 1989, pp. 1479–1509
Lowe, C. U., Terrey, M. and MacLachlan, E. A. Organic aciduria, decreased renal ammonia production, hydrophthalmos and mental retardation. *Am. J. Dis. Child.* 83 (1952) 164–184
Luzzatto, L. and Mehta, A. Glucose-6-phosphate dehydrogenase deficiency. In Scriver, C. R., Beaudet, A. L., Sly, W. S. and Valle, D. (eds.), *The Metabolic Basis of Inherited Disease*, McGraw-Hill, New York, 1989, pp. 2237–2265
Mason, H. H. and Turner, M. E. Chronic galactosemia. *Am. J. Dis. Child.* 50 (1935) 359–374
Merin, S. and Crawford, J. S. Hypoglycemia and infantile cataract. *Arch. Ophthalmol.* 86 (1971) 495–498
Monteleone, J. A., Beutler, E., Monteleone, P. L., Utz, C. L. and Casey, E. C. Cataracts,

galactosuria and hypergalactosemia due to galactokinase deficiency in a child. *Am. J. Med.* 50 (1971) 403–407

Öckerman, P.-A. A generalized storage disease resembling Hurler's syndrome. *Lancet* 2 (1967) 239–241

Prchal, J. T., Conrad, M. E. and Skalka, H. W. Association of presenile cataracts with heterozygosity for galactosaemic states and with riboflavin deficiency. *Lancet* 1 (1978) 12–13

Rinaldi, E., Costagliola, C., Albini, L., de Rosa, G., Auricchio, G., de Vizia, B. and Auricchio, S. High frequency of lactose absorbers among adults with idiopathic senile and presenile cataract in a population with a high prevalence of primary adult lactose malabsorption. *Lancet* 1 (1984) 355–357

Sakano, T., Okuda, N., Yoshimitsu, K., Hatano, S., Nishi, Y., Tanaka, T. and Usui, T. A case of Menkes' syndrome with cataracts. *Eur. J. Pediatr.* 138 (1982) 357–358

Sardharwalla, I. B., Wraith, J. E., Bridge, C., Fowler, B. and Roberts, S. A. A patient with severe type of epimerase deficiency galactosaemia. *J. Inher. Metab. Dis.* 11, Suppl. 2 (1988) 249–251

Schatz, H. Alport's syndrome in a negro kindred. *Am. J. Ophthalmol.* 71 (1971) 1236–1240

Segal, S. Disorders of galactose metabolism. In Scriver, C. R., Beaudet, A. L., Sly, W. S. and Valle, D. (eds.), *The Metabolic Basis of Inherited Disease*, McGraw-Hill, New York, 1989, pp. 453–480

Sengers, R. C. A., ter Haar, B. G. A., Trijbels, J. M. F., Willems, J. L., Daniels, O. and Stadhouders, A. M. Congenital cataract and mitochondrial myopathy of skeletal and heart muscle associated with lactic acidosis after exercise. *J. Pediatr.* 86 (1975) 873–880

Shin, Y. S., Rieth, M., Endres, W. and Haas, P. Sorbitol dehydrogenase deficiency in a family with congenital cataracts. *J. Inher. Metab. Dis.* 7, Suppl. 2 (1984) 151–152

Shin, Y. S., Endres, W., Rieth, M., Kruse, K. and Jakobs, C. Metabolite patterns and clinical expressions of uridine diphosphogalactose epimerase deficiency. *Pediatr. Res.* 19 (1985a) 1075

Shin, Y. S., Endres, W., Schmid, K.-M., Völcker, H. E. and Jakobs, C. Elevated plasma sorbitol levels in cataract patients with sorbitol dehydrogenase deficiency. *Pediatr. Res.* 19 (1985b) 1082

Similä, S. and Käär, M.-L. Hyperglycinuria in a family with autosomal dominantly inherited cataract. *Clin. Genet.* 6 (1974) 138–141

Thalhammer, O., Gitzelmann, R. and Pantlitschko, M. Hypergalactosemia and galactosuria due to galactokinase deficiency in a newborn. *Pediatrics* 42 (1968) 441–445

Vaca, G., Ibarra, B., Bracamontes, M., Garcia-Cruz, D., Sánchez-Corona, J., Medina, C., Wunsch, C., González-Quiroga, G. and Cantú, J. M. Red blood cell sorbitol dehydrogenase deficiency in a family with cataracts. *Hum. Genet.* 61 (1982) 338–341

Valle, D. and Simell, O. The hyperornithinemias. In Scriver, C. R., Beaudet, A. L., Sly, W. S. and Valle, D. (eds.), *The Metabolic Basis of Inherited Disease*, McGraw-Hill, New York, 1989, pp. 599–627

Varma, S. D. and Kinoshita, J. H. Sorbitol pathway in diabetic and galactosemic rat lens. *Biochim. Biophys. Acta* 338 (1974) 632–640

Winder, A. F., Fielder, A. R., Mount, J. N. and Menzies, J. S. Direct and maternal aspects of the risk of cataract with partial disorders of galactose metabolism. *Clin. Genet.* 28 (1985) 199–206.

J. Inher. Metab. Dis. 13 (1990) 517–522

Plasma Polyol Levels in Patients with Cataract

C. Jakobs[1], A. C. Douwes[1], M. Brockstedt[1], F. Stellaard[1], W. Endres[2] and Y. S. Shin[2]
[1]*Department of Paediatrics, Free University Hospital, de Boelelaan 1117, 1007 MB, Amsterdam, the Netherlands;* [2]*Children's Hospital, University of Munich, Munich, FRG*

Summary: Galactitol and sorbitol concentrations in plasma were determined in patients (with or without cataract) in whom homo- or heterozygosity for galactokinase, galactose-1-phosphate uridyltransferase, systemic or peripheral UDP-galactose epimerase and sorbitol dehydrogenase deficiency was confirmed. For the above disorders it can be concluded that elevation of plasma polyols is not always related to the presence or absence of cataract. In all cases with cataract, however, the plasma galactitol or sorbitol levels were elevated. In another group of patients with unexplained congenital or infantile cataracts, but without apparent enzyme defects, mild to moderately elevated concentrations of plasma galactitol or sorbitol were found in about 45%. In 8% of this group the cataract and the elevated plasma galactitol concentration could possibly have been related to partial maternal enzyme deficiency. In all the other cases the elevated plasma polyol concentration remains unexplained but could indicate a further cause of cataract formation due to a hitherto unknown galactose or glucose metabolic aberration.

Three genetically determined disorders involving an enzymatic defect in the galactose metabolic pathway are associated with cataracts. They are galactokinase (EC 2.7.1.6) deficiency, galactose-1-phosphate uridyltransferase (EC 2.7.7.12) deficiency and UDP-galactose epimerase (EC 5.1.3.2) deficiency. All are autosomal recessive inherited traits. Recently, patients with sorbitol dehydrogenase (EC 1.1.1.14) deficiency have also been described with cataracts (Vaca *et al.*, 1982; Shin *et al.*, 1984). In contrast to the multiple systems affected in transferase deficiency and in the generalized form of the epimerase deficiency (Holton *et al.*, 1981), cataract formation is usually the sole manifestation in galactokinase and sorbitol dehydrogenase deficiency and in some of the patients with the peripheral epimerase deficiency (Shin *et al.*, 1985). Early diagnosis and dietary control of these disorders can prevent cataracts and even achieve regression in some cases. The mechanism of cataract formation involves the reduction of galactose to galactitol by the enzyme aldose reductase within the lens.

This polyol cannot diffuse out of the lens and exerts an osmotic effect leading to disruption of the lens fibres (Stambolian, 1988). In the case of sorbitol dehydrogenase deficiency, accumulation of sorbitol in the lens possibly causes the cataract.

We routinely screen patients with congenital and/or infantile cataracts for kinase, transferase, epimerase and sorbitol dehydrogenase in erythrocytes, using the plasma from the same blood specimen for polyol determination. In most of the cases of congenital cataracts, however, no specific cause can be detected, although partial deficiency of maternal enzyme of galactose metabolism has been suggested to play a role in inexplicable congenital or infantile cataracts (Harley *et al.*, 1974; Winder *et al.*, 1983).

We present here our findings of elevated galactitol and sorbitol levels in plasma from a number of defined disorders in galactose metabolism as well as in cases with inexplicable congenital infantile cataracts. A preliminary report of this latter study has been published elsewhere (Jakobs *et al.*, 1988).

MATERIALS AND METHODS

Blood samples were received from several centres and enzyme activities in erythrocytes were determined according to the method of Shin *et al.* (1976, 1977, 1982 and 1984).

Plasma samples were frozen at $-20^{\circ}C$ prior to analysis. Galactitol and sorbitol in plasma samples were determined by a stable isotope dilution gas chromatographic–mass spectrometric assay (Jakobs *et al.*, 1984).

RESULTS AND DISCUSSION

Samples were received from numerous different centres and unfortunately were therefore not always accompanied by data on age, date of sampling and the status of the parents. In the cases with inexplicable congenital or infantile cataracts, little data were available on feeding habits at the time of sampling and the types of cataract.

Table 1 shows the plasma galactitol and sorbitol concentrations of patients with galactokinase, transferase and epimerase deficiency as well as those of a family with sorbitol dehydrogenase deficiency. Of the patients with transferase deficiency and cataract the highest values of galactitol (78.9–120 μmol/L) were found in the patients prior to treatment. On treatment, possibly started too late to obtain complete regression of the cataract, the concentrations were lower (12.9–19.8 μmol/L). However, even in patients without cataract the galactitol concentrations (7.15–18.8 μmol/L) were higher than normal on treatment. It is interesting to note that the heterozygous patient for the transferase deficiency with cataract had lower concentrations of galactitol than the treated homozygote patients who did not have cataracts. For kinase deficiency the trend is in general comparable with the transferase deficiency but the elevations of galactitol are less pronounced.

There is a clear difference between the plasma concentrations of galactitol in the systemic epimerase deficiency and the peripheral epimerase deficiency with cataract. Certainly the liver involvement in the case of systemic epimerase deficiency contributes

Table 1 Plasma galactitol and sorbitol concentrations in defined disorders

Disorder	*Galactitol* (μmol/L)			
	Homozygote		*Heterozygote*	
With (+) or without (−) cataract	+	−	+	−
Transferase deficiency	12.9–120 ($n = 9$)	7.15–18.8 ($n = 12$)	4.01 ($n = 1$)	0.09–0.43 ($n = 3$)
Kinase deficiency	27.5 ($n = 1$)	2.72–4.66 ($n = 3$)	1.26 ($n = 1$)	0.09 ($n = 1$)
Peripheral epimerase deficiency	1.10–3.43 ($n = 7$)	0.14–0.49 ($n = 6$)	1.92–6.90 ($n = 3$)	0.21–0.51 ($n = 3$)
Systemic epimerase deficiency*	99.1 ($n = 1$)			
	Sorbitol (μmol/L)			
Sorbitol dehydrogenase deficiency	5.58; 12.9 ($n = 2$)			

Controls ($n = 20$): galactitol = 0.08–0.86 μmol/L; sorbitol = 0.21–3.75 μmol/L
*The diagnosis was not confirmed by the analysis of liver or cultured fibroblasts

a great deal to the circulating galactitol. The galactitol concentrations in the patients with peripheral epimerase deficiency and cataract (homozygous as well as heterozygous) are only mildly elevated. However, they are higher than in the patients with this disorder without cataract who have absolutely normal concentrations. In the family (father and son) with sorbitol dehydrogenase deficiency (Shin *et al.*, 1984) relatively mild elevations of sorbitol level were found.

From the study of plasma galactitol and sorbitol concentrations in the defined disorders it can be concluded that the magnitude of elevation in the plasma is not always related to the presence or absence of cataract. In all patients with cataract, however, the plasma galactitol or sorbitol concentrations were elevated. The blood values do not necessarily reflect the situation in the lens but may in some cases give an indication that patients are at risk of developing a cataract. This is also true for the group of patients with inexplicable congenital or infantile cataracts (Jakobs *et al.*, 1988).

We investigated 82 patients (aged 1 week–2 years) with congenital or infantile cataract without other clinical abnormalities who had normal activity of transferase, epimerase and kinase, as well as of the sorbitol dehydrogenase. Out of these 82 patients we found 39 cases with mild to moderate elevations of galactitol or sorbitol concentration (Table 2). The concentrations of galactose-1-phosphate were not significantly elevated in the same blood samples. Urinary galactitol or sorbitol excretions have not been measured. The elevated galactitol concentrations were mostly in the same range as the levels in patients with peripheral epimerase deficiency with cataract or those with heterozygosity for the other disorders. The elevated levels of sorbitol in 11 cases were of the order of magnitude of the levels in both patients with sorbitol dehydrogenase deficiency.

Conflicting data have been reported on whether or not partial maternal deficiencies, particularly of galactokinase activity, can contribute to the formation of congenital cataracts in patients who are enzymatically normal (Harley *et al.*, 1974; Winder *et al.*, 1983; 1985; Brivet *et al.*, 1986). In these studies, however, no data on epimerase activity were available. Recent reports of variable forms of epimerase deficiency

Table 2 Plasma galactitol and sorbitol concentrations in 82 patients with cataract but no apparent enzyme defect

	Galactitol (μmol/L)	*Sorbitol* (μmol/ L)
43 Cases	Normal	Normal
2 Cases mother heterozygote peripheral epimerase deficiency	1.17; 1.23	Normal
1 Case mother heterozygote transferase deficiency	1.17	Normal
25 Cases	0.98–7.57	Normal
11 Cases	Normal	5.44–16.10
Controls (n = 20)	0.08–0.86	0.21–3.75

(Holton *et al.*, 1982; Shin *et al.*, 1984) indicate the importance of determination of this enzyme in cataract patients. In addition, none of the studies of inexplicable cataracts included the determination of galactitol concentrations in plasma. In our study we found the cataract and the elevated galactitol concentrations in plasma to coincide with heterozygosity of the mother in only three cases. In the other cases heterozygosity of the mother for these disorders as well as for the epimerase was ruled out. It appears that many infants with congenital cataracts do have increased blood galactitol which cannot be attributed to a known enzyme defect in these children or their mothers. Our finding could indicate a further cause for cataract formation due to a galactose or glucose (sorbitol) metabolic aberration.

The following possibilities are indicated:

(a) a variant form of a known enzyme defect eventually due to isoenzymes with different kinetic characteristics not measured in the *in vitro* assays;

(b) an individual fluctuation (increased activity) of the aldose reductase;

(c) other causes for galactose and glucose (sorbitol) intolerance;

(d) an isolated enzyme defect in the lens with secondary changes of plasma polyol concentrations.

Although further studies are necessary to elucidate the significance of our findings, we suggest that determination of galactitol and sorbitol in plasma may help in finding the cause of inexplicable congenital or infantile cataracts and consequently the possible therapy for these patients. Studies involving galactose loading tests and galactitol and sorbitol measurements in lenses, as well as the effect of dietary lactose-galactose restriction on prevention and regression of cataracts in these patients should be considered.

ACKNOWLEDGEMENT

Mr S. Persad, S. Langelaar and R.M. Kok are gratefully acknowledged for their excellent analytical support. This work is supported in part by Deutsche Forschungsgemeinschaft Grant Sh17/1–1.

REFERENCES

Brivet, M., Abadie, V., Soni, T., Cheron, G. and Dufier, J. L. Inexplicable infantile cataracts and partial maternal galactose disorder. *Arch. Dis. Child.* 61 (1986) 445–448

Harley, J. D., Mutton, P., Irvine, S. and Gupta, J. D. Maternal enzymes of galactose metabolism and the 'inexplicable' infantile cataract. *Lancet* 2 (1974) 259–261

Holton, J. B., Gillett, M. G., MacFaul, R. and Young, R. Galactosaemia: a new severe variant due to uridine diphosphate galactose-4-epimerase deficiency. *Arch. Dis. Child.* 56 (1981) 885–887

Jakobs, C., Warner, T. G., Sweetman, L. and Nyhan, W. L. Stable isotope dilution analysis of galactitol in amniotic fluid: an accurate approach to the prenatal diagnosis of galactosemia. *Pediatr. Res.* 18 (1984) 714–718

Jakobs, C., Douwes, A. C., Kok, R. M., De Jong, A., Endres, W. and Shin, Y. S. Elevated plasma galactitol levels in patients with congenital cataracts without enzyme defects. *Eur. J. Pediatr.* 147 (1988) 446

Shin, Y. S., Osang, M., Ziegler, R. and Schaub, J. A method for galactose-1-phosphate uridyltransferase assay and the separation of its isoenzymes by DEAE-cellulose column chromatography. *Clin. Chim. Acta* 70 (1976) 371–377

Shin, Y. S., Osang, M., Ziegler, R. and Schaub, J. A simple assay for galactokinase using DEAE-cellulose column chromatography. *Clin. Chim. Acta* 74 (1977) 1–5

Shin, Y. S., von Rucker, A., Rieth, M. and Endres, W. Assay of UDP-galactose-4-epimerase. *Clin. Chem.* 28 (1982) 2332–2333

Shin, Y. S., Rieth, M., Endres, W. and Haas, P. Sorbitol dehydrogenase deficiency in a family with congenital cataracts. *J. Inher. Metab. Dis.* 7 Suppl. 2 (1984) 151–152

Shin, Y. S., Endres, W., Rieth, M., Kruse, K. and Jakobs, C. Metabolite patterns and clinical expressions of uridine diphosphogalactose epimerase deficiency. *Pediatr. Res.* 19 (1985) 1075A

Stambolian, D. Galactose and cataract. *Survey Ophthalmol.* 32 (1988) 333–348

Vaca, G., Ibarra, B., Bracamontes, M., Garcia-Cruz, D., Sanchez-Corona, J., Medina, C., Wunsch, C., Gonzalez-Quiroga, G. and Cantu, J. M. Red blood cell sorbitol dehydrogenase deficiency in a family with cataracts. *Hum. Genet.* 61 (1982) 338–341

Winder, A. F., Claringbold, L. J., Jones, R. B., Jay, B. S., Rice, N. S. C., Kissun, R. D., Menzies, I. S. and Mount, J. N. Partial galactose disorders in families with premature cataracts. *Arch. Dis. Child.* 58 (1983) 362–366

Winder, A. F., Fielder, A. R., Mount, J. N. and Menzies, I. S. Direct and maternal aspects of the risk of cataract with partial disorders of galactose metabolism. *Clin. Genet.* 28 (1985) 199–206

J. Inher. Metab. Dis. 13 (1990) 523–537

Disorders of Glycoprotein Degradation

M. CANTZ and B. ULRICH-BOTT
Institute of Pathochemistry and General Neurochemistry, University of Heidelberg, Im Neuenheimer Feld 220/221, D-6900 Heidelberg, FRG

Summary: The intracellular degradation of glycoproteins occurs predominantly in the lysosomes through the concerted action of proteases and glycosidases. Genetic defects in any of the enzymes cleaving the oligosaccharide side chains lead to specific diseases because of an excessive lysosomal accumulation of partially degraded material, mostly oligosaccharides.

This paper presents an overview of the biochemistry and the clinical spectrum of this group of diseases including sialidosis, galactosialidosis, α- and β-mannosidosis, fucosidosis, aspartylglucosaminuria, and α-N-acetylgalactosaminidase deficiency (Schindler disease). In addition, the sialic acid storage disorder (Salla disease) which is caused by a defect in the lysosomal transport of this acidic monosaccharide is included because of functional and clinical correlations.

This article briefly reviews genetic defects in the lysosomal catabolism of glycoproteins. Clinically, the diseases resemble a milder form of a mucopolysaccharidosis and are inherited in an autosomal recessive fashion. They are mostly caused by the deficiency of a specific lysosomal hydrolase. Biochemistry and clinical features of this group of storage diseases have been delineated in greater detail elsewhere (Durand and O'Brien, 1982; Beaudet and Thomas, 1989).

Glycoproteins are important and ubiquitous constituents of cells, extracellular structures and fluids. They are made up of oligosaccharide chains which are covalently attached to a polypeptide backbone. Depending on the mode of biosynthesis, two main classes of glycoproteins can be differentiated (Berger *et al.*, 1982). In the group with so-called mucin-type sugar chains, the oligosaccharides are linked O-glycosidically to serine or threonine residues and are synthesized by the sequential addition of single sugars from sugar nucleotides. Examples of this type are shown in Figure 1; structure VII represents a blood group substance. The other class of glycoproteins is characterized by oligosaccharides which are linked N-glycosidically to asparagine residues. Here, the oligosaccharide chains are synthesized as lipid-linked intermediates before they are attached to the peptide backbone. Further trimming and elongation steps lead to final structures of the 'high mannose' or 'complex' types, examples of which are shown in Figure 2.

As cells and tissues turn over, their constituent glycoproteins, like other complex carbohydrates and lipids, are eventually degraded. This is accomplished in an intracellular digestive system, the lysosomes, by the combined action of hydrolytic

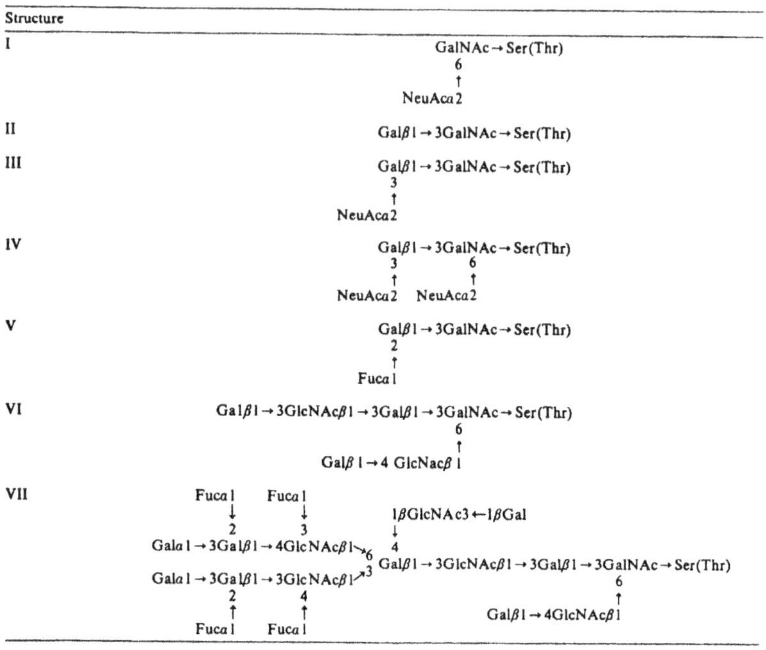

Figure 1 Examples of oligosaccharide chains linked O-glycosidically to serine or threonine residues. Modified from Berger *et al.* (1982).

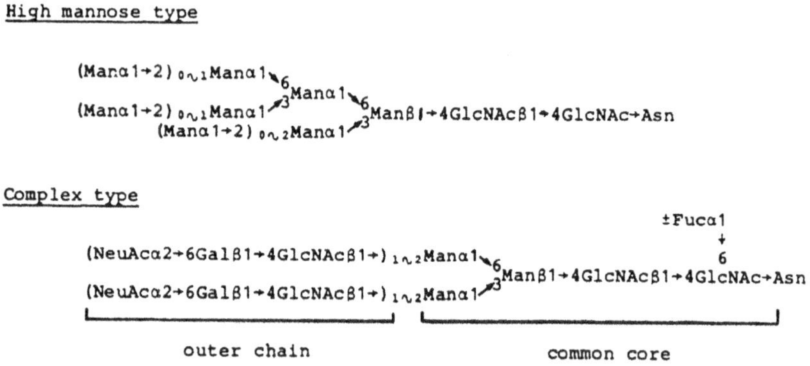

Figure 2 Oligosaccharide chains linked N-glycosidically to asparagine residues. Modified from Berger *et al.* (1982).

enzymes with an acidic pH optimum. The majority of the lysosomal enzymes are themselves glycoproteins which have been channelled to 'primary lysosomes' by means of a mannose-6-phosphate signal attached to them which is recognized by specific membrane receptors (von Figura and Hasilik, 1986).

The glycoproteins which are to be degraded may reach the lysosomes through endocytic or autophagic processes, thereby forming 'secondary lysosomes'. The protein portion is degraded by a number of proteases. The oligosaccharide chains are cleaved by specific glycosidases such as sialidase (α-neuraminidase), β-galactosidase, β-N-acetylhexosaminidase, α-mannosidase, β-mannosidase, α-fucosidase, and α-N-acetylgalactosaminidase. These are exo-enzymes which can only act on the respective residue if it is exposed at the non-reducing end of the chain. The N-glycosidic linkage between N-acetylglucosamine and asparagine is hydrolysed by a specific aspartylglycosaminidase. After some initial uncertainty, there is now good evidence for the existence of lysosomal endo-β-N-acetylglucosaminidases which hydrolyse the chitobiosyl linkage between the two GlcNAc residues of asparagine-linked oligosaccharides (Kuranda and Aronson, 1985; De Gasperi *et al.*, 1989). The final products of glycoprotein degradation are amino acids and monosaccharides which are released from the lysosome for further utilization. Recent work has shown that this release occurs not via simple diffusion but may involve specific transport mechanisms.

A genetic mutation leading to a functional deficit in any of the enzymes or proteins required for glycoprotein catabolism will prevent further breakdown, with lysosomal accumulation of partially degraded material (Figure 3). The resulting clinical symptoms develop progressively and range from coarse facial features, bone changes and organomegaly to neurological problems and psychomotor retardation. A list of the diseases known so far is presented in Table 1. It contains disorders where the accumulation of oligosaccharides and glycopeptides appears to be the predominant pathogenetic mechanism and which have therefore sometimes been called 'oligosaccharidoses'; diseases such as GM1 or GM2 gangliosidoses, where the oligosaccharide storage is but a minor feature of the much more prominent glycolipid storage, are not included. The major clinical features of the disorders of glycoprotein degradation are summarized in Table 2.

ASPARTYLGLUCOSAMINURIA

In 1968, Pollitt and colleagues in England first described aspartylglucosaminuria (McKusick 20840) in two siblings who had severe mental retardation. There was an abnormal urinary excretion of aspartylglucosamine, 2-acetamido-1-(β-L-aspartamido)-1,2-dideoxyglucose, which could be explained on the basis of a deficiency of the enzyme aspartylglycosaminidase (EC 3.5.1.26).

More than 100 patients have been described so far, most of them in Finland. The clinical course is fairly uniform in most patients (Aula *et al.*, 1982). After normal development during the first months of life, there may be frequent upper respiratory tract infections and the appearance of herniae. After about one year of age, clumsiness,

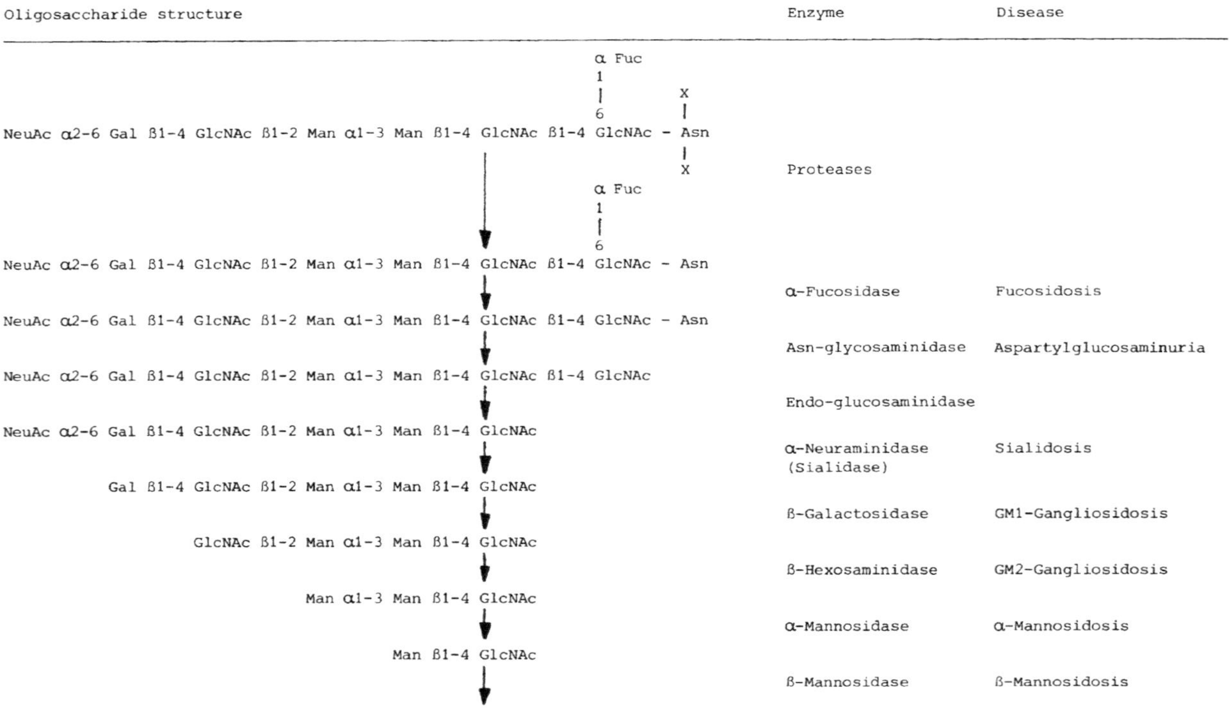

Figure 3 Scheme of genetic defects in the lysosomal degradation of the glycan portion of glycoproteins: (a) 'Complex' type oligosaccharide chains.

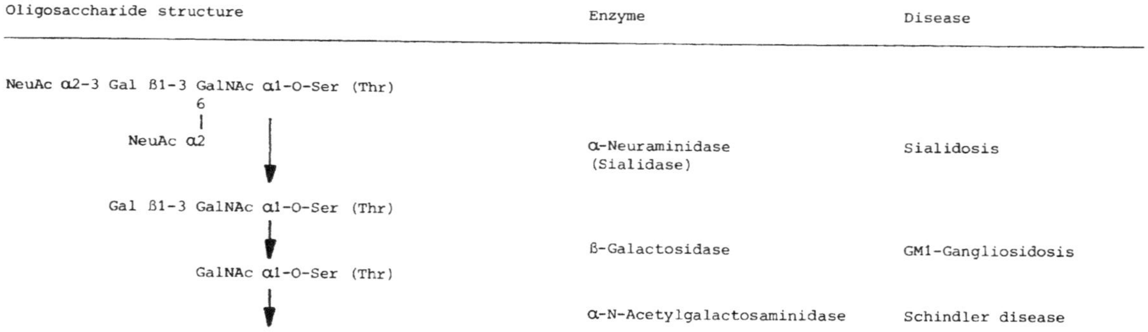

Figure 3 *continued* (b) O-glycosidically linked oligosaccharide chains.

Table 1 Disorders of glycoprotein degradation

Disease	*Biochemical defect*	*Chromosomal location*[a]
Aspartylglucosaminuria	Aspartylglycosaminidase deficiency	4q21-ter
Fucosidosis	α-Fucosidase deficiency	1p34
α-Mannosidosis	α-Mannosidase deficiency	19p13.2-q12
β-Mannosidosis	β-Mannosidase deficiency	
Sialidosis	α-Neuraminidase (sialidase) deficiency	10pter-q23
Galactosialidosis	Combined α-neuraminidase/β-galactosidase deficiency due to 'protective protein' defect	20
Schindler disease	α-N-Acetylgalactosaminidase deficiency	22q11
Sialic acid storage disease (Salla disease)	Defective lysosomal transport of sialic acid	

[a] Reviewed in Beaudet and Thomas, 1989

muscular hypotonia and slight mental retardation may develop. By about 10 years, there are coarse facial features, moderate to severe mental retardation, increased clumsiness, excitable behaviour and skeletal dysplasia. The disease progresses with impairment of speech and of motor functions and often leads to death in the third or fourth decade.

Electron microscopic investigations of biopsy or autopsy material showed the presence of enlarged lysosomes in all organs studied. The storage lysosomes usually contained amorphous fibrillogranular material on a clear background (Aula *et al.*, 1982). Storage phenomena were also observed upon light microscopy, e.g. there was abnormal vacuolation of lymphocytes in blood smears.

Biochemical studies on the nature of the storage material in tissues showed that it consisted mainly of aspartylglucosamine, with minor contributions from other glycoasparagines (Aula *et al.*, 1982). Such compounds are formed in the course of glycoprotein catabolism and are normally cleaved to asparagine and N-acetylglucosamine before being released from the lysosome. As uncleaved aspartylglucosamine is unable to pass through the lysosomal membrane, it accumulates in the absence of sufficient aspartylglycosaminidase activity.

The biochemical diagnosis of aspartylglucosaminuria is made by the demonstration of an increased excretion of aspartylglucosamine in the urine, e.g. on a thin layer chromatogram, and of a deficient aspartylglycosaminidase activity in plasma, leukocytes, lymphocytes or cultured fibroblasts; prenatal diagnosis and carrier detection are also possible by use of the enzyme assay (Aula *et al.*, 1982).

FUCOSIDOSIS

Fucosidosis (McKusick 23000) was first recognized as a disease entity by Durand and colleagues in 1966. Ultrastructural and biochemical studies then led to the elucidation of the basic metabolic defect (Durand *et al.*, 1982). The deficiency of the lysosomal α-fucosidase (EC 3.2.1.51) leads to the intracellular accumulation of fucose-containing oligosaccharides and glycolipids in most of the patients' tissues.

Table 2 Major clinical findings in disorders of glycoprotein degradation

	Age of onset	*Psychomotor retardation*	*Coarse facies*	*Dysostosis multiplex*	*Eye findings*	*Neurological*	*Other*
Aspartylglucosaminuria	1–5 y	++	+	+	Lens opacities	Clumsiness, muscular hypotonia	Excitable behaviour
Fucosidosis							
Type I	5–12 mon	+++	(+)	(+)	—	Muscle spasticity, seizures	
Type II	1–2 y	++	+	+	Vascular abnormalities	Ataxia, spasticity, seizures	Angiokeratoma
α-Mannosidosis	1–2 y	+	+	+	Cataracts, corneal opacities	Ataxia	Hearing loss, frequent infections
β-Mannosidosis	1–2 y	+	(+)	(+)	—	Hypotonia	Angiokeratoma, hearing loss, infections
Sialidosis							
Type I	8–25 y	(+)	(+)	(+)	Cherry-red spots	Myoclonus, seizures, ataxia	Occasionally renal disease
Type II	0–10 mon	+	+	+	Cherry-red spots	Seizures, myoclonus	Occasionally hydrops fetalis
Galactosialidosis	0–6 y	+	+	+	Cherry-red spots, corneal clouding	Ataxia, myoclonus	Angiokeratoma
Sialic acid storage disease (Salla disease) (possibly different types)	0–1 y	++	+	+	—	Ataxia, spasticity	Organomegaly, occasionally hydrops fetalis
Schindler disease	8 mon	+++	–	–	Blindness	Seizures, spasticity, myoclonus	Neuroaxonal dystrophy

There is considerable clinical heterogeneity in fucosidosis which has led to the delineation of two disease types (Durand *et al.*, 1982). Type I, the more severe one, usually begins during the first year of life with repeated respiratory infections, feeding difficulties, muscular hypotonia and failure to thrive. Thereafter, there is progressive psychomotor retardation ending in dementia and a vegetative state. There may be slight coarsening of the face and sometimes bony changes. The patients usually die from pneumonia before the age of six. Fucosidosis type II is less severe, beginning after the first year of life with walking difficulties, ataxia, emotional disturbances, and general psychomotor retardation. After three or four years, the patients develop the characteristic angiokeratoma corporis diffusum on the scrotum, the extremities, the abdomen, and the back, and there is hypohidrosis or anhidrosis. In addition, there is growth retardation and skeletal dysplasia. The progression of the clinical course is much slower than in type I, and survival to adulthood is possible.

Ultrastructural studies in a variety of tissues revealed the presence of typical storage lysosomes containing material suggestive of oligosaccharides, glycoproteins, and glycolipids; the nature of the storage material was subsequently identified and found to be fucose-containing oligosaccharides and glycolipids (Durand *et al.*, 1982).

A profound deficiency of α-fucosidase can be detected in all tissues of the patients. Recently, evidence for molecular heterogeneity among patients with fucosidosis has been presented. Thus, while fibroblasts from one group of patients had no detectable fucosidase enzyme protein, the cells from another group synthesized the 53 kDa enzyme precursor but had no mature 50 kDa enzyme, while another patient had small amounts of cross-reacting material in his cells (Johnson and Dawson, 1985).

For diagnostic purposes, cultured skin fibroblasts, leukocytes or lymphocytes are suitable sources for fucosidase determinations. Serum or plasma are not adequate because there are individuals with very low serum α-fucosidase who do not have fucosidosis (Beaudet and Thomas, 1989). Thin layer chromatography of urine samples can demonstrate an abnormal excretion of oligosaccharides, but may occasionally be negative.

α-MANNOSIDOSIS AND β-MANNOSIDOSIS

In 1967, Öckerman in Sweden described a patient with a generalized storage disorder resembling a mucopolysaccharidosis but without mucopolysacchariduria (Öckerman, 1967). There was a severe deficiency of an α-mannosidase (EC 3.2.1.24) in the patient's tissues leading to the lysosomal storage and urinary excretion of mannose-containing oligosaccharides. Since then, many more patients with α-mannosidosis (McKusick 24850) have been detected in different parts of the world.

As in other lysosomal storage disorders, the severity of the disease may vary considerably (Chester *et al.*, 1982; Beaudet and Thomas, 1989), but it is at present not clear if a distinction of different forms is justified. Early non-specific symptoms are frequent respiratory and ear infections. Between 1 and 4 years, delayed mental and motor functions become apparent and progressive ataxia and clumsiness are noted. In most patients there are coarse facial features and skeletal dysplasia, and hepatosplenomegaly is frequent. A sensorineural hearing loss is often observed and is a characteristic sign.

The oligosaccharides accumulating in the patients' tissues were found to be of different size, but all had α-glycosidically linked mannose residues on their non-reducing ends and structures compatible with fragments of high-mannose type oligosaccharide chains of glycoproteins (Chester *et al.*, 1982). The α-mannosidase involved is a lysosomal enzyme with an acidic pH optimum; other α-mannosidases with different subcellular localization (cytoplasm, Golgi) and properties are of normal activity in the patients (Chester *et al.*, 1982).

Besides human α-mannosidosis, there are genetic animal models in Angus cattle and in a domestic cat (Beaudet and Thomas, 1989).

In 1986, Wenger and colleagues and Cooper and colleagues (see also the contribution of Cooper *et al.* on pages 538–548) independently described patients with marked deficiencies of β-mannosidase (EC 3.2.1.25) activity and increased urinary excretion of the disaccharide Man-β-GlcNAc. The patient of Wenger and colleagues also had a low level of heparan sulphamidase (EC 3.10.1.1) activity and an increased urinary excretion of heparan sulphate. An additional two brothers with β-mannosidosis were recently reported by Dorland *et al.* (1988). All of the patients showed psychomotor retardation and frequent infections; in some, there were hearing problems or angiokeratoma. In the patient of Wenger and colleagues, there were additional dysmorphic features but the relationship, if any, between the two enzyme deficiencies is unclear.

Before it was described in humans, β-mannosidosis was discovered in goats, where the disease is fatal and involves demyelination (Jones and Dawson, 1981).

SIALIDOSIS, GALACTOSIALIDOSIS AND SIALIC ACID STORAGE DISEASE (SALLA DISEASE)

Sialidosis (McKusick 25655) and galactosialidosis (McKusick 25654) have in common a defect in the catabolism of sialic acid-containing glycoconjugates, whereas sialic acid storage disease (McKusick 26874 and 26992) is a disorder of the lysosomal transport of free sialic acid.

The biochemical defect which is characteristic of sialidosis was elucidated in 1977 in two groups of patients. Cantz and colleagues (1977) demonstrated an increased accumulation of sialic acid-containing compounds and a profound deficiency of an 'acid' α-neuraminidase (sialidase EC 3.2.1.18) in cultured fibroblasts of a mentally retarded, dysmorphic boy who had previously been classified as having mucolipidosis I. Deficiency of α-neuraminidase was also observed in an infant with Hurler-like somatic features but normal mental development by Kelly and Graetz (1977). Another group of young adults with normal intelligence and skeletal system, but with impaired vision, cherry-red macular spots and muscle cramps who had been classified as cherry-red spot-myoclonus syndrome (Durand *et al.*, 1977; O'Brien, 1977; Thomas *et al.*, 1978; Rapin *et al.*, 1978) had been found to have an increased urinary excretion of sialyloligosaccharides and a deficiency of α-neuraminidase. Sialidosis has therefore been subdivided into two types: a normosomatic one, and a dysmorphic one which is clinically more severe (Lowden and O'Brien, 1979).

Sialidosis type I presents between 8 and 25 years with decreasing visual acuity and/or myoclonus. The patients are usually of normal intellect and have normal somatic features. Cherry-red spots are observed in the macular region of the fundi of both eyes. The myoclonus is progressive and may become debilitating, and seizures are frequent; some patients have severe renal disease (Lowden and O'Brien, 1979; O'Brien, 1982; Harzer *et al.*, 1986).

Patients with type II sialidosis show a more variable spectrum of symptoms. In some, the disease is congenital and presents with hydrops fetalis and ascites. Other patients appear normal at birth, first symptoms being noted in infancy or even later. All patients have coarse facial features and skeletal dysplasia and there is organomegaly and mental retardation. Myoclonus and cherry-red spots become evident when the children are older.

In the patients' urine there is a massive excretion of a great number of sialyloligosaccharides, the structures of which have been elucidated (Strecker *et al.*, 1977; van Pelt *et al.*, 1988a) and which are derived from N-linked as well as O-glycosidically linked oligosaccharide chains of glycoproteins. Such sialyloligosaccharides undoubtedly represent the material stored intralysosomally in the tissues and have been identified in cultured fibroblasts of a sialidosis patient (van Pelt, 1988b). Occasionally there are adult patients with residual sialidase activity where the urinary oligosaccharide excretion is normal (Harzer *et al.*, 1986).

As part of the sialyloligosaccharide structures is identical to structures of parts of a number of gangliosides, there was the question of an additional ganglioside storage in the patients. Early studies in sialidosis fibroblasts on the sialidase activity towards suitable ganglioside substrates showed nearly normal values, indicating the ganglioside sialidase to be a genetically separate enzyme (Cantz and Messer, 1979). Ganglioside analyses of brain tissue from sialidosis patients gave no abnormal results either (O'Brien, 1982). It was therefore surprising to find a marked elevation of gangliosides GM4, GM3 and GM2 in visceral organs obtained at autopsy from such a patient (Ulrich-Bott *et al.*, 1987); in the brain, however, there was again a normal level. Further work on the ganglioside sialidase activity of cultured fibroblasts then yielded evidence for two separate activities: a Triton X-100-stimulated enzyme which was situated on the plasma membrane and was active in sialidosis, and a cholate-activated enzyme which was localized in lysosomes and was deficient in sialidosis cells (Lieser *et al.*, 1989). Taken together, these findings indicate that in sialidosis there is a catabolic derangement of both classes of compounds, sialyloligosaccharides and gangliosides.

The biochemical diagnosis of sialidosis is based on the demonstration of an isolated sialidase deficiency in cultured fibroblasts or lymphocytes; leukocytes should not be used as there may be interference from another sialidase (Beaudet and Thomas, 1989). β-Galactosidase activity is normal or sometimes slightly decreased. In cultured fibroblasts, increased levels of 'bound' sialic acid are demonstrable. The excessive excretion of oligosaccharides in the urine can be detected by thin layer chromatography or colorimetric determination. Occasionally, there are adult patients with residual sialidase activity in whom there is no abnormal sialyloligosacchariduria (Harzer *et al.*, 1986).

Galactosialidosis was recognized as a distinct entity only recently. Clinically, it resembles a sialidosis (O'Brien, 1989). There is, however, a combined deficiency of lysosomal sialidase (α-neuraminidase) and β-galactosidase (EC 3.2.1.23) which, according to the eminent studies of Galjaard and colleagues, is due to the primary genetic defect of a 'protective protein' (D'Azzo *et al.*, 1982). This protein is needed for sialidase activity and the protection of β-galactosidase from inactivation and is closely associated with both enzymes in a complex (Galjaard *et al.*, 1987). As the amino acid sequence of the protein bears homology to yeast proteases, it may function as a processing enzyme for sialidase and β-galactosidase (Galjart *et al.*, 1988).

In the patients' urine and cells there are excessive amounts of sialyloligosaccharides of the same structures as in sialidosis (van Pelt *et al.*, 1988b). The final diagnosis is based on the demonstration of a simultaneous and profound deficiency of lysosomal sialidase and β-galactosidase activities in cultured fibroblasts.

Sialic acid storage disease was first described by Aula *et al.* (1979) in patients with severe psychomotor retardation. The disorder was named Salla disease after the area of Finland from which the patients originated. After this first report, many more patients were discovered, most of them Finnish. The patients accumulate in their tissues and excrete in the urine excessive amounts of free N-acetylneuraminic acid (sialic acid). Clinically, the disease is variable and ranges from severely affected newborns with ascites, hepatosplenomegaly and coarse facial features, recurrent infections and early death to intermediate or milder forms with psychomotor retardation, skeletal dysplasia, seizures and ataxia; patients with the Finnish form (Salla disease) generally reach a normal life span (Gahl *et al.*, 1989).

Recent work on the biochemistry of this disease suggested that the intralysosomal storage of free sialic acid was due to a defective transport through the lysosomal membrane (reviewed in Gahl *et al.*, 1989). Thus, it became clear that the sialic acid which was liberated from glycoproteins and glycolipids by the sialidase could not simply diffuse out of the lysosome but needed some sort of a carrier mechanism. Indeed, when cultured fibroblasts from sialic acid storage disease patients were allowed to incorporate the glycoprotein fetuin which was radioactively labelled in its sialic acid residues, there was an intralysosomal accumulation of radioactive free sialic acid which was much higher than in control cells (Mendla *et al.*, 1988); interestingly, there was also an abnormal accumulation of sialyloligosaccharides which was interpreted as being caused by partial inhibition of the sialidase by sialic acid, a known competitive inhibitor. Increased amounts of 'bound' in addition to free sialic acid had indeed been found in tissues of a sialic acid storage disease patient (Baumkötter *et al.*, 1985), suggesting that storage of such compounds besides sialic acid may contribute to the pathogenesis of the disorder.

The biochemical diagnosis of sialic acid storage disease is made by the demonstration of increased amounts of free sialic acid in cultured fibroblasts and in the urine. Additionally, more detailed studies regarding the lysosomal transport of sialic acid may be considered to differentiate the disease from patients with sialuria (McKusick 26992), where there is no concomitant lysosomal storage of sialic acid (Gahl *et al.*, 1989). A prenatal diagnosis of an affected fetus with sialic acid storage disease has been accomplished by the use of such methods (Vamos *et al.*, 1986).

SCHINDLER DISEASE: α-N-ACETYLGALACTOSAMINIDASE DEFICIENCY (McKUSICK 10417)

Recently, van Diggelen and colleagues (1988) and Schindler and colleagues (1989) described two German brothers with progressive psychomotor deterioration, bilateral pyramidal tract signs, hypotonia, marked visual impairment and neuropathological changes characteristic of patients with neuroaxonal dystrophy (see also the article by Desnick and Wang on pages 549–559). In their urine, they excreted abnormal glycopeptides as detected by thin layer chromatography. A structural analysis of some of the major ones revealed the presence of the blood group A trisaccharide as well as several O-linked glycopeptides. Besides GalNAc α1-O-serine or threonine, there were GalNAc-containing sialoglycopeptides, which also accumulate in sialidosis. In the patients' cells and plasma there was a virtually complete deficiency of α-N-acetylgalactosaminidase (EC 3.2.1.49) activity, whereas the parents showed intermediate values suggestive of heterozygosity. Further studies showed that no immunologically detectable enzyme protein was present in cell extracts of both patients, suggesting that the mutation resides in the gene coding for α-N-acetylgalactosaminidase (Schindler *et al.*, 1989).

CONCLUSION

All but one of the diseases discussed in this article have in common a primary genetic defect in the lysosomal degradation of the glycan portion of glycoproteins, with subsequent abnormal oligosaccharide or glycopeptide storage. An exception is sialic acid storage disease, where one of the end products of glycoprotein catabolism, i.e. free sialic acid, accumulates due to a block in a carrier system in the lysosomal membrane. It is possible that the greatly increased lysosomal sialic acid concentration in this disease leads to secondary storage of sialoglycoconjugates, as sialic acid is an inhibitor of the lysosomal sialidase.

In some disorders there is not only an accumulation of oligosaccharides but also of glycolipids. This is found in fucosidosis and sialidosis and is due to the fact that the deficient glycosidases are specific not only for oligosaccharides but also for glycolipids with the same kind of sugar linkage. It is perhaps for this reason that these diseases are among the most severe of the whole group.

As in other lysosomal diseases, the clinical spectrum of each of the disorders of glycoprotein degradation may vary greatly. In some cases this has been correlated with the amount of residual enzyme activity present in the tissues. The existence of adult forms in most of the diseases necessitates appropriate diagnostic considerations which have not been customarily applied to this group of patients.

In all of the disorders, prenatal diagnosis is theoretically feasible and has been performed in most of them using amniotic fluid, cultured amniotic cells, or chorionic villi (Beaudet and Thomas, 1989; Gahl *et al.*, 1989; O'Brien, 1989).

Attempts at therapy by way of enzyme replacement have been made, but have remained largely experimental. Before such treatment may eventually become generally available through bone marrow transplantation or gene therapy, quite a number of problems need to be solved. Several animal models exist which are of great importance for the development of successful therapeutic strategies.

ACKNOWLEDGEMENT

We thank Miss Evelyn Becker for the preparation of the manuscript.

REFERENCES

Aula, P., Autio, S., Raivio, K. O., Rapola, J., Thoden, C.-J., Koskela, S.-L. and Yamashina, J. 'Salla disease', a new lysosomal storage disorder. *Arch. Neurol.* 36 (1979) 88–94

Aula, P., Autio, S., Raivio, K. O. and Rapola, J. Aspartylglucosaminuria. In Durand, P. and O'Brien, J. S. (eds.), *Genetic Errors of Glycoprotein Metabolism*, edi ermes, Milano, Springer-Verlag, Berlin, Heidelberg, New York, 1982, pp. 123–152

Baumkötter, J., Cantz, M., Mendla, K., Baumann, W., Friebolin, H., Gehler, J. and Spranger, J. N-Acetylneuraminic acid storage disease. *Hum. Genet.* 71 (1985) 155–159

Beaudet, A. L. and Thomas, G. H. Disorders of glycoprotein degradation: mannosidosis, fucosidosis, sialidosis, and aspartylglycosaminuria. In Scriver, C. R., Beaudet, A. L., Sly, W. S. and Valle, D. (eds.), *The Metabolic Basis of Inherited Disease*, 6th edn., McGraw-Hill, New York, 1989, pp. 1603–1621

Berger, E. G., Buddecke, E., Kamerling, J. P., Kobata, A., Paulson, J. C. and Vliegenthart, J. F. G. Structure, biosynthesis and functions of glycoprotein glycans. *Experientia* 38 (1982) 1129–1258

Cantz, M. and Messer, H. Oligosaccharide and ganglioside neuraminidase activities of mucolipidosis I (sialidosis) and mucolipidosis II (I-cell disease) fibroblasts. *Eur. J. Biochem.* 97 (1979) 113–118

Cantz, M., Gehler, J. and Spranger, J. Mucolipidosis I: increased sialic acid content and deficiency of an α-N-acetylneuraminidase in cultured fibroblasts. *Biochem. Biophys. Res. Commun.* 74 (1977) 732–738

Chester, M. A., Lundblad, A., Öckerman, P. A. and Autio, S. Mannosidosis. In Durand, P. and O'Brien, J. S. (eds.), *Genetic Errors of Glycoprotein Metabolism*, edi ermes, Milano, Springer-Verlag, Berlin, Heidelberg, New York, 1982, pp. 89–122

Cooper, A., Sardharwalla, I. B. and Roberts, M. M. Human β-mannosidase deficiency. *N. Engl. J. Med.* 315 (1986) 1231

D'Azzo, A., Hoogeveen, A., Reuser, A. J. J., Robinson, D. and Galjaard, H. Molecular defect in combined β-galactosidase and neuraminidase deficiency in man. *Proc. Natl. Acad. Sci. USA* 79 (1982) 4535–4539

De Gasperi, R., Li, Y.-T. and Li, S.-C. Presence of two endo-β-N-acetylglucosaminidases in human kidney. *J. Biol. Chem.* 264 (1989) 9329–9334

Dorland, L., Duran, M., Hoefnagels, F. E. T., Breg, J. N., Fabery de Jonge, H., Cransberg, K., van Sprang, F. J. and van Diggelen, O. P. β-Mannosidosis in two brothers with hearing loss. *J. Inher. Metab. Dis.* 11, Suppl. 2 (1988) 255–258

Durand, P. and O'Brien, J. S. (eds.), *Genetic Errors of Glycoprotein Metabolism*, edi ermes, Milano, Springer-Verlag, Berlin, Heidelberg, New York, 1982

Durand, P., Gatti, R., Cavalieri, S., Borrone, C., Tondeur, M., Michalski, J.-C. and Strecker, G. Sialidosis (mucolipidosis I). *Helv. Paediatr. Acta* 32 (1977) 391–400

Durand, P., Gatti, R. and Borrone, C. Fucosidosis. In Durand, P. and O'Brien, J. S. (eds.), *Genetic Errors of Glycoprotein Metabolism*, edi ermes, Milano, Springer-Verlag, Berlin, Heidelberg, New York, 1982, pp. 49–87

Gahl, W. A., Renlund, M. and Thoene, J. G. Lysosomal transport disorders: Cystinosis and sialic acid storage disorders. In Scriver, C. R., Beaudet, A. L., Sly, W. S. and Valle, D. (eds.), *The Metabolic Basis of Inherited Disease*, 6th edn., McGraw-Hill, New York, 1989, pp. 2619–2647

Galjaard, H., Willemsen, R., Hogeveen, A. T., Mancini, G. M. S., Palmeri, S., Verheijen, F. W. and D'Azzo, A. Molecular heterogeneity in human β-galactosidase and neuraminidase deficiency. *Enzyme* 38 (1987) 132–143

Galjart, N. J., Gillemans, N., Harris, A., van der Horst, G. T. J., Verheijen, F. W., Galjaard, H. and D'Azzo, A. Expression of cDNA encoding the human 'protective protein' associated with lysosomal β-galactosidase and neuraminidase: homology to yeast proteases. *Cell* 54 (1988) 755–764

Harzer, K., Cantz, M., Sewell, A. C., Dhareshwar, S. S., Roggendorf, W., Heckl, R. W., Schofer, O., Thumler, R., Peiffer, J. and Schlote, W. Normomorphic sialidosis in two female adults with severe neurologic disease and without sialyl oligosacchariduria. *Hum. Genet.* 74 (1986) 209–214

Johnson, K. and Dawson, G. Molecular defect in processing α-fucosidase in fucosidosis. *Biochem. Biophys. Res. Commun.* 133 (1985) 90

Jones, M. Z. and Dawson, G. Caprine β-mannosidosis. Inherited deficiency of β-D-mannosidase. *J. Biol. Chem.* 256 (1981) 5185–5188

Kelly, T. E. and Graetz, G. Isolated acid neuraminidase deficiency: a distinct lysosomal storage disease. *Am. J. Med. Genet.* 1 (1977) 31–46

Kuranda, M. J. and Aronson, N. N. Use of active site-directed inhibitors to study *in situ* degradation of glycoproteins by the perfused rat liver. *J. Biol. Chem.* 260 (1985) 1856–1866

Lieser, M., Harms, E., Kern, H., Bach, G. and Cantz, M. Ganglioside GM3 sialidase activity in fibroblasts of normal individuals and of patients with sialidosis and mucolipidosis IV. Subcellular distribution and some properties. *Biochem. J.* 260 (1989) 69–74

Lowden, J. A. and O'Brien, J. S. Sialidosis: A review of human neuraminidase deficiency. *Am. J. Hum. Genet.* 31 (1979) 1–18

Mendla, K., Baumkötter, J., Rosenau, C., Ulrich-Bott, B. and Cantz, M. Defective lysosomal release of glycoprotein-derived sialic acid in fibroblasts from patients with sialic acid storage disease. *Biochem. J.* 250 (1988) 261–267

O'Brien, J. S. Neuraminidase deficiency in the cherry-red spot-myoclonus syndrome. *Biochem. Biophys. Res. Commun.* 79 (1977) 1163–1241

O'Brien, J. S. Sialidosis. In Durand, P. and O'Brien, J. S. (eds.), *Genetic Errors of Glycoprotein Metabolism*, edi ermes, Milano, Springer-Verlag, Berlin, Heidelberg, New York, 1982, pp. 33–48

O'Brien, J. S. β-Galactosidase deficiency (GM1 gangliosidosis, galactosialidosis, and Morquio syndrome type B); ganglioside sialidase deficiency (mucolipidosis IV). In Scriver, C. R., Beaudet, A. L., Sly, W. S. and Valle, D. (eds.), *The Metabolic Basis of Inherited Disease*, 6th edn., McGraw-Hill, New York, 1989, pp. 1797–1806

Öckerman, P.-A. A generalized storage disorder resembling Hurler's syndrome. *Lancet* 2 (1967) 239–241

Pollitt, R. J., Jenner, F. A. and Merskey, H. Aspartylglycosaminuria: an inborn error of metabolism associated with mental defect. *Lancet* 2 (1968) 253

Rapin, I., Goldfischer, S., Katzman, R., Engel, J. and O'Brien, J. S. The cherry-red spot-myoclonus syndrome. *Ann. Neurol.* 3 (1978) 234–242

Schindler, D., Bishop, D. F., Wolfe, D. E., Wang, A. M., Egge, H., Lemieux, R. U. and Desnick, R. J. Neuroaxonal dystrophy due to lysosomal α-N-acetylgalactosaminidase deficiency. *N. Engl. J. Med.* 320 (1989) 1735–1740

Strecker, G., Peers, M. C., Michalski, J. C., Hondi-Assah, T., Fournet, B., Spik, G., Montreuil, J., Farriaux, J. P., Marteaux, P. and Duran, P. Structure of nine sialyloligosaccharides accumulated in nine of eleven patients with three different types of sialidosis. *Eur. J. Biochem.* 75 (1977) 391–398

Thomas, G. H., Tipton, R. E., Chien, L. T., Reynolds, L. W. and Miller, C. S. Sialidase (α-N-acetylneuraminidase) deficiency: the enzyme defect in an adult with macular cherry-red spots and myoclonus without dementia. *Clin. Genet.* 13 (1978) 369–379

Ulrich-Bott, B., Klem, B., Kaiser, R., Spranger, J. and Cantz, M. Lysosomal sialidase deficiency: increased ganglioside content in autopsy tissues of a sialidosis patient. *Enzyme* 38 (1987) 262–266

Vamos, E., Libert, J., Elkhazen, N., Jauniaux, E., Hustin, J., Wilkin, P., Baumkötter, J., Mendla, K. and Cantz, M. Prenatal diagnosis and confirmation of infantile sialic acid storage disease. *Prenat. Diagn.* 6 (1986) 437–446

van Diggelen, O. P., Schindler, D., Willemsen, R., Boer, M., Kleijer, W. J., Huijmans, G. M., Blom, W. and Galjaard, H. α-N-acetylgalactosaminidase deficiency, a new lysosomal storage disorder. *J. Inher. Metab. Dis.* 11 (1988) 349–357

J. Inher. Metab. Dis. 13 (1990) 538–548

α- and β-Mannosidoses

A. Cooper, C. E. Hatton, M. Thornley and I. B. Sardharwalla
Willink Biochemical Genetics Unit, Royal Manchester Children's Hospital, Pendlebury, Manchester M27 1HA, UK

Summary: Clinical, pathological and biochemical findings in the mannosidoses are described. Family studies showed granulocyte-rich white cell fractions to be the tissue of choice for carrier detection in β-mannosidosis. Metabolic labelling studies using [^{3}H] mannose demonstrated accumulation of Manβ1-4GlcNAc in cultured skin fibroblasts from a patient with this condition. Alternative methods of egress from lysosomes were suggested for this compound by its secretion into culture medium and apparent reduction of storage with time in cultures. β-mannosidase deficient goats are not thought to be a true animal model of the human condition, as although they showed a similar enzyme deficiency, the clinical presentation is much more severe and the major storage material (Manβ1-4GlcNAcβ1-4GlcNAc) is different.

Defective lysosomal catabolism of glycopeptides has been widely described (Beaudet and Thomas, 1989). Deficiencies of lysosomal enzymes lead to accumulation of undegraded storage products. The mannosidoses are two such diseases due to deficiencies of α-mannosidase (EC 3.2.1.24) and β-mannosidase (EC 3.2.1.25). In α-mannosidosis, oligosaccharides containing α1-3 and α1-6 linkages accumulate (Strecker *et al.*, 1976; Yamashita *et al.*, 1979), whereas in human β-mannosidosis the major storage material is a disaccharide, Manβ1-4GlcNAc (Cooper *et al.*, 1988; Dorland *et al.*, 1988b). α-Mannosidosis is the more severe disorder (Beaudet and Thomas, 1989), with symptoms resembling the mucopolysaccharidoses, whilst in β-mannosidosis the major findings are mental retardation, deafness, and in older patients, angiokeratoma (Cooper *et al.*, 1986; Dorland *et al.*, 1988a). Pathological findings in both conditions include cytoplasmic vacuolation due to lysosomal storage (Kjellman *et al.*, 1969; Sung *et al.*, 1977; Cooper, unpublished observation). Animal models are known for both conditions. Bovine α-mannosidosis resembles the human disorder (Whittem and Walker, 1957; Jolly and Thompson, 1978) but caprine β-mannosidosis (Jones *et al.*, 1983) is more severe. Results of family studies and metabolic labelling experiments will be described for β-mannosidosis and the differences between the human condition and the animal analogue will be discussed.

Materials and methods

White cells and plasma were prepared and skin fibroblasts cultured as previously described (Cooper *et al.*, 1987; Cooper *et al.*, 1988). Bio-Gel P-2 chromatography, oligosaccharide TLC and mannosidase assays were accomplished as reported (Cooper *et al.*, 1988). Lymphocyte-rich and granulocyte-rich fractions were isolated from heparanized blood by centrifugation on Histopaque (Sigma). Metabolic labelling studies were performed in 25 cm^2 tissue culture flasks. Cultures of controls and mutant cells were subcultured into 10 flasks and just prior to confluence culture medium was replaced with medium supplemented with 10 μCi/ml (D[2 − ^{3}H]mannose (Amersham International). After a four day 'pulse', labelled medium was removed and cells were washed three times with phosphate buffered saline (PBS). Cultures were maintained in unlabelled medium and flasks harvested in duplicate, immediately (day 0), and at days 1,3,5 and 11 (chase). Cells were harvested by scraping, washed three times with PBS, and disrupted by sonication as previously described (Cooper *et al.*, 1988). After centrifugation (4000 *g*, 10 min), supernatants were applied to Bio-Gel P-2 columns (1.5 × 100 cm) and eluted with water. 1 ml fractions were collected and the radioactivity in 25 μl aliquots in 4 ml Unisolve (Koch-Light) was determined in a Rack-Beta 1216 scintillation counter (Pharmacia-LKB). Culture medium from the chase period was deproteinized by addition of an equal volume of 5% (w:v) trichloroacetic acid. The supernatant obtained by centrifugation was chromatographed on Bio-Gel P-2 as described. Mutant cells were also labelled with medium containing 1 μCi/ml D-[U-^{14}C] glucosamine (Amersham International) and 10 μCi/ml tritiated mannose for a seven day pulse and harvested after a one day chase in unlabelled medium. Dual-labelled trisaccharide was digested for 24 h with endoglycosidase H (Sigma) in 0.1 mmol/L citrate/0.2 mmol/L phosphate buffer, pH 4.0. Reaction products were isolated by Bio-Gel P-2 chromatography. Undigested trisaccharide was further incubated with α-mannosidase (Sigma) under identical conditions.

ANIMAL MODELS OF THE MANNOSIDOSES

Animal models of α-mannosidosis include Aberdeen Angus cattle (Whittem and Walker, 1957; Jolly *et al.*, 1980) and cats (Burditt *et al.*, 1980b). The former is of considerable economic importance. α-Mannosidosis may also be induced by ingestion of Swainsonine, a potent α-mannosidase inhibitor (Daniel *et al.*, 1984).

A deficiency of β-mannosidase in anglo-nubian goats was first described in 1981 (Jones *et al.*, 1981; Healy *et al.*, 1981), five years prior to the disorder being detected in man (Cooper *et al.*, 1986; Wenger *et al.*, 1986). In the caprine species the presentation is much more severe. Findings include facial dysmorphism involving doming of the skull, ocular abnormalities, folding of the ears, and extensive demyelination of the central nervous system; severe neurological symptoms, including intention tremor and inability to stand; joint hyperextension, muscle atrophy, mental retardation, nerve deafness and death in the neonatal period (Jones *et al.*, 1983). There is marked cytoplasmic vacuolation of all tissues, including the brain (Lovell and Jones, 1983; Malachowski and Jones, 1983; Render *et al.*, 1988).

CLINICAL FINDINGS IN HUMAN MANNOSIDOSES

α-Mannosidosis was first described in 1967 (Ockermann, 1967). The condition is divided into severe and mild forms designated as types I and II respectively. The clinical features of both types are presented in Table 1. Type I resembles the mucopolysaccharidoses and differentiation on clinical grounds is often impossible. The most obvious findings are facial dysmorphism, organomegaly, dysostosis multiplex and early death. Type II patients show a milder presentation in which deafness is prominent and they may survive to adulthood (Beaudet and Thomas, 1989). There is considerable clinical heterogeneity with adult forms described (Montgomery *et al.*, 1982) and mild and severe forms occurring in the same family (Mitchell *et al.*, 1981).

The findings in the four patients with an isolated deficiency of β-mannosidase described to date are illustrated in Table 2. The presentation is much less severe than α-mannosidosis, with survival into the fifth decade. Our proband was diagnosed at 44 years of age. He is the first male child of unrelated Hindu parents. His mother describes the pregnancy and neonatal development as normal. Mental retardation was suspected on first attending school in East Africa and no further formal education has been attempted. To date the patient has been maintained within the family. A 29-year-old brother was subsequently found to be affected by the same condition.

Common findings in patients so far reported are mental retardation and nerve

Table 1 Clinical features of α-mannosidosis types I and II

	Type I	*Type II*
Facial dysmorphism	+ + +	+ −
Skeletal deformities	+ + +	+ −
Organomegaly	+ + +	+ −
Nerve deafness	+ + +	+ + +
Mental retardation	+ + +	+ −
Hernia	+ + +	−
Angiokeratoma	+ −	−
Early death	+ + +	−
Ocular abnormalities	+ + +	+ −

Table 2 Clinical findings in reported cases of β-mannosidosis

	Adults	*Children*
Facial dysmorphism	−	−
Skeletal deformities	−	−
Organomegaly	−	−
Nerve deafness	+ + +	+ + +
Mental retardation	+ + +	+ +
Hernia	−	−
Angiokeratoma	+ + +	−
Early death	−	−
Aggression	+ −	−
Lymphoedema	+ −	−

deafness (Cooper *et al.*, 1986; Dorland *et al.*, 1988a). A sloping sensorineural hearing loss was demonstrated in our proband (Table 3). IQs of both our patients were assessed using the Griffiths Mental Development Scale as adult tests proved beyond their capabilities. For both brothers, hearing-speech, hand-eye co-ordination and performance were at the 6–7 year level, whilst practical reasoning was at the 7–8 year level. Angiokeratoma has only been described in two affected adults, the second of whom also exhibited aggressive behaviour resulting in institutionalization (Cooper *et al.*, 1986). This patient also had diabetes mellitus, and cellulitis and lymphoedema of the legs necessitating dual amputations. Whether this lymphoedema is related to β-mannosidase deficiency is unclear. There was no evidence of lymphatic involvement in the proband.

A patient with dual deficiencies of β-mannosidase and sulphamidase has also been described (Wenger *et al.*, 1986). The clinical picture in this patient is that of Sanfilippo syndrome. Three unreported affected children are at present under investigation in Holland and France (personal communications). These include the first affected female patient to be discovered. In contrast to human α-mannosidosis and the animal model, human β-mannosidosis does not involve facial dysmorphism, organomegaly, severe neurological involvement or demyelination (Table 2); a CT scan of our patient's brain showed normal myelination.

PATHOLOGICAL FINDINGS

A common finding in α-mannosidosis is vacuolation of marrow cells and peripheral lymphocytes. Electron microscopy of organs and the central nervous system shows enlargement of lysosomes due to storage of mannose-rich oligosaccharides (Kjellmann *et al.*, 1969; Sung *et al.*, 1977).

In β-mannosidosis, electron microscopy demonstrated cytoplasmic vacuolation of varying degrees in different cell types. Marked cytoplasmic vacuolation of fibroblasts and pericytes was observed, and proliferation of endothelial cells into the lumen of vessels was also seen. Presumably it is this which causes the angiokeratoma in our patients. Following amputation of our second patient's leg, vacuolation of lymph

Table 3 Audiology findings in the proband using pure tone audiometry

Right side: Sloping sensorineural hearing loss with significant high frequency loss						
Frequency	250 Hz	500 Hz	1 kHz	2 kHz	4 kHz	8 kHz
Thresholds:						
Air conduction	25 dBA	25	40	55	70	80
Bone conduction	20 dBA	30	35	65	70	65
Left side: No response except vibrotactile frequency of 250 Hz						
Air conduction	65 dBA	110	110	NR	NR	NR
Bone conduction	70 dBA	NR	NR	NR	NR	NR
Brain stem evoked response: Threshold of 65 dBHL on right, no response on left						

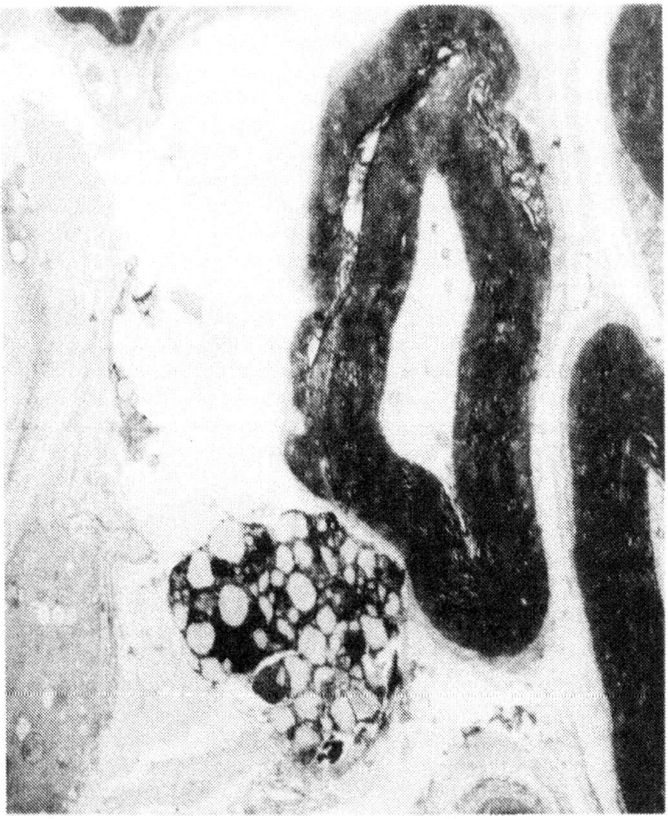

Figure 1 Electron-lucent intracytoplasmic vacuoles in Schwann cell of peripheral nerve

nodes, muscle fibres and blood vessel walls was observed. Nerves showed more discrete vacuolation of some Schwann cells. Only isolated cells were involved; however, in some vacuolation was extensive (Figure 1). Pathological findings will be described in more detail elsewhere.

BIOCHEMICAL FINDINGS

α-Mannosidosis is characterized by deficient lysosomal α-mannosidase activity. Considerable residual activity is present in some tissues, although this is thought not to be lysosomal in origin (Winchester *et al.*, 1989). This remaining activity differs from normal enzyme with respect to its much elevated K_m, reduced stability to heating at 60°C and stimulation rather than inhibition by cobalt ions (Burditt *et al.*,

1980a). Urinary excretion of mannose-rich oligosaccharides can be demonstrated by TLC or HPLC (Sewell, 1981; Warren *et al.*, 1984). The major component is the trisaccharide Manα1-3Manβ1-4GlcNAc but up to 16 other larger compounds containing α1-3 and α1-6 linkages have been described (Matsuura *et al.*, 1981). Prenatal diagnosis of this condition has been reported using cultured amniocytes (Poenaru *et al.*, 1979) and first trimester diagnosis is also possible as the enzyme is present in uncultured chorionic villi (Fowler *et al.*, 1989).

β-Mannosidosis is characterized by deficient β-mannosidase activity. Our original patient was diagnosed by assay of plasma β-mannosidase activity (Cooper *et al.*, 1986; Cooper *et al.*, 1987). Subsequently deficient activity was demonstrated in leukocytes, cultured skin fibroblasts and urine of the proband and his brother (Cooper *et al.*, 1988). TLC of urinary oligosaccharides showed a single prominent band with the mobility of a disaccharide. Mass spectrometry of the permethylated compound and digestion with snail β-mannosidase indicated a structure of Manβ1-4GlcNAc (Cooper *et al.*, 1988). Further purification by adsorption, size exclusion and descending paper chromatography revealed a second compound with a similar mobility on TLC (Cooper *et al.*, 1988). This compound has been identified as Manβ1-4GlcNAc complexed with urea (Dorland *et al.*, 1988b). The novel minor storage tetra- and pentasaccharides described in goats (Matsuura and Jones, 1985) have not so far been detected in man, although a sialylated oligosaccharide N-acetylneuraminyl-α-(2-6)-mannosyl-β-(1-4)-N-acetylglucosamine has recently been described (Hokke *et al.*, 1989). First trimester prenatal diagnosis is theoretically possible as β-mannosidase is present in uncultured chorionic villi (Fowler *et al.*, 1989).

In an attempt to identify carriers of the mutant gene in relatives of our patients, we undertook family studies. Initally we investigated plasma β-mannosidase activity, but this proved to be a less than ideal enzyme source due to marked variation of activity with age (Cooper *et al.*, 1987). The enzyme is most active in the neonatal period and declines steadily thereafter. Similar findings have been described in goats (Dunstan *et al.*, 1983).

White cell β-mannosidase assay gave more promising results, particularly in isolated cell types (Figure 2). Activity in granulocyte-rich fractions was considerably higher than in lymphocytes. The obligate heterozygote parents Ia and Ib showed reduced activity compared to controls in both cell types, the difference being more marked in granulocytes. Two siblings of the affected patients IIc and IId showed reduced β-mannosidase activity in both cell types; again differentiation from controls was best seen in granulocytes. Relatives IIIa, b, c and d had activities indistinguishable from control values in both granulocytes and lymphocytes, and are presumed not to carry the mutation.

To demonstrate storage in mutant cells we undertook metabolic labelling studies. Following culture in labelled medium, cell extracts were fractionated on Bio-Gel P-2 columns. Figure 3(a) shows the composition of fibroblast extracts after a four day pulse in labelled medium. In mutant cells large amounts of labelled material were present at the void volume, and in the position of Manβ1-4GlcNAc and mannose. Lesser amounts were also present in control cells. Following a one day chase in unlabelled medium (Figure 3(b)), several additional peaks of mannose-

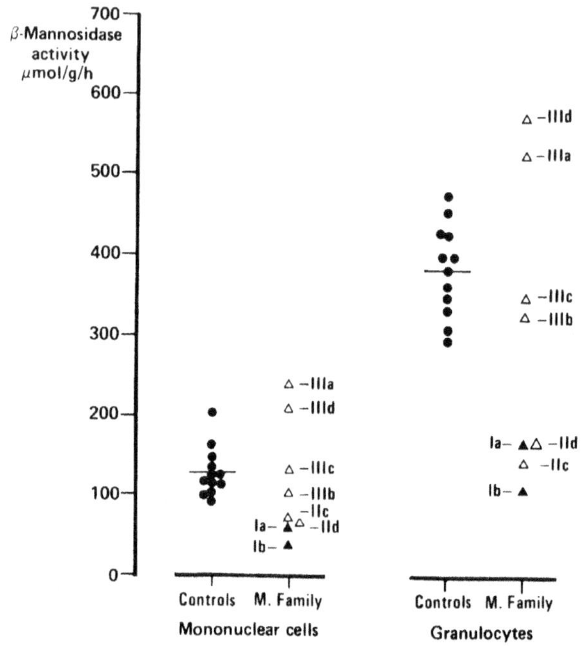

Figure 2 β-Mannosidase activity of granulocyte-rich and lymphocyte fractions from controls, obligate heterozygotes and putative heterozygotes

rich oligosaccharides were observed, presumably due to metabolism of labelled glycoproteins. In both control and mutant cells a prominent peak of trisaccharide was seen. Dual labelling experiments using tritiated mannose and ^{14}C-glucosamine followed by digestion with endoglycosidase H and α and β-mannosidase showed this peak to be a mixture of Manα1-3Manβ1-4GlcNAc and Manβ1-4GlcNAcβ1-4GlcNAc (results not shown). After three days chase, di- and trisaccharides were still present (Figure 3(c)), but after five days (data not shown) and 11 days (Figure 3(d)), tritiated oligosaccharides were no longer detectable in control cells. In contrast, in mutant cells, a disaccharide peak persisted, demonstrating intracellular storage of this material, although the amount decreased steadily. Enzymic digestion with snail β-mannosidase showed this compound to contain mannose and N-acetylglucosamine. As has been described in goats (Hancock *et al.*, 1986), mutant cells secreted labelled disaccharide and lesser amounts of trisaccharide into culture medium during the chase period. This was not observed in control cell lines (Figure 4).

DISCUSSION AND CONCLUSIONS

α-Mannosidosis is a well documented condition (Beaudet and Thomas, 1989), in which considerable clinical heterogeneity has been described (Mitchell *et al.*, 1981;

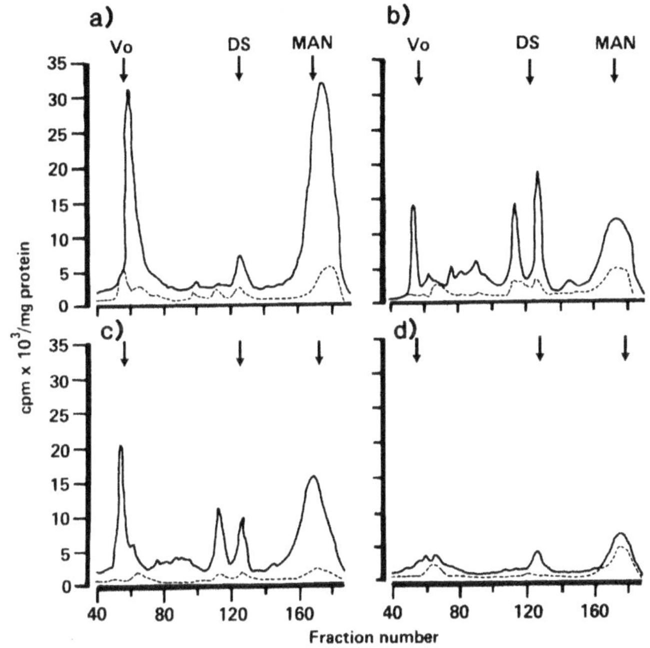

Figure 3 Bio-Gel P-2 chromatography of control ---- and β-mannosidosis ——— fibroblast extracts. (a) Day 0, (b) Day 1, (c) Day 3 and (d) Day 11 (a similar pattern was observed at Day 5)

Montgomery *et al.*, 1982). The clinical consequences are severe and no adequate treatment is at present available. Bone marrow transplantation has been described in one case (Will *et al.*, 1987), but the outcome was unfavourable. The best management at present is genetic counselling and the ready availability of prenatal diagnosis (Poenaru *et al.*, 1979; Fowler *et al.*, 1989).

In contrast, the clinical presentation of β-mannosidosis is mild both compared to human α-mannosidosis and to the caprine condition. Indeed, the term animal model is perhaps a misnomer for the disorder in goats. Not only the phenotypic expression but also the major storage material differs. Extrapolation of results from animal experiments to man, such as treatment by bone marrow transplantation, would be difficult to interpret. It would perhaps be better to apply the term 'animal analogue' to the caprine disorder. The prospect of carrier detection in the human condition appears promising. Plasma results should be interpreted with caution (Cooper *et al.*, 1987). In contrast, the results in granulocyte-rich fractions (Figure 2) indicate this to be the tissue of choice.

Why is the presentation of β-mannosidosis mild compared to both the animal model and to human α-mannosidosis? It may simply be due to the smaller size of the stored material. Alternative methods of egress from lysosomes may be available

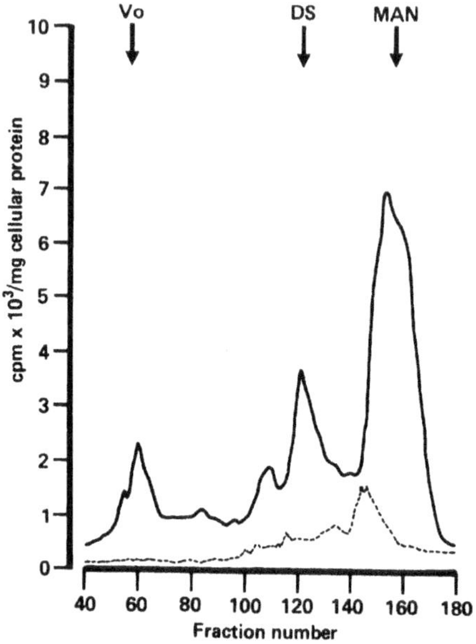

Figure 4 Bio-Gel P-2 chromatography of culture medium of control ---- and β-mannosidosis ——— fibroblast cultures 1 day post-labelling with tritiated mannose

to a disaccharide, but not to the larger storage materials found in α-mannosidosis and caprine β-mannosidosis. This is supported by findings in our metabolic labelling studies. Throughout the chase period, Manβ1-4GlcNAc was secreted into culture medium (Figure 4). Whilst this may be attributed to cell death, it could also reflect efflux from intact lysosomes. The steady reduction in the amount of disaccharide present in mutant cells (Figure 3) would also suggest removal of disaccharide from lysosomes. There may also be a sparing effect brought about by selective excretion by the kidney as postulated for α-mannosidosis (Lott and Daniel, 1981). Manβ1-4GlcNAc is certainly found in large amounts (64 mg/mmol creatinine) in the urine of our patients. The variation between human and caprine β-mannosidosis may also simply be due to interspecies differences.

The delayed discovery of β-mannosidosis in man after its detection in goats in 1981 (Jones *et al.*, 1981; Healy *et al.*, 1981) may have been due to the clinical dissimilarities of the two conditions. Studies of dysmorphic or severely affected individuals proved fruitless (Panday *et al.*, 1984). The non-specific features of mental retardation and nerve deafness present difficulties for clinical diagnosis in the future. Whether clinical heterogeneity will be discovered in future cases is impossible to predict, but it seems likely that human β-mannosidosis will be one of the least severe of the lysosomal storage diseases. The existence of a dual deficiency of β-mannosidase and sulphamidase (Wenger *et al.*, 1986) has not yet been adequately explained. The production of antibody to β-mannosidase, localization of the gene to a specific chromosome and isolation of complementary DNA will provide more information in the future. These studies are at present in progress.

REFERENCES

Beaudet, A. L. and Thomas, G. H. Disorders of glycoprotein degradation : mannosidosis, fucosidosis, sialidosis and aspartylglycosaminuria. In Scriver, C. R., Beaudet, A. L., Sly, W. S. and Valle, D. (eds.), *The Metabolic Basis of Inherited Disease*, McGraw-Hill, New York, 1989, pp 1603–1621

Burditt, L., Chotai, K., Halley, D. and Winchester, B. Comparison of the residual acidic α-D-mannosidase in three cases of mannosidosis. *Clin. Chim. Acta* 104 (1980a) 201–209

Burditt, L. J., Chotai, K., Hirani, S., Nugent, P. G., Winchester, B. G. and Blakemore, W. F. Biochemical studies on a case of feline mannosidosis. *Biochem. J.* 189 (1980b) 467–473

Cooper, A., Sardharwalla, I. B. and Roberts, M. M. Human β-mannosidase deficiency. *N. Engl. J. Med.* 315 (19) (1986) 1231

Cooper, A., Hatton, C. and Sardharwalla, I. B. Acid β-mannosidase of human plasma: influence of age and sex on enzyme activity. *J. Inher. Metab. Dis.* 10 (3) (1987) 229–233

Cooper, A., Hatton, C., Thornley, M. and Sardharwalla, I. B. Human β-mannosidase deficiency: biochemical findings in plasma, fibroblasts, white cells and urine. *J. Inher. Metab. Dis.* 11 (1) (1988) 17–29

Daniel, P. F., Warren, C. D. and James, L. F. Swainsonine-induced oligosaccharide excretion in sheep. *Biochem. J.* 221 (1984) 601–607

Dorland, L., Duran, M., Hoefnagels, F. T. E., Breg, J. N., Fabery de Jonge, H., Cranzberg, K., van Sprang, F. J. and van Diggelen, O. P. β-Mannosidosis in two brothers with hearing loss. *J. Inher. Metab. Dis.* 11 Suppl. 2 (1988a) 255–258

Dorland, L., van Rhee, A. M., van Pelt, J., Duran, M., Dallinga, J., Heerma, W. and de Waard, P. Mannosyl-β(1-4)-N-acetylglucosaminyl-β(1-N)-urea, a compound isolated from the urine of patients with β-mannosidosis. *Glycoconjugate J.* 5 (3) (1988b) 215–222

Dunstan, R. W., Cavanagh, K. and Jones, M. Z. Caprine α and β-mannosidase activities: Effect of age, sex and reproductive status and potential use in heterozygote detection of β-mannosidosis. *Am. J. Vet. Res.* 44 (4) (1983) 685–689

Fowler, B., Giles, L., Cooper, A. and Sardharwalla, I. B. Chorionic villus sampling: uses and limitations of enzyme assays. *J. Inher. Metab. Dis.* 12 Suppl. 1 (1989) 105–117

Hancock, L. W., Jones, M. Z. and Dawson, G. Glycoprotein metabolism in normal and β-mannosidase-deficient cultured goat skin fibroblasts. *Biochem. J.* 234 (1986) 175–183

Healy, P. J., Seaman, J. T., Gardner, I. A. and Sewell, C. A. β-Mannosidase deficiency in anglo-nubian goats. *Austr. Vet. J.* 57 (1981) 504–507

Hokke, C. E., Duran, M., Dorland, L., van Pelt, J. and van Sprang, F. J. Novel storage products in human β-mannosidosis. *Abstracts of the 27th Annual Symposium of the Society for the Study of Inborn Errors of Metabolism*, Munich, 1989, Abstract No. 114.

Jolly, R. D. and Thompson, K. G. The pathology of bovine mannosidosis. *Vet. Pathol.* 15 (1978) 141–152

Jones, M. Z. and Laine, R. A. Caprine oligosaccharide storage disease: accumulation of β-mannosyl (1-4)β-N-acetylglucosamine β-N-acetylglucosamine in brain. *J. Biol. Chem.* 256 (1981) 5181–5184

Jones, M. Z., Cunningham, J. G., Dade, A. W., Alessi, D. M., Mostoski, U. V., Vorro, J. R., Benitez, J. T. and Lovell, K. L. Caprine β-mannosidosis: clinical and pathological features. *J. Neuropathol. Exp. Neurol.* 421 (1983) 268–285

Kjellman, B., Gamstorp, I., Brun, A., Ockerman, P-A. and Palmgren, B. Mannosidosis: a clinical and histopathological study. *J. Pediatr.* 75 (1969) 366–373

Lott, I. T. and Daniel, P. F. Serum and urinary trisaccharides in mannosidosis. *Neurology* 31 (1981) 1159–1162

Lovell, K. L. and Jones, M. Z. Distribution of central nervous system lesions in β-mannosidosis. *Acta Neuropathol.* (Berlin) 62 (1983) 121–126
Malachowski, J. A. and Jones, M. Z. β-Mannosidosis: lesions of the distal peripheral nervous system. *Acta Neuropathol.* (Berlin) 61 (1983) 95–100
Matsuura, F. and Jones, M. Z. Structural characterization of novel complex oligosaccharides accumulating in the caprine β-mannosidosis kidney. *J. Biol. Chem.* 260 (28) (1985) 15239–15245
Matsuura, F., Nunez, H. A., Grabowski, G. A. and Sweeley, C. C. Structural studies of urinary oligosaccharides from patients with mannosidosis. *Arch. Biochem. Biophys.* 207 (2) (1981) 337–352
Mitchell, M. L., Erickson, R. P., Schmid, D., Hieber, V., Poznanski, A. K. and Hicks, S. P. Mannosidosis: two brothers with different degrees of disease severity. *Clin. Genet.* 20 (1981) 191–202
Montgomery, T. R., Thomas, G. H. and Valle, D. L. Mannosidosis in an adult. *The Johns Hopkins Medical J.* 151 (1982) 113–121
Okermann, P. A. A generalised storage disease resembling Hurler's syndrome. *Lancet* 2 (1967) 239–241
Panday, R. S., van Diggelen, O. P., Kleijer, W. J. and Niermeijer, M. F. β-Mannosidase in human leukocytes and fibroblasts. *J. Inher. Metab. Dis.* 7 (1984) 155–156
Poenaru, L., Girard, S., Thepot, F., Madelenat, P., Huraux-Rendu, H., Vinet, M. and Dreyfus, J. Antenatal diagnosis in three pregnancies at risk for mannosidosis. *Clin. Genet.* 16 (1979) 428–432
Render, J. A., Lovell, K. L. and Jones, M. Z. Otic pathology of caprine β-mannosidosis. *Vet. Pathol.* 25 (1988) 437–442
Sewell, A. C. An improved thin-layer chromatographic method for urinary oligosaccharide screening. *Clin. Chim. Acta.* 92 (1979) 411–414
Strecker, G., Fournet, B., Bouquelet, S., Montreuil, J., Dhondt, J. L. and Farariaux, J. P. Etude chimique des mannosides urinaires excretes au cours de la mannosidosis. *Biochimie* 58 (1976) 578–586
Sung, J. H., Hayano, M. and Desnick, R. J. Mannosidosis: pathology of the nervous system. *J. Neuropathol. Exp. Neurol.* 36 (1977) 807–820
Warren, T. G., Mock, A. K., Nyhan, W. L. and O'Brien, J. S. α-Mannosidosis: analysis of urinary oligosaccharides with high performance liquid chromatography and diagnosis of a case with unusually mild presentation. *Clin. Genet.* 25 (1984) 248–255
Wenger, D. A., Sujanski, E., Fennesaey, P. V. and Thompson, J. N. Human β-mannosidase deficiency. *N. Engl. J. Med.* 315 (1986) 1201–1205
Whittem, J. M. and Walker, D. 'Neuronopathy' and 'Pseudolipidosis' in Aberdeen Angus calves. *J. Pathol. Bacteriol.* 74 (1957) 281–288
Will, A., Cooper, A., Hatton, C., Sardharwalla, I. B. Evans, D. I. K. and Stevens, R. F. Bone marrow transplantation in the treatment of α-mannosidosis. *Arch. Dis. Child.* 62 (1987) 1044–1049
Winchester, B., Cenci di Bello, I. and Willemsen, R. The molecular basis of the enzymic defect in α-mannosidosis. *Abstracts of the 27th Annual Symposium of the Society for the Study of Inborn Errors of Metabolism*, Munich, 1989, Abstract No. 112
Yamashita, K., Tachibana, Y., Mihara, K., Okada, S., Yabuuchi, H. and Kobata, A. Urinary oligosaccharides of mannosidosis. *J. Biol. Chem.* 255 (1979) 5126–5133

J. Inher. Metab. Dis. 13 (1990) 549–559

Schindler Disease: an Inherited Neuroaxonal Dystrophy due to α-*N*-Acetylgalactosaminidase Deficiency

R. J. Desnick and A. M. Wang
Division of Medical and Molecular Genetics, Mount Sinai School of Medicine, New York, NY 10029, USA

Summary: The clinical, pathological and biochemical features of a neuroaxonal dystrophy resulting from the deficient activity of lysosomal α-*N*-acetylgalactosaminidase are described. This neurodegenerative disorder was recognized in two brothers who had the typical clinical manifestations and neuropathological lesions observed in patients with Seitelberger disease, the infantile form of neuroaxonal dystrophy. Axonal 'spheroids' were observed histologically in the grey matter, and ultrastructural examination revealed the characteristic formations in dystrophic axons in the myenteric plexus and neocortex. Using a newly synthesized fluorogenic substrate, 4-methylumbelliferyl-α-*N*-acetylgalactosaminide, the markedly deficient activity of α-*N*-acetylgalactosaminidase was demonstrated in the affected brothers while their consanguineous parents had intermediate activities, consistent with the autosomal recessive transmission of this disease. No detectable α-*N*-acetylgalactosaminidase was seen in immunoblots using monospecific rabbit antihuman α-*N*-acetylgalactosaminidase antibodies. Abnormally increased amounts of urinary glycopeptides were observed by high resolution thin layer chromatography. Analytical studies identified four of the accumulating urinary compounds, the blood group A trisaccharide GalNAcα1→3(Fucα1→2)Gal and three *O*-linked glycopeptides, GalNAcα1→*O*-serine and -threonine, NeuNAcα2→3Galβ1→3(NeuNAcα2→6)GalNAcα1→*O*-serine and -threonine, and NeuNAcα2→3Galβ1→4GlcNAcβ1→6(NeuNAcα2→3Galβ1→3)GalNAcα1→*O*-serine and -threonine. Of eight unrelated patients diagnosed as having infantile neuraxonal dystrophy by pathological studies, none had deficient α-*N*-acetylgalactosaminidase activity, emphasizing the biochemical heterogeneity underlying this diagnostic entity. These findings document the first delineation of a metabolic defect in an inherited neuroaxonal dystrophy and suggest that the axonal pathology in this disorder, and perhaps in the other neuroaxonal dystrophies, results from abnormal glycoprotein metabolism involving *O*-linked glycopeptides.

PURSUIT AND PERSISTENCE, A MEDICAL PARADIGM

> Nature is nowhere accustomed more openly to display her secret mysteries than in cases where she shows traces of her workings apart from the beaten path; nor is there any better way to advance the proper practice of medicine than to give our minds to the discovery of the usual law of nature, by the careful investigation of cases of rare forms of disease (Harvey, 1657).

> The concept of metabolism in blocks is giving place to that of metabolism in compartments. The view is daily gaining ground that each successive step in the building up and breaking down, not merely of proteins, carbohydrates, and fats in general, but even of individual fractions of proteins and of individual sugars is the work of special enzymes set apart for each particular purpose (Garrod, 1908).

The recent identification and rapid delineation of Schindler disease, an infantile neuroaxonal dystrophy due to α-*N*-acetylgalactosaminidase deficiency (van Diggelen *et al.*, 1987, 1988; Schindler *et al.*, 1989), illustrates two current themes in medicine: (1) That suspicion and/or supposition concerning a possible new disease entity, diagnostic method or treatment modality should be *pursued*, and that *persistence* in this pursuit is required for success, and (2) that the application of modern biochemical, somatic cell and molecular biological techniques can facilitate the rapid delineation of the cellular and/or molecular defects in newly discovered disease entities.

William Harvey and Sir Archibald E. Garrod both understood the concept of *pursuit and persistence* and their accomplishments were seminal in the history of medicine. Both men were practising physicians and experimentalists and both appreciated the importance of investigating 'rarer forms of disease' to gain understanding of 'nature's ways'. For over a decade, Harvey sought to prove that blood circulated continuously within a closed system. His persistence, against a large and influential opposition based in the tradition of Galenic physiology (i.e., blood was produced in the liver and flowed to the periphery), led to one of the most significant of the early advances in physiology and medicine. Garrod sought to understand the nature of the 'biochemical individuality' that caused the specific metabolic defects in the disorders he designated as 'inborn errors of metabolism'. Today, the spirit of *pursuit and persistence* continues. However, modern medical science has become so sophisticated that an innovative thought or reasoned suspicion requires not only a stubborn commitment to pursuit, but also a team of resourceful and persistent investigators to bring a given hypothesis to fruition.

Physicians and scientists strive to identify and delineate new disease entities. The application of modern ultrastructural, biochemical and cell culture techniques has facilitated the identification of a variety of new inherited metabolic disorders and disease variants. Of the recently described lysosomal disorders, galactosialidosis (Wenger *et al.*, 1978), Salla disease (Aula *et al.*, 1979), and β-mannosidosis (Cooper *et al.*, 1986; Wenger *et al.*, 1986), it is notable that each had prominent visceral manifestations similar to those found in other lysosomal storage diseases which led to their elucidation (e.g., dysostosis multiplex, cherry-red maculae and/or organomegaly). The key to the recognition of these disorders was physician suspicion, phenotypic clues and the diligent pursuit of the pathological and biochemical defects. Such was the brief historical trail that led Dr Detlev Schindler, a human geneticist at the University of Würzburg in West Germany, to identify and delineate a new neurological disease. He saw the index family in 1985 when the parents sought genetic counselling concerning the prognosis for their two affected sons and the possible reproductive risks for their normal son and other relatives. Although the affected brothers had been evaluated by many specialists, the absence of visceral manifestations did not provide the diagnostic clues suggesting a storage disease. No diagnosis had been made other than 'psychomotor delay'. Dr Schindler suspected that the two affected brothers had an autosomal recessive metabolic disease since they experienced a remarkably similar regressive course and since the parents came from a small, inbred village. With parental consent, renewed efforts were undertaken to establish a diagnosis.

Dr Schindler began systematically: cultured lymphoblast and fibroblast lines were established, and urine and blood were collected for biochemical analyses. Initially, he had a variety of metabolic screening tests performed by various expert laboratories in Europe. The first positive finding was the abnormal urinary oligosaccharide profile observed by Dr Helen Christomanou in Munich. This pattern has not been previously seen in the known storage diseases with oligosacchariduria. This finding led Dr Schindler to determine the activities of the lysosomal enzymes whose deficiencies result in oligosacchariduria. He arranged for his colleagues Drs Christomanou, Klaus Harzer in Tübingen, Rudolf Sengers in Nijmegen and Adrian Sewell in Mainz to assay various lysosomal enzyme activities in the leukocytes of the affected brothers. All the activities were normal. Subsequently, Dr Michael Cantz of Heidelberg determined that the neuraminidase activity, free and bound neuraminic acid content, and the mucopolysaccharide ^{35}S incorporation studies were normal in cultured fibroblasts from the propositi. He also repeated the urinary oligosaccharide screening studies and confirmed the original findings. Since Dr Schindler was eager to characterize the nature of the abnormal oligosaccharides, he was referred to Dr Heinze Egge, a glycoconjugate expert at the University at Bonn. Urines from the two brothers were analysed, and the markedly increased amount of the blood group A trisaccharide GalNAc(1→3)Gal(2→1)αFuc was detected in the older sib with blood group A. This finding focused attention on α-*N*-acetylgalactosaminidase, the enzyme that normally hydrolyses the terminal α-*N*-acetylgalactosaminyl linkage of the blood group A trisaccharide, as a candidate for the metabolic defect in this disease.

Dr Schindler also informed Dr Hans Galjaard in Rotterdam of the status of the diagnostic pursuit and requested additional suggestions. Dr Galjaard's colleague, Dr Otto van Diggelen, responded with an offer to assay the α-*N*-acetylgalactosaminidase activity, one of the few lysosomal enzyme activities which had not been determined previously. Dr Schindler sent blood and cultured fibroblasts from the affected brothers for assay, and Dr van Diggelen found the marked deficiency of enzymatic activity, using *p*-nitrophenyl-α-*N*-acetylgalactosaminide as substrate. Thus, Dr Schindler's suspicion, pursuit, and persistence were rewarded in June 1986 by the identification of the specific enzyme defect, which documented the discovery of a new inborn error of metabolism.

Word of this discovery reached our laboratory in May 1987. We had already microsequenced homogeneous human α-*N*-acetylgalactosaminidase, had produced monospecific antibodies against it, and were isolating the cDNA for this enzyme. We therefore contacted Dr Schindler and established a collaboration. The affected brothers were evaluated at the General Clinical Research Center of the Mount Sinai School of Medicine in November 1987. The neurological findings were documented, the enzymatic defect was characterized further, and biopsies were performed for pathological examination by Dr David E. Wolfe. A significant finding was the ultrastructural observation of 'tubulovesicular' material in terminal axons in the myenteric plexus of a rectal biopsy. In March 1988, a cortical biopsy was performed in the older brother with the informed consent of both parents. Histological and ultrastructural examination revealed the presence of unique deposits in terminal axons, particularly in grey matter. These neuronal alterations resembled the spheroids seen in patients with Seitelberger and Hallervorden–Spatz diseases (Seitelberger, 1986), the infantile and juvenile forms of neuroaxonal dystrophy, respectively. However, cultured fibroblasts from several patients with Seitelberger disease, who had been diagnosed definitively at autopsy, had normal levels of α-*N*-acetylgalactosaminidase activity. Since the ultrastructural abnormalities are similar, it is possible that the neuroaxonal dystrophies and Schindler disease share common pathophysiological alterations, presumably in the fast axonal transport pathway (Griffin and Watson, 1988). It is likely that patients with α-*N*-acetylgalactosaminidase deficiency may have been diagnosed as having Seitelberger or Hallervorden–Spatz diseases in the past, consistent with the phenotypic heterogeneity observed in the neuroaxonal dystrophies.

Since it is cumbersome to refer to this disease as α-*N*-acetylgalactosaminidase deficiency, and since the parents of the propositi preferred not to name the disease after their village or by their surname, it seems only fitting to designate this disorder as *Schindler disease*, an appropriate eponym acknowledging the unusual persistence of a physician who successfully pursued a diagnosis in a family suffering from a previously unrecognized neurodegenerative disorder. In this communication we review the pathological, biochemical and molecular findings in two affected siblings with this newly recognized form of infantile neuroaxonal dystrophy due to α-*N*-acetylgalactosaminidase deficiency.

CLINICAL MANIFESTATIONS

The first described cases of this disease are brothers, the offspring of fourth cousins of German descent (Figure 1) (van Diggelen *et al.*, 1987, 1988; Schindler *et al.*, 1989). Clinical onset occurred in the first year of life when developmental delay and regression of developmental milestones were noted. Grand mal seizures, muscular weakness, incoordination, strabismus and nystagmus were early manifestations. Subsequently, each child experienced a rapid neurodegenerative course with loss of all previously acquired mental and motor skills by three to four years of age. Later neurological signs included spastic quadriplegia, cortical blindness, deafness, myoclonus, rigidity and a decorticate state with little, if any, contact with the environment. Imaging studies revealed generalized atrophy of the brain, especially of the cerebellum and brainstem. The clinical findings were essentially identical to

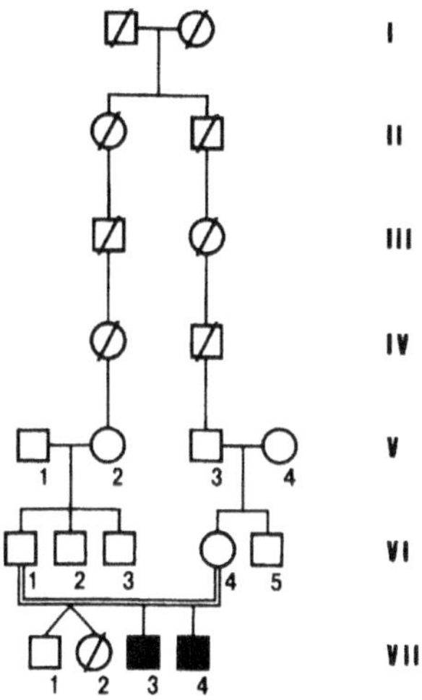

Figure 1 Pedigree: the parents were fourth cousins of German ancestry.

those of the infantile form of neuroaxonal dystrophy or Seitelberger disease (Seitelberger, 1986).

CHARACTERIZATION OF THE ENZYMATIC DEFECT

The deficient activity of α-*N*-acetylgalactosaminidase was demonstrated in the affected siblings using the new, specific and highly sensitive fluorogenic substrate, 4-methylumbelliferyl-α-*N*-acetylgalactosaminide. Residual activities of 0.5 to 2% of mean normal values were observed in plasma and cultured cell extracts from the affected siblings. The residual activities were not due to assay variability or background fluorescence since they were linear with time and protein concentration. Mixing experiments with fibroblast extracts from an affected sibling and an unrelated normal control revealed the expected intermediate activity, thereby excluding the presence of an inhibitor or the absence of an activator as the cause of the enzymatic defect. Intermediate levels of α-*N*-acetylgalactosaminidase activity were demonstrated in the parents, consistent with the deficiency being inherited as an autosomal recessive trait.

To further characterize the nature of the enzymatic defect, immunoblot studies were performed with purified enzyme and fibroblast extracts from family members and unrelated normal individuals. Using monospecific rabbit anti-α-*N*-acetylgalactosaminidase antibodies, two immunoreactive bands ($\sim$48 and 117 kDa) were detected in preparations of the homogenous enzyme (Figure 2, lane 7). The same two bands were present in fibroblast extracts from an unrelated normal individual, the unaffected brother and the heterozygous parents of the affected siblings (Figure 2, lanes 1–3 and 6). Neither immunoreactive band was detected in extracts from the affected siblings (Figure 2, lanes 4 and 5). Furthermore, no immunologically detectable enzyme

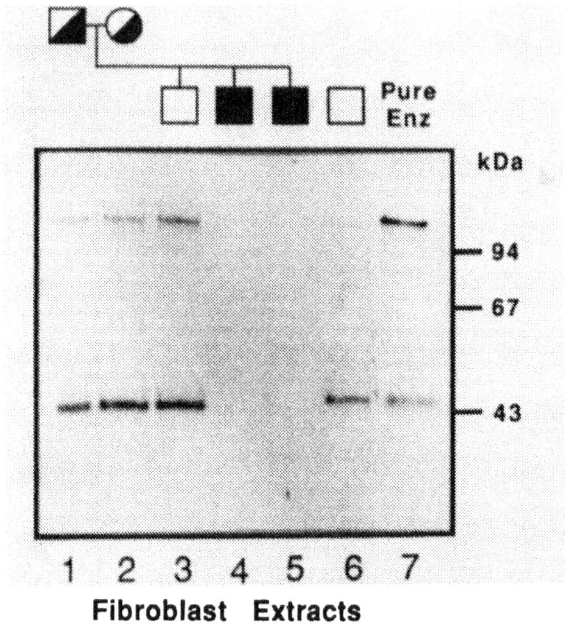

Figure 2 Immunoblot of α-*N*-acetylgalactosaminidase. When antihuman α-*N*-acetylgalactosaminidase antibodies were used, two reactive peptide species (molecular weights, 48 and 117 kDa) were detected in fibroblast extracts from the father (lane 1), the mother (lane 2), the unaffected brother (lane 3), and an unrelated control (lane 6) and in the purified enzyme (lane 7). No immunoreactive enzyme protein bands were seen in extracts from the patients (lanes 4 and 5). See Schindler *et al.*, (1989) for details.

protein was observed in concentrated fibroblast extracts. The fact that the 48 and 117 kDa forms of the purified enzyme had the identical N-terminal amino acid sequences (27 residues determined by microsequencing, data not shown) and that both forms were immunologically undetectable in the affected siblings, indicated that both forms of α-*N*-acetylgalactosaminidase in normal human tissues were encoded by a single gene. Thus, the enzyme defect in this family is due to a mutation in the gene encoding α-*N*-acetylgalactosaminidase which results in the absence of immunologically detectable enzyme protein.

NATURE OF THE ACCUMULATING SUBSTRATES

Since the deficient activity of α-*N*-acetylgalactosaminidase should result in the accumulation of compounds containing α-*N*-acetylgalactosaminyl moieties, qualitative and quantitative analyses of neutral glycosphingolipids, oligosaccharides and glycopeptides were performed. The concentrations of the individual neutral glycosphingolipids in the plasma, erythrocytes, and urinary sediments from both affected siblings and in cortical tissue from the older affected sibling were normal (data not shown). In contrast, the abnormal accumulation of urinary glycopeptides was demonstrated by a new screening procedure designed to resolve and identify oligosaccharides and glycopeptides by thin layer chromatography and selective stains (Schindler *et al.*, 1990). As shown in Figures 3(A) and 3(B), several urinary compounds were present only in the affected siblings which stained positive with both orcinol-$FeCl_3$ and ninhydrin, suggesting their glycopeptide composition. Although it was difficult to identify abnormally accumulated compounds in the chromatogram stained for oligosaccharides (orcinol-$FeCl_3$), the presence of three major and several minor components in the urines of the affected siblings was readily detected when the chromatogram was stained with ninhydrin. The three major bands were also positive with orcinol-$FeCl_3$ indicating their glycopeptide nature. The major ninhydrin-positive components were not detected in desalted urines from the other family members, twelve age- and sex-matched unrelated normal individuals, or in the urines of patients with other oligosaccharide or glycoprotein storage diseases with the exception of sialidosis (van Pelt *et al.*, 1988; Schindler *et al.*, 1990).

Subsequent structural analysis of the accumulated urinary compounds from the affected siblings revealed the glycopeptide structures, NeuNAcα2→3Galβ1→3(NeuNAcα2→6)GalNAcα1→*O*-serine and -threonine, NeuNAcα2→3Galβ1→

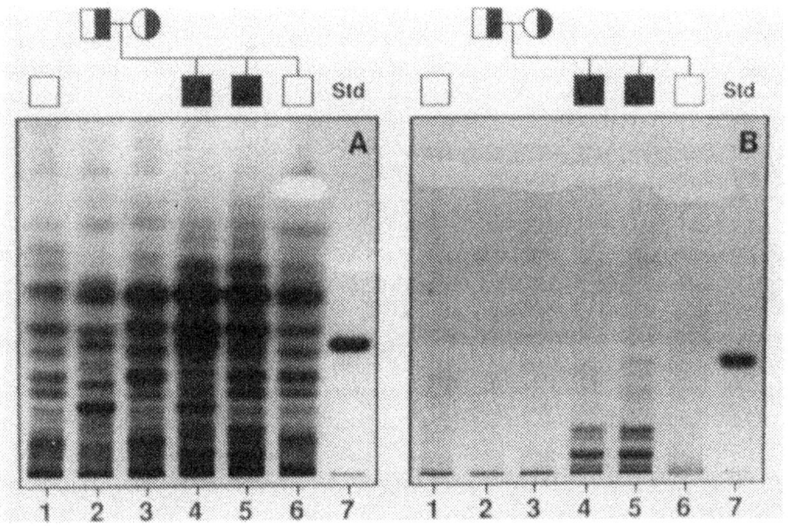

Figure 3 Urinary glycopeptide profiles. Thin layer chromatograms of desalted urine samples which were applied to duplicate plates, developed simultaneously, and then stained separately for oligosaccharides (A) and peptides (B). Additional peptide bands were present only in the samples from the affected brothers (lanes 4 and 5). Lane 1, normal control; lanes 2 and 3, parents; lane 6, unaffected brother; lane 7A, blood group A trisaccharide, GalNAcα1→3[Fucα1→2]Gal as standard (std); and lane 7B, GalNAcα1→*O*-Ser/Thr as standard (std). See Schindler *et al.* (1990) for details.

4GlcNAcβ1$\rightarrow$6(NeuNAcα2$\rightarrow$3Galβ1$\rightarrow$3)-GalNAcα1$\rightarrow$*O*-serine and -threonine, and GalNAcα1$\rightarrow$*O*-serine and -threonine. Only the older affected sibling, who was blood group type A positive, excreted the blood group A trisaccharide, GalNAcα1$\rightarrow$3(Fucα1$\rightarrow$2)Gal (Linden *et al.*, 1989). Thus, the analysis of the urinary components demonstrated the accumulation of glycoconjugates with terminal and internal α-*N*-acetylgalactosaminyl residues.

NEUROPATHOLOGICAL STUDIES

Ultrastructural studies of biopsied rectal tissue from the younger affected sibling detected abnormal tubulovesicular material free in the cytoplasm in only a few preterminal and terminal (intraganglionic) axons in the myenteric plexus. Subsequently, examination of frontal lobe brain biopsy tissue from the older affected sibling showed the characteristic neuropathology of neuroaxonal dystrophy (Wolfe *et al.*, 1989). Histologically, there was no obvious nerve cell loss. There were numerous, large, dense axonal swellings or 'spheroids' throughout the neocortex with no apparent laminar distribution; very few of these formations were observed in axons in the white matter. The deposits were sharply demarcated, rounded or polygonal structures which contained prominent angular or curving clefts in a darker amorphous background (Figure 4). Ultrastructurally, these abnormal formations were exclusively within preterminal and terminal axons and were not observed in neuronal perikarya, dendrites, axons in white matter, small axon terminals in the cortical neuropil, astrocytes, oligodendrocytes, microglia, endothelial, or arachnoid cells. The accumulations were morphologically heterogeneous, comprising dense labyrinthine membranous tubulovesicular formations, looser membranous whorls, regular or even paracrystalline vesicular arrays, and angular electron-lucent clefts, all admixed with a few mitochondria, lysosomes, and occasional microtubules. These aggregates were free in the axoplasm and were limited by a plasmalemma facing a narrow interspace.

Since the clinical and neuropathological findings in the older affected sibling clearly classified this disease as an infantile neuroaxonal dystrophy, efforts were directed to determine the α-*N*-acetylgalactosaminidase activity in unrelated patients with Seitelberger disease (Schindler *et al.*, 1989). In eight biopsy- or autopsy-proven cases, the α-*N*-acetylgalactosaminidase activities in plasma, cultured cells or cortical tissue were within the normal range. Thus, α-*N*-acetylgalactosaminidase deficiency is not the enzymatic defect in these unrelated patients with infantile neuroaxonal dystrophy, and the phenotype of infantile neuroaxonal dystrophy is biochemically heterogeneous.

NATURE OF THE MOLECULAR DEFECT

The cDNA encoding human α-*N*-acetylgalactosaminidase has been isolated, sequenced and expressed (Wang *et al.*, in press). To investigate the nature of the genetic lesion in the brothers with α-*N*-acetylgalactosaminidase deficiency, a series of molecular studies were performed using the α-*N*-acetylgalactosaminidase cDNA as a probe (Wang *et al.*, 1988). Southern analyses did not detect any gene rearrangements. Northern analyses showed transcripts of normal size and abundancy, excluding the possibility of splice junction mutations or transcriptional mutations. In order to

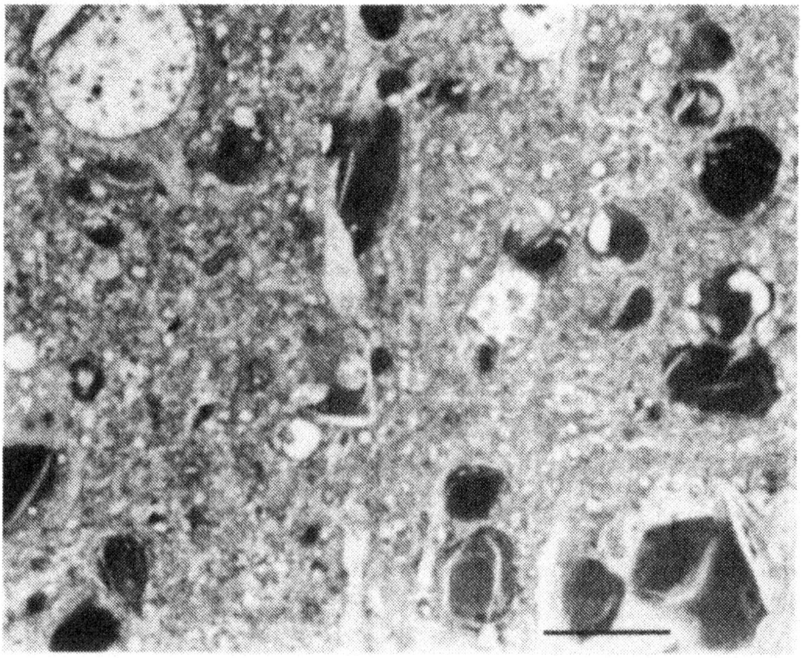

Figure 4 Light photomicrograph of neocortex. Abundant discrete deposits of axonal swellings appear throughout the cortical neuropil (toluidine-blue-stained semithin plastic section). Bar = 10 μm. See Schindler *et al.* (1989) for details.

identify a mutation due to a single base pair substitution within the coding region of the gene, total RNA was isolated from the lymphoblastoid line of one affected sibling, reverse transcribed and amplified by the polymerase chain reaction (PCR) using α-*N*-acetylgalactosaminidase specific primers. The PCR products were sequenced and revealed the presence of a single base pair substitution which was confirmed in PCR-amplified genomic DNA using allele-specific oligonucleotide probes.

CONCLUSION

Among inherited neurological diseases, the neuroaxonal dystrophies constitute a group of neurodegenerative disorders characterized by a common axonal lesion (Seitelberger, 1986). These disorders include the infantile form of neuroaxonal dystrophy (Seitelberger disease), late-infantile and juvenile forms of neuroaxonal dystrophy, neuroaxonal leukodystrophy, and Hallervorden–Spatz disease which has late-infantile-, juvenile- and adult-onset forms. The morphological hallmark of these disorders is the presence of swellings or 'spheroids' which are observed histologically in the terminal endings and/or in the distal portions of axons in the central nervous system. Ultrastructurally, these axonal swellings contain densely packed layers of smooth endoplasmic reticulum and other membranous arrays into which mitochondria, lysosomes, and a variety of other organelles and granular particles are interspersed. Presumably, the common neuropathology in these disorders results from abnormalities in axonal transport and/or metabolism. However, neither the pathogenesis nor the metabolic basis for any of these disorders has been elucidated previously.

The studies described here led to the identification of the enzymatic defect in a family with one form of infantile neuroaxonal dystrophy. The pursuit and delineation of this new disease entity was the result of collaborative clinical, pathological, biochemical and molecular investigations. The predominant neuroaxonal dystrophy and the paucity of lysosomal storage in α-*N*-acetylgalactosaminidase deficiency implicate a causal relationship between the deficiency of this enzyme and the resultant axonal pathology. Seitelberger proposed that the dystrophic axons resulted from defective retrograde axonal transport (Seitelberger, 1986). However, little is known about the nature of the transport vesicles, their membrane receptors or the lysosomal- and Golgi-mediated events involved in retrograde transport. Further pursuit, including the characterization of the role of neuronal α-*N*-acetylgalactosaminidase and the metabolism of α-*N*-acetylgalactosaminyl-containing compounds, may provide insight into the mechanisms of axonal transport as well as into the biochemical basis of the other forms of neuroaxonal dystrophy.

ACKNOWLEDGEMENTS

This work was supported in part by a grant (5 R01 DK34045) from the National Institutes of Health, a grant (1-578) from the March of Dimes Birth Defects Foundation, and a grant (RR-71) for the General Clinical Research Center from the Division of Research Resources, National Institutes of Health. AMW is the recipient of a predoctoral fellowship in medical genetics from the National Institutes of Health (5 T32 HD07105).

REFERENCES

Aula, P., Autio, S., Raivio, K. O., Rapola, J., Thoden, D. J., Koskela, W. L. and Yamashina, I. Salla disease: a new lysosomal storage disorder. *Arch. Neurol.* 36 (1979) 88–94

Cooper, A., Sardharwalla, I. B. and Roberts, M. M. Human β-mannosidase deficiency. *N. Engl. J. Med.* 315 (1986) 1231

Garrod, A. E. Inborn errors of metabolism (Croonian Lectures). *Lancet* 2 (1908) 1, 73, 142, 214

Griffin, J. W. and Watson, D. F. Axonal transport in neurological disease. *Ann. Neurol.* 68 (1988) 65–73

Harvey, W. Opera Omnia: a collegio medicorum londinensi edita: MDCCLXVI Epistola Octava Londoni excudebal. Bowyer, G., London, 1766, pp. 634–635

Linden, H. U., Klein, R. A., Egge, H., Peter-Katalinic, J., Dabrowski, J. and Schindler, D. Isolation and structural characterization of sialic acid-containing glycopeptides of the O-glycosidic type from the urine of two patients with an hereditary deficiency in α-*N*-acetylgalactosaminidase activity. *Biol. Chem. Hoppe-Seyler* 370 (1989) 661–672

Schindler, D., Bishop, D. F., Wolfe, D. E., Wang, A. M., Egge, H., Lemieux, R. U. and Desnick, R.J. A neuroaxonal dystrophy due to lysosomal α-*N*-acetylgalactosaminidase deficiency. *N. Engl. J. Med.* 320 (1989) 1735–1740

Schindler, D., Kanzaki, T. and Desnick, R. J. A method for the rapid detection of urinary glycopeptides in α-*N*-acetylgalactosaminidase deficiency and other lysosomal storage diseases. *Clin. Chim. Acta* (in press)

Seitelberger, F. Neuroaxonal dystrophy: its relation to aging and neurological disease. In: Vinken, P. J., Bruyn, G. W. and Klawans, H. L. (eds.), *Handbook of Clinical Neurology*, Vol. 49, 1986, pp. 391–415

van Diggelen, O. P., Schindler, D., Kleijer, W. J., Huijmans, J. M. G., Galjaard, H., Linden, H. U., Peter-Katalinic, J., Egge, H., Dabrowski, U. and Cantz, M. Lysosomal α-*N*-acetylgalactosaminidase deficiency. A new inherited metabolic disease. *Lancet* 2 (1987) 804

van Diggelen, O. P., Schindler, D., Willemsen, R., Boer, M., Kleijer, W. J., Huijmans, J. G. M., Blom, W. and Galjaard, H. α-*N*-Acetylgalactosaminidase deficiency, a new lysosomal storage disorder. *J. Inher. Metab. Dis.* 11 (1988) 349–357

van Pelt, J., van Bilsen, G. J. L., Kamerling, J. P. and Vliegenthart, J. F. G. Structural analysis of O-glycoside type of sialyloglycosaccharide-alditols derived from urinary glycopeptides of a sialidosis patient. *Eur. J. Biochem.* 174 (1988) 183–187

Wang, A. M., Schindler, D., Bishop, D. F., Lemieux, R. U. and Desnick, R. J. Schindler disease: Biochemical and molecular characterization of a new neuroaxonal dystrophy due to α-*N*-acetylgalactosaminidase deficiency. *Am. J. Hum. Genet* 43 (1988) A99

Wang, A. M., Bishop, D. F. and Desnick, R. J. Human α-*N*-acetylgalactosaminidase: Isolation, nucleotide sequence and expression of the full-length cDNA., in press

Wenger, D. A., Targy, J. F. and Wharton, C. Macular cherry-red spots and a myoclonus with dementia: Co-existent neuraminidase and β-galactosidase deficiencies. *Biochem. Biophys. Res. Commun.* 82 (1978) 589–59

Wenger, D. A., Sujansky, E., Fennessey, P. F. and Thompson, J. N. Human β-mannosidase deficiency. *N. Engl. J. Med.* 315 (1986) 1201–1205

Wolfe, D., Schindler, D., Desnick, R. J. and Perl, D. Infantile neuroaxonal dystrophy (INAD) associated with a lysosomal enzyme deficiency. *J. Neuropathol. Exp. Neurol.* 48 (1989) 349

J. Inher. Metab. Dis. 13 (1990) 560–571

Advances in the Molecular Genetics of Metachromatic Leukodystrophy

V. GIESELMANN and K. VON FIGURA
Georg August University, Biochemie II, Gosslerstrasse 12d, D-3400 Göttingen, FRG

Summary: Metachromatic leukodystrophy is a lysosomal storage disorder caused by the deficiency of arylsulphatase A (EC 3.1.6.1). This results in the intralysosomal storage of cerebroside sulphate, which leads to a progressive demyelination of the nervous system. The patients usually die within a few years from the onset of symptoms. Clinically, there are different forms of the disease and the molecular basis for this heterogeneity is unknown. The gene for arylsulphatase A has recently been cloned and provides a necessary tool for the exact description of the molecular defects occurring in the different forms of metachromatic leukodystrophy. Metachromatic leukodystrophy can also be caused by the deficiency of an arylsulphatase A activator protein (sphingolipid activator protein B). The cDNA for the precursor of this protein has been isolated and a mutant cDNA of one patient has been analysed. A substantial arylsulphatase A deficiency can also occur in healthy individuals, a phenotype termed pseudodeficiency. Two concurrent mutations have been identified in this low arylsulphatase A activity allele. This permitted the development of a rapid assay which allows the detection of the pseudodeficiency allele. Bone marrow transplantation has been tried in several metachromatic leukodystrophy patients and there is evidence that this treatment might slow or even halt the progression of the disease. A final conclusion as to whether bone marrow transplantation is a suitable therapy for metachromatic leukodystrophy cannot be drawn yet.

Metachromatic leukodystrophy is a recessively inherited disease, the frequency of which is estimated to be 1:40000 (Gustavson *et al.*, 1971). The disease was first recognized as an entity by Scholz in 1925 who described his pathological findings in three affected children from one family (Scholz, 1925). However, due to the particular staining procedure he used, he missed the typical metachromatic glycolipid inclusions in the nervous system which later gave the disease its name (Peiffer, 1959). Two groups independently identified the material stored in these inclusions as cerebroside sulphate (Jatzkewitz, 1958; Austin, 1959) and some years later arylsulphatase A deficiency was recognized as the genetic defect causing metachromatic leukodystrophy (Austin, 1963; Mehl *et al.*, 1965).

Arylsulphatase A catalyses the first step in the degradation pathway of galactosyl-3-sulphate ceramide (cerebroside sulphate), one of the major membrane lipids of the myelin sheaths. When this desulphation step does not occur due to arylsulphatase A deficiency the substrate accumulates.

The storage of cerebroside sulphate has been described in many tissues of metachromatic leukodystrophy patients. The storage mainly affects the nervous system, where it is associated with a progressive demyelination. The clinical symptoms are a delay in neurological development, weakness, ataxia, progressive spastic tetraparesis, optic atrophy and dementia (Kolodny *et al.*, 1983). The disease is lethal. Based on the age of onset and the severity of the symptoms, three different clinical forms are distinguished: a late infantile form (about 60% of all cases), a juvenile form (30%), and an adult form (10%) (Kolodny *et al.*, 1983). The molecular basis for this heterogeneity is unknown, although low levels of enzyme activity can be detected in samples from the later onset cases.

A rare form of metachromatic leukodystrophy is caused by the deficiency of a sphingolipid activator protein which physiologically solubilizes the hydrophobic substrates for the enzymatic action of arylsulphatase A. The clinical picture resembles that of a juvenile (Shapiro *et al.*, 1979) or late infantile (Wenger *et al.*, 1989) form of metachromatic leukodystrophy.

Occasionally, low arylsulphatase A activities are observed in individuals who are clinically healthy (Dubois *et al.*, 1977). This condition has been designated as arylsulphatase A pseudodeficiency. The frequent occurrence of these low activity alleles creates a problem in the pre- and postnatal diagnosis of metachromatic leukodystrophy. Metachromatic leukodystrophy and pseudodeficiency cannot be distinguished reliably by measurement of enzyme activity with commonly employed arylsulphatase A substrates.

This article will review the progress which has been made during the last few years in the molecular biology and treatment of metachromatic leukodystrophy. This includes the cloning of the arylsulphatase A gene and the cDNA for the activator protein. It will discuss the mutations occurring in the arylsulphatase A pseudodeficiency allele and approaches to treating metachromatic leukodystrophy by bone marrow transplantation.

MOLECULAR BIOLOGY OF ARYLSULPHATASE A

The cloning of an arylsulphatase A cDNA has been described recently (Stein *et al.*, 1989). The structure of this arylsulphatase A cDNA is shown in Figure 1. It is 2027 bp long and has an open reading frame of 1521 bp. The 5′ untranslated region is 363 bp long and the 3′ untranslated region is 140 bp. A canonical polyadenylation signal AATAAC is present at position 1621 of the cDNA. The coding region starts with a putative 18 amino acid signal peptide, followed by a sequence which codes for a protein of 489 amino acids. The calculated molecular weight of this protein is in good agreement with the 62 kDa for arylsulphatase A polypeptides found in biosynthesis studies (Waheed *et al.*, 1982). Besides this 62 kDa polypeptide, an additional 54–59 kDa form of arylsulphatase A can be detected in metabolic labelling experiments (Waheed *et al.*, 1982) or Western blot analysis (Hohenschutz *et al.*, 1988). It is most likely that the 62 kDa polypeptide represents the precursor of arylsulphatase A, which is proteolytically processed to the smaller 54–57 kDa forms. However, a

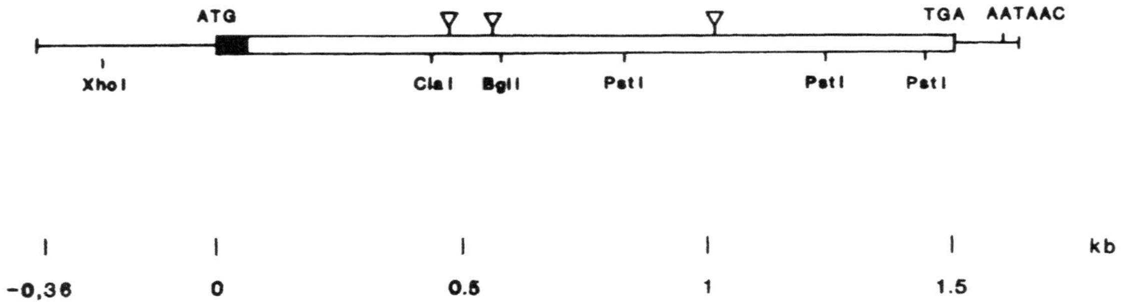

Figure 1 Structure of the arylsulphatase A cDNA. The bar shows the coding regions of the cDNA, the filled part of the bar the signal peptide. ATG and TGA indicate the initiation or stop codon, respectively. AATAAC is the sequence of the polyadenylation signal. Y shows potential glycosylation sites. The numbers at the bottom indicate kb.

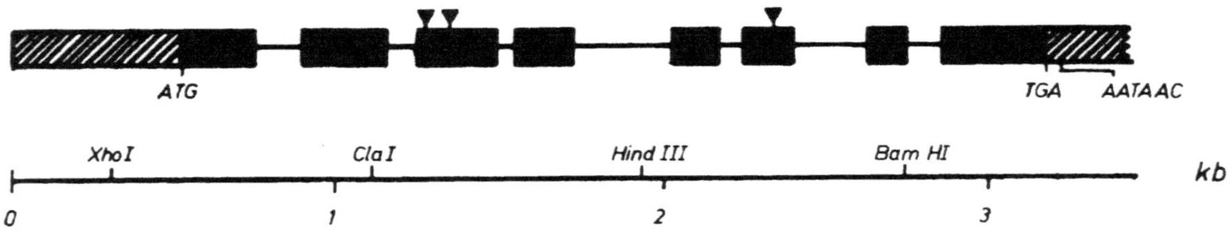

Figure 2 Structure of the arylsulphatase A gene. Bars indicate exons, hatched parts of the bars 5' or 3' untranslated regions. Y shows potential glycosylation sites. The positions of start codon (ATG), stop codon (TGA) and the first polyadenylation signal (AATAAC) downstream of the stop codon are shown. A scale in kb and the positions of unique restriction sites are shown below.

precursor product relationship between these products has not yet been proven.

Three potential N-glycosylation sites are found in the arylsulphatase A cDNA. It has been shown earlier that arylsulphatase A has only two oligosaccharide side chains (Waheed *et al.*, 1983). Which of the three potential sites are actually used is not known, although there is evidence that site 2 (position 550–558) might not be glycosylated (Gieselmann, unpublished observations). The arylsulphatase A cDNA was used to clone the arylsulphatase A gene from a human genomic library (Kreysing *et al.*, 1989). One of the clones isolated had a 14 kb insert. The entire arylsulphatase A gene was present on a 6 kb EcoRI fragment contained in this insert. Sequencing and restriction mapping of the 6 kb fragment revealed the arylsulphatase A gene structure, which is depicted in Figure 2. The entire coding sequence of the gene encompasses just 3.2 kb and is divided into eight exons. The cap site of the mRNA has been mapped about 365 bp upstream of the ATG start codon. Knowing the structure of the gene and its restriction sites, we have analysed 34 different metachromatic leukodystrophy cell lines by Southern blot analysis. None of these had major deletions or rearrangements, suggesting that in most of the cases a defect in metachromatic leukodystrophy alleles is due to point mutations or small insertions or deletions. This is in good agreement with our finding that out of seven metachromatic leukodystrophy cell lines tested by Northern blot analysis for the presence of arylsulphatase A mRNAs, only one failed to show any arylsulphatase A RNA (Gieselmann, unpublished observations).

In normal human fibroblasts three different arylsulphatase A RNA species of 2.1, 3.7 and 4.8 kb are found (Stein *et al.*, 1989). The 2.1 kb mRNA accounts for about 30–40% and the 3.7 and 4.8 kb species for 60–70% of total arylsulphatase A RNA. Upon purification of poly A^+ RNA, most of the two larger RNA species is lost, suggesting that those forms are poorly polyadenylated. The translational efficiencies of the different arylsulphatase A RNA species are unknown. They probably arise from the use of different polyadenylation signals, although the signals for the 3.7 and 4.8 kb species have not been identified as yet.

So far no mutant metachromatic leukodystrophy arylsulphatase A allele has been characterized. The availability of an arylsulphatase A cDNA probe and the knowledge of the gene structure will allow the molecular characterization of these alleles in the near future.

MOLECULAR BIOLOGY OF THE ARYLSULPHATASE A ACTIVATOR PROTEIN (SPHINGOLIPID ACTIVATOR PROTEIN B)

Several different sphingolipid activator proteins have been identified. In different publications these proteins have been given different names resulting in a rather confusing nomenclature. Here we will use the nomenclature suggested by Morimoto and colleagues (1988). The alternative names of the activator proteins discussed here are given in Table 1, which summarizes the major properties of the different proteins.

Sphingolipid activator protein B activates the hydrolysis of cerebroside sulphate, G_{M1}-ganglioside and globotriaosyl ceramide by arylsulphatase A (EC 3.1.6.1), β-galactosidase (EC 3.2.1.23) and α-galactosidase (EC 3.2.1.2), respectively (see Morimoto *et al.*, 1988 for detailed references). The protein interacts with the substrate

Table 1 Summary of the properties of the sphingolipid activator proteins derived from the precursor protein encoded by the cDNA discussed in the text and shown in Figure 3

	Alternative names	*Activated enzymes*	*Mode of activation*
SAP A	Saposin A	β-glucosylceramidase β-galactosylceramidase	Increases V_{max}
SAP B	Saposin B SAP 1 Cerebroside sulphatase activator G_{M1} activator Dispersion non-specific activator protein	Arylsulphatase A β-galactosidase α-galactosidase	Solubilizes hydrophobic substrates for enzyme hydrolysis
SAP C	Saposin C SAP 2 Factor P Glucocerebrosidase activator Coglucosidase A_1 activator	β-glucosylceramidase β-galactosylceramidase Sphingomyelinase	Increases V_{max}
SAP D	Saposin D Component C	Sphingomyelinase	Increases V_{max}

SAP = sphingolipid activator protein

and solubilizes it for enzymatic hydrolysis (Fischer *et al.*, 1977). It was recently shown that sphingolipid activator protein B has a broad substrate specificity acting on many different glycolipids (Li *et al.*, 1988). It functions as a detergent and this mode of action is likely to be less specific than that of other sphingolipid activator proteins which act on the enzymes directly. The deficiency of this protein causes a disease resembling juvenile or late infantile metachromatic leukodystrophy (Shapiro *et al.*, 1979; Wenger *et al.*, 1989). The nucleotide sequence of a sphingolipid activator protein B cDNA was reported in 1986 and 1987 (Dewji *et al.*, 1986, 1987). Clones were isolated by screening an expression library in λgt11 with an antibody against sphingolipid activator protein B. Full-length cDNA clones coding for a protein of 527 amino acids have been isolated by two groups (O'Brien *et al.*, 1988; Nakano *et al.*, 1989). From biosynthesis studies it was known that sphingolipid activator protein B is synthesized as a large 70 kDa precursor so that extensive proteolytic processing was thought to occur to yield the mature, rather small 9–11 kDa activator protein (Fujibayashi *et al.*, 1986).

The same group (O'Brien *et al.*, 1988) cloned the cDNA of sphingolipid activator protein C, which is involved in the degradation of glycosyl ceramide, galactosyl ceramide and sphingomyelin by β-glucosyl ceraminidase (EC 3.2.1.45), galactosyl ceramide β-galactosidase (EC 1.2.1.46) and sphingomyelinase (EC 1.1.4.12) (see Morimoto *et al.*, 1988 for detailed references). By taking the same approach as for sphingolipid activator protein B they found that the nucleotide sequence of sphingolipid activator protein C was colinear with that of sphingolipid activator protein B (O'Brien, 1988). The coding sequence of sphingolipid activator protein C was on the same cDNA located 3′ of that of sphingolipid activator protein B. Both sequences are separated by 108 nucleotides which are in the same open reading frame. This showed that sphingolipid activator protein B and sphingolipid activator protein C are products of the same genetic locus and are derived from the same precursor protein by proteolytic processing. When the coding region of the entire cDNA was analysed for homologous sequences, four sphingolipid activator protein-like domains of about 80 amino acids each were identified. The homology was based on the identical placement of cysteines, conserved prolines and positions of potential glycosylation sites. Thus, the cDNA codes for a precursor protein with four domains separated by regions which are cleaved proteolytically to yield the four sphingolipid activator proteins. The structure of the cDNA is shown in Figure 3.

Before the sphingolipid activator protein C cDNA was cloned and its colinearity with the sphingolipid activator protein B cDNA was revealed, the amino acid sequence of the fourth sphingolipid activator protein-like domain was published (Fürst *et al.*, 1988). During the purification of the G_{M2}-ganglioside activator, this group isolated a protein they called component C, which showed homology to sphingolipid activator protein B, and they noticed that the amino acid sequence of component C was contained in the cDNA deduced amino acid sequence of the C-terminal part of sphingolipid activator protein B, which at that time was thought to be processed proteolytically and to be without function. Based on their amino acid sequence data and the cDNA sequence published by Dewji *et al.* (1987), they suggested that both proteins – component C and sphingolipid activator protein B – are derived from the same precursor, which was then confirmed by the sphingolipid activator protein C cDNA cloning (O'Brien *et al.*, 1988). When the colinearity of the sphingolipid activator proteins was revealed the functions of the sphingolipid activator protein A and sphingolipid activator protein D proteins derived from domains 1 and 4 of the precursor protein were unknown, but they have been elucidated in the meantime.

Sphingolipid activator protein A was found to activate β-glucosylceramidase and β-galactosylceramidase by increasing the maximal velocity of the reaction. Its action resembles that of sphingolipid activator protein C, but sphingolipid activator protein A does not activate sphingomyelinase (Morimoto *et al.*, 1989). Sphingolipid activator protein D only stimulates the activity of sphingomyelinase, again by increasing the

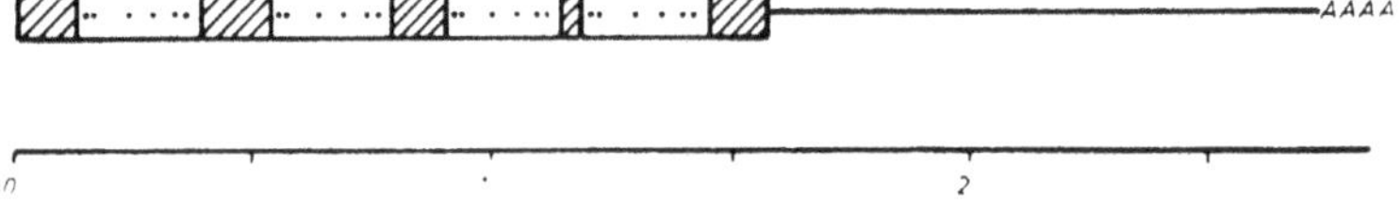

Figure 3 Structure of the sphingolipid activator precursor proteins cDNA. Coding regions are shown as a bar; hatched parts are regions separating the sphingolipid activator proteins. ▼ shows potential glycosylation sites and points show conserved cysteine residues, the patterns of which are very similar in all four domains (modified from Fürst *et al.*, 1988; O'Brien *et al.*, 1988; Nakano *et al.*, 1989).

maximal velocity (Morimoto *et al.*, 1988). The properties of all the sphingolipid activator proteins are summarized in Table 1.

In a patient suffering from metachromatic leukodystrophy caused by sphingolipid activator protein B deficiency, a C → T transition has been described recently (Kretz *et al.*, 1989). This changes a threonine which is part of a potential glycosylation site to isoleucine. The loss of this glycosylation site might alter sphingolipid activator protein B stability or processing pattern. Increased degradation or altered proteolytic processing might render the molecule non-functional.

THE ARYLSULPHATASE A PSEUDODEFICIENCY ALLELE

Low activity of arylsulphatase A can occur in individuals who are clinically healthy. This phenotype has been designated as arylsulphatase A pseudodeficiency. The existence of these pseudodeficiency alleles poses a serious problem (Baldinger *et al.*, 1987) in genetic counselling and prenatal diagnosis of families at risk for metachromatic leukodystrophy. Based on enzyme activity determinations, patients homozygous for metachromatic leukodystrophy alleles cannot be reliably distinguished from those who are homozygous for the pseudodeficiency allele or who carry one pseudodeficiency and one metachromatic leukodystrophy allele. The problem is aggravated by the high frequency of the pseudodeficiency allele in the population, which has been estimated to be between 7% and 15% (Herz *et al.*, 1984; Hohenschutz *et al.*, 1989).

Discrimination between metachromatic leukodystrophy and pseudodeficiency is possible by using the so-called cerebroside sulphate loading test (Kihara *et al.*, 1980), in which the cells are exposed to the radioactively labelled natural substrate of arylsulphatase A and the turnover of this substrate is measured. Pseudodeficiency fibroblasts catabolize this substrate at almost normal rates, whereas metachromatic leukodystrophy fibroblasts do not. However, this assay is time-consuming and the results are very sensitive to culture conditions (Tonnessen *et al.*, 1984), restricting the application of this assay to laboratories with particular experience.

The low arylsulphatase A activity of individuals homozygous for the pseudodeficiency allele is apparently sufficient to prevent the development of a disease. Individuals carrying one metachromatic leukodystrophy allele and one pseudodeficiency allele might have a residual arylsulphatase A activity too low to prevent lysosomal storage of cerebroside sulphate and neurological or psychiatric symptoms might occur later in life. One such patient was described recently (Hohenschutz *et al.*, 1988), in whom such symptoms were associated with compound heterozygosity for the metachromatic leukodystrophy and pseudodeficiency alleles. The patient had a residual arylsulphatase A activity of 5%, intermediate between adult metachromatic leukodystrophy (2.5%) and pseudodeficiency (23%). At the age of 52 she was diagnosed as having encephalomyelitis disseminata with various neuropsychiatric symptoms. The identification of this single patient does not establish a causal relationship between symptoms and metachromatic leukodystrophy/pseudodeficiency genotype: the association of the symptoms with the arylsulphatase A genotype may be coincidental. In order to establish whether this genotype bears any health risk, more such individuals have to be identified and examined clinically. If metachromatic leukodystrophy/pseudodeficiency compound heterozygosity does implicate the development of a disease, it would be one of the most frequently inherited disorders. Given the gene frequencies of the metachromatic leukodystrophy and pseudodeficiency alleles, the frequency of compound heterozygotes should be approximately 1 : 1000. However, it is hard to imagine that a genetic disorder of such a high frequency would not yet have been discovered. It therefore seems more likely that the compound heterozygosity predisposes for the development of other neurological diseases or has no effect at all.

The arylsulphatase A polypeptides found in pseudodeficiency fibroblasts are about 2.5 kDa smaller in size and are reduced in quantity when compared to normal fibroblasts (Bach *et al.*, 1983; Fluharty *et al.*, 1983). The reduced size is due to the loss of an N-glycosylation site, which has been thought to alter the stability of the molecule leading to an attenuated activity. Recently, our group has shown that in pseudodeficiency fibroblasts the synthesis of arylsulphatase A and not the stability is reduced. It was unclear how the loss of an N-glycosylation site could account for reduced synthesis of arylsulphatase A.

To allow a further molecular characterization of the pseudodeficiency allele, the arylsulphatase A gene was cloned from a library made of size-selected DNA from an individual homozygous for the pseudodeficiency allele, and the gene was sequenced. Two A → G transitions were found. One changes an asparagine at cDNA position 1049 to serine and causes the loss of a N-glycosylation site. Introduction of this mutation into a normal cDNA by site-directed mutagenesis and its expression in BHK cells showed that neither the catalytic activity nor the stability of the underglycosylated pseudodeficiency arylsulphatase A was altered when compared to normal arylsulphatase A. The loss of the N-glycosylation site does not therefore contribute to the attenuated arylsulphatase A activity in pseudodeficiency fibroblasts. The second A → G transition changes the sequence of the first polyadenylation signal downstream of the stop codon from AATAAC to AGTAAC. The loss of this polyadenylation signal does not allow the proper termination of the 2.1 kb arylsulphatase A mRNA species, which is therefore deficient in pseudodeficiency fibroblasts. The absence of one of the arylsulphatase A RNA species provides an explanation for the reduced synthesis of arylsulphatase A polypeptides in the pseudodeficiency (Gieselmann *et al.*, 1989).

Thus, the pseudodeficiency allele carries two mutations (see Figure 4), only one of which causes the attenuation of arylsulphatase A activity. It is reasonable to expect that alleles might exist in which only one of these mutations is present. Based on the knowledge of these two mutations an assay is now available which allows the rapid detection of the pseudodeficiency allele by using polymerase chain reaction and oligonucleotide specific hybridization. This assay will facilitate the pre- and postnatal diagnosis of metachromatic leukodystrophy and the genetic counselling of families at risk for metachromatic leukodystrophy.

METACHROMATIC LEUKODYSTROPHY AND BONE MARROW TRANSPLANTATION

During the last few years several attempts have been made to treat metachromatic leukodystrophy with bone marrow transplantation. There were several rationales for

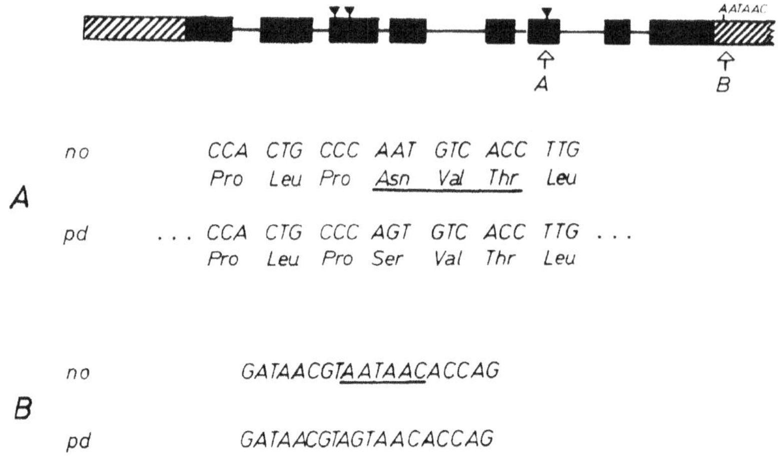

Figure 4 Mutations in the arylsulphatase A pseudodeficiency allele. At the top a map of the arylsulphatase A gene is shown. Arrows label parts of the gene in which the mutations shown below are located. no = normal allele. pd = pseudodeficiency allele. The potential glycosylation site and the polyadenylation signal in the wild type allele are underlined.

the use of this therapy in metachromatic leukodystrophy. Arylsulphatase A-deficient cells from metachromatic leukodystrophy patients can be supplemented by endocytosis of arylsulphatase A added to the medium (Porter *et al.*, 1971). Microglial cells were suspected to be derived from bone marrow cells and were thus thought to be suitable for delivering the enzyme across the blood–brain barrier. That microglial cells are indeed of bone marrow origin was recently proven (Hoogerbrugge *et al.*, 1988a). The delivery of deficient enzymes to the brain was demonstrated after bone marrow transplantation of dogs deficient in fucosidase (Taylor *et al.*, 1986), and of mice deficient in β-galactocerebroside-β-galactosidase (twitcher mouse – a model of Krabbe's globoid cell leukodystrophy in humans) (Hoogerbrugge *et al.*, 1988b). After transplantation the enzyme activity in the brains of the deficient animals was between 15% (twitcher mouse) and 35% (fucosidosis dog) of normal brain enzyme levels. In both animal models a reduction in the storage lesions was found histologically after bone marrow transplantation. The twitcher mouse showed a retardation in the development of the symptoms; however, in both animal models the fatal outcome of the disease could not be prevented (Yeager *et al.*, 1984; Taylor *et al.*, 1986; Hoogerbrugge *et al.*, 1988b).

Several patients with metachromatic leukodystrophy treated by bone marrow transplantation have been reported (Bayerer *et al.*, 1985; Krivit *et al.*, 1987). After bone marrow transplantation the clinical symptoms and the neurophysiological parameters did not improve but progression appeared to be abated. The clinical neurophysiological parameters measured pre- and post-transplantation included nerve conduction velocities, sural nerve biopsies, ophthalmic examinations, several neuropsychological tests, brainstem auditory evoked potentials and CT scans. When transplanted patients were compared to non-transplanted metachromatic leukodystrophy-affected siblings it was apparent that the development of symptoms was slowed (Bayerer *et al.*, 1985), and in one case deterioration due to the disease was prevented for several years (Krivit *et al.*, 1987). The disease usually progresses slowly over a period of several years and it is still too early to decide whether the disease process in the patients who have undergone bone marrow transplantation has been stopped or whether deterioration has just been delayed. Concern remains that bone marrow transplantation might convert a late infantile form of the disease into a juvenile or adult form. It is now under investigation whether a transplantation performed before the onset of symptoms can prevent the appearance of all disease symptoms, or at least provide an acceptable non-fatal outcome of the disease process.

ACKNOWLEDGEMENT

We thank Dr A. L. Fluharty for critical comments on the manuscript.

REFERENCES

Austin, J. Metachromatic sulfatides in cerebral white matter and kidney. *Proc. Soc. Exp. Biol. Med.* 100 (1959) 361

Austin, J. H., Balasubramanian, A. S., Patabiramen, T. N., Saraswathi, S., Basu, D. K.and Bachhawat, B. K. A controlled study of enzymatic activities in three human disorders of glycolipid metabolism. *J. Neurochem.* 10 (1963) 805

Bach, G. and Neufeld, E. F. Synthesis and maturation of cross reactive glycoprotein in fibroblasts deficient in arylsulfatase A activity. *Biochem. Biophys. Res. Commun.* 112 (1983) 198–205

Baldinger, S., Pierpont, M. E. and Wenger, D. A. Pseudodeficiency of arylsulfatase A: a counselling dilemma. *Clin. Genet.* 31 (1987) 70–76

Bayerer, E., Ladisch, S., Philippart, M., Brill, N., Nuwer, M., Sparkes, R. S. and Feig, S. A. Bone marrow transplantation for metachromatic leukodystrophy. *Lancet* 1 (1985) 471–473

Dewji, N. N., Wenger, D. A., Fujibayashi, S., Donoviel, M., Esch, F., Hill, F. and O'Brien, J. S. Molecular cloning of the sphingolipid activator protein-1 (SAP 1). The sulfatide sulfatase activator. *Biochem. Biophys. Res. Commun.* 134 (1986) 989–994

Dewji, N. N., Wenger, D. A. and O'Brien, J. S. Nucleotide sequence of cloned cDNA for human sphingolipid activator protein precursor. *Proc. Natl. Acad. Sci. USA* 84 (1987) 8652–8656

Dubois, G., Harzer, K. and Baumann, N. Very low arylsulfatase A and cerebroside sulfatase activities in leukocytes of healthy members of a metachromatic leukodystrophy family. *Am. J. Hum. Genet.* 29 (1977) 191–194

Fischer, G. and Jatzkewitz, H. The activator of cerebroside sulphatase. Binding studies with enzyme and substrate demonstrating the detergent function of the activator protein. *Biochim. Biophys. Acta* 481 (1977) 561–572

Fluharty, A. L., Meek, W. E. and Kihara, H. Pseudoarylsulfatase A deficiency: evidence for a structurally altered enzyme. *Biochem. Biophys. Res. Commun.* 112 (1983) 191–197

Fujibayashi, S. and Wenger, D. A. Biosynthesis of the sulfatide/G_{M1} activator protein (SAP-1) in control and mutant cultured skin fibroblasts. *Biochim. Biophys. Acta* 875 (1986) 554–562

Fürst, W., Machleidt, W. and Sandhoff, K. The precursor of sulfatide activator protein is processed to three different proteins. *Biol. Chem. Hoppe-Seyler* 369 (1988) 317–328

Gieselmann, V., Polten, A., Kreysing, J. and von Figura, K. Arylsulfatase pseudodeficiency:

Loss of a polyadenylation signal and N-glycosylation site. *Proc. Natl. Acad. Sci. USA* 86 (1989) 9436–9440

Gustavson, K. H. and Hagberg, B. The incidence and genetics of MLD in Northern Sweden. *Acta Pediatr. Scand.* 60 (1971) 585–590

Herz, B. and Bach, G. Arylsulfatase A in pseudodeficiency. *Hum. Genet.* 661 (1984) 147–150

Hohenschutz, C., Friedl, W., Schlör, K. H., Waheed, A., Conzelmann, E., Sandhoff, K. and Propping, P. Probable metachromatic leukodystrophy/pseudodeficiency compound heterozygote at an arylsulfatase A locus with neurologic and psychiatric symptomatology. *Am. J. Med. Genet.* 31 (1988) 169–175

Hohenschutz, C., Eich, P., Friedl, W., Waheed, A., Conzelmann, E. and Propping, P. Pseudodeficiency of arylsulfatase A: a common genetic polymorphism with possible disease implications. *Hum. Genet.* 82 (1989) 45–48

Hoogerbrugge, P. M., Suzuki, K., Suzuki, K. *et al.* Donor derived cells in the central nervous system of twitcher mice after bone marrow transplantation. *Science* 239 (1988a) 1035–1038

Hoogerbrugge, P. M., Poorthuis, B. J., Romme, A. E., van de Kamp, J. J., Wagemaker, G. and von Bekkum, D. W. Effect of bone marrow transplantation on enzyme levels and clinical course in the neurologically affected twitcher mouse. *J. Clin. Invest.* 81 (1988b) 1790–1794

Jatzkewitz, H. Zwei Typen von Cerebrosidschwefelsäureestern als sog. Prälipoide und Speichersubstanzen bei der metachromatischen Leukodystrophie. *Z. Physiol. Chem.* 311 (1958) 279

Kihara, H., Chen-Kung, H., Fluharty, A. L., Tsay, K. K., Hartlage, P. L. Prenatal diagnosis of metachromatic leukodystrophy in a family with pseudodarylsulfatase A deficiency by the cerebroside sulfate loading test. *Pediatr. Res.* 14 (1980) 224–227

Kolodny, E. H., Moser, H. W. Sulfatide lipidosis: metachromatic leukodystrophy. In Stanbury, J. B., Wyngaarden, J. B., Fredrickson, D. S., Goldstein, J. L. and Brown, M. S. (eds.) *The Metabolic Basis of Inherited Diseases*, McGraw-Hill, New York, 1983, pp. 881–905

Kretz, K., Ginns, E., Carson, G., Morimoto, S., Kishimoto, Y., Fluharty, A. L. and O'Brien, J. S. Characterization of a mutation in a family with saposin B deficiency. *Am. Soc. Hum. Genet.* (1989) abstract

Kreysing, J., von Figura, K. and Gieselmann, V. The structure of the human arylsulfatase A gene. *ESGLD Meeting (1989)*, Ittingen, abstract

Krivit, W., Lipton, M. E., Lockman, L. A., Tsai, M., Dyck, P. J., Smith, S., Ramsay, N. K. C. and Kersey, J. Prevention of deterioration in metachromatic leukodystrophy by bone marrow transplantation. *Am. J. Med. Sci.* 294 (1987) 80–85

Li, S. C., Sonnino, S., Tettamanti, G. and Li, Y. T. Characterization of a non-specific activator protein for the enzymatic hydrolysis of glycolipids. *J. Biol. Chem.* 263 (1988) 6588–6591

Mehl, E. and Jatzkewitz, H. Evidence for the genetic block in metachromatic leukodystrophy. *Biochem. Biophys. Res. Commun.* 19 (1965) 407

Morimoto, S., Martin, B. M., Kishimoto, Y. and O'Brien, J. S. Saposin D: A sphingomyelinase activator. *Biochem. Biophys. Res. Commun.* 156 (1988) 403–410

Morimoto, S., Martin, B. M., Yamamoto, Y., Kretz, K. A., O'Brien, J. S. and Kishimoto, Y. Saposin A: Second cerebrosidase activator protein. *Proc. Natl. Acad. Sci. USA* 86 (1989) 3389–3393

Nakano, T., Sandhoff, K., Stümper, J., Christomanou, H. and Suzuki, K. Structure of full length cDNA coding for sulfatide activator, a co-β-glucosidase and two other homologous proteins: Two alternate forms of the sulfatide activator. *J. Biochem. Tokyo* 105 (1989) 152–154

O'Brien, J. S., Kretz, K. A., Dewji, N. N., Wenger, D. A., Esch, F. and Fluharty, A. L. Coding of two sphingolipid activator proteins (SAP 1 and SAP 2) by the same genetic locus. *Science* 234 (1988) 1098–1101

Peiffer, J. Über die metachromatischen Leukodystrophien (Typ Scholz). *Arch. Psychiatr. Nervenkr.* 199 (1959) 386

Porter, N. T., Fluharty, A. L. and Kihara, H. Correction of abnormal cerebroside sulfate metabolism in cultured metachromatic leukodystrophy fibroblasts. *Science* 172 (1971) 1263–1265

Scholz, W. Klinische, pathologisch anatomische und erbbiologische Untersuchungen bei familiärer diffuser Hirnsklerose im Kindesalter. *Z. Gesamte Neurol. Psychiatr.* 99 (1925) 42

Shapiro, L. J., Aleck, K. A., Kaback, M. M., Itabashi, H., Desnick, R. J., Brand, N., Stevens, R. L., Fluharty, R. L. and Kihara, H. Metachromatic leukodystrophy without arylsulfatase A deficiency. *Pediatr. Res.* 13 (1979) 1179

Stein, C., Gieselmann, V., Kreysing, J., Schmidt, B., Pohlmann, R., Waheed, A., Meyer, E. H., O'Brien, J. S. and von Figura, K. Cloning and expression of human arylsulfatase A. *J. Biol. Chem.* 264 (1989) 1252–1259

Taylor, R. M., Farrow, B. R., Stewart, G. J., Healy, P. J. Enzyme replacement in nervous tissue after allogeneic bone marrow transplantation for fucosidosis in dogs. *Lancet* 1 (1986) 772–774

Tonnesen, T., Vrang, C., Wiesmann, U., Christomanou, H. and Lou, H. O. Atypical metachromatic leukodystrophy? *Hum. Genet.* 67 (1984) 170–173

Waheed, A., Hasilik, A. and von Figura, K. Synthesis and processing of arylsulfatase A in human skin fibroblasts. *Hoppe-Seyler's Z. Physiol. Chem.* 363 (1982) 425–430

Waheed, A., Steckel, F., Hasilik, A. and von Figura, K. Two allelic forms of human arylsulfatase A with different numbers of asparagine linked oligosaccharides. *Am. J. Hum. Genet.* 35 (1983) 228–233

Wenger, D. A., De Gala, G., Williams, C., Taylor, H. A., Stevenson, R. E., Pruitt, J. R., Miller, J., Garen, P. D. and Balentine, J. D. Clinical pathological and biochemical studies on an infantile case of sulfatide/G_{M1} activator protein deficiency. *Am. J. Med. Genet.* 33 (1989) 255–265

Yeager, A. M., Brennan, S., Tiffany, C., Moser, H. W. and Santos, W. G. Prolonged survival and remyelination after hematopoietic cell transplantation in the twitcher mouse. *Science* 225 (1984) 1052–1054

J. Inher. Metab. Dis. 13 (1990) 572–596

Displacement Bone Marrow Transplantation for Some Inborn Errors

J. R. HOBBS
Westminster Bone Marrow Team, Charing Cross and Westminster Medical School, Westminster Hospital, 17 Page Street, London SW1, UK

Summary: The initial simple bone marrow transplants for genetic immunodeficiency diseases could hardly be rejected by the host, but required matched sibling donors, only available for about 1 in 5 patients. Improved inductions enabled alternative donors from the family or unrelated volunteers to be used. Measurement of the extent of engraftment by donor cell markers or their normal enzymes showed the need for displacement, which aims to obtain 100% donor-type marrow so that the future immune responses of the recipient become those of the donor and tolerant to donor cells or their products. Immunoprophylaxis can prevent residual host immune cells from surviving to impair the graft. The concept of DBMT with immunoprophylaxis has evolved either to replace abnormal host cells or to confer a component transferable from donor cells to deficient host tissues. Within 10 years over 40 previously fatal genetic diseases have been satisfactorily corrected and seven partially corrected, but for five there has been inadequate delivery of component to genetically defective tissues such as heart, cartilage and brain. The principles can be applied to some 40 other genetic diseases for which no suitable alternative treatments yet exist.

The objective of displacement bone marrow transplantation (DBMT) is to obtain 100% healthy donor-type marrow which can correct an inborn error which was expressed in the bone marrow of the recipient and, at the same time, to endow the recipient with the immunology of the donor so that the healthy gene product will enjoy immune tolerance. Humoral or cellular reactions by the host could be the major problem when gene transfer is undertaken *in vivo* after birth. DBMT is not a panacea, being only applicable to about 7% of understood genetic diseases, where it is possible to devise *in vitro* tests to predict the *in vivo* outcome of installing a donor bone marrow as a 'component factory' which might last the lifetime of the recipient. The importance of immunoprophylaxis will be stressed, and using it, worthwhile correction has been achieved for over 40 previously fatal genetic diseases; partial correction has been achieved for another seven, but there has been failure in five diseases. Following the introduction of simple BMT (no induction) by Gatti *et al* (1968), the need for a displacement induction was demonstrated by work done in 1970–1973 at the Westminster Hospital, London (see Figure 1 and Table 1) where

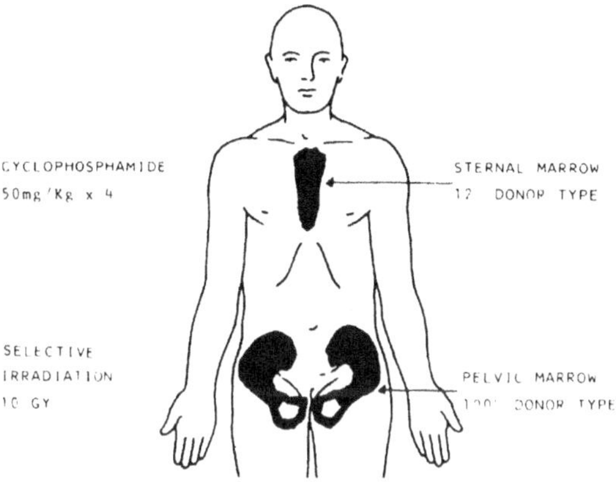

Figure 1 The need for displacement bone marrow transplantation. Cyclophosphamide alone achieved only 12% donor phagocytes (illustrated by the sternal marrow in two patients with chronic granulomatous disease) but in the second patient, prior selective radiation of the pelvis achieved there 100% donor phagocytes. Today, busulphan is preferred.

Table 1 Incomplete engraftment due to lack of inductions yielding adequate displacement (extracted from the literature)

	No. of Patients
Wiskott–Aldrich syndrome	6
T-cell defects; B-cells present	60
Phagocyte errors	10
Osteopetrosis	18
Antibody deficiency; B-cells present	20
Red cell errors	46

it was also first successfully extended to include other family members (Hobbs *et al.*, 1976, 1985) and volunteer unrelated donors (Foroozanfar *et al.*, 1977) needed for the four out of five patients who do not have a healthy matched sibling.

BMT can correct genetic diseases in two main ways: (i) by replacing genetically deranged or absent blood cells (as when Steinmuller and Motulsky (1967) corrected spherocytosis in an animal, or Gatti *et al.* (1968) installed helper T-cells in a boy); (ii) by implanting bone marrow cells which will deliver a normal protein to the tissues of the host, as I discovered in 1970 when the lymphocytes of a healthy brother transferred the capacity to the cells of an elder brother to produce migration inhibitory factor (MIF), both *in vitro* and *in vivo* by the transplant (Valdimarsson *et al.*, 1972). Others have similarly discovered corrective factors (e.g. Porter, 1971), but did not prove their potential by transplant. The evolution of this latter work led to the displacement concept and I proposed in 1978 to a Working Party of the European Bone Marrow Transplant organization that over 30 previously fatal genetic diseases might respond to DBMT. The introduction of busulphan for BMT induction in rats

(Tutschka and Santos, 1977) encouraged its successful use in a boy with Hurler's disease, and the proposal was then published (Hobbs, 1981). Since then, DBMT with immunoprophylaxis has been extensively used and reviewed (Hobbs, 1987). The principles are given in Table 2; the need for immunoprophylaxis is explained in Figure 2, and the treatable diseases are listed in Tables 3 and 4; Table 5 summarizes how best to refer patients for elective DBMT. The present review outlines the procedures undertaken when a patient is referred to our team and then considers results which have been obtained using this form of treatment for genetic diseases, always remembering that the most serious complications of infection and graft-versus-host diseases (GVHD) can cause serious morbidity so that the therapy is used only for otherwise fatal inborn errors for which no better treatment has yet been established.

PROCEDURE

It is good ethical practice that the clinical condition of a patient referred for BMT should be assessed by at least two teams, the referring team and one other, usually our own; when the disease is not familiar to us, we seek an expert opinion elsewhere. This should be done as early as possible for best results (see Table 5). The assessment will indicate any urgency, or permit an extensive donor search, *in vitro* assays of potential transfers and testing for any binding antibodies already generated in the patient by previous exposures to normal components. We store in viable form the cells of the patient, parents, siblings and donors, their sera, and extracts of DNA so that as molecular biology progresses, referral back to stored material may better categorize disorders in relation to DBMT outcome. In about half of the patients we have seen in the past five years, it was decided not to proceed with a transplant for a variety of reasons: (a) the disease had progressed too far; (b) white cell or enzyme therapy had generated secondary antibody responses in nine patients, likely to persist postgraft (Riches *et al*., 1986); (c) the condition had not been accurately diagnosed; (d) the missing enzyme was not transferable to the right site; (e) no suitable donor could be found, etc.

A donor search begins within the family with full tissue typing and blood grouping, as well as tests for the carrier or affected state of the disease; in recent years, three prospective compatible siblings turned out to have preclinical forms of the same

Table 2 Principles for correcting inborn errors by DBMT

1.	The inborn error should be expressed in bone marrow stem cells
2.	The patient's abnormal marrow should be displaced
3.	Install a healthy donor marrow factory to produce the normal gene product
4.	The host must be immunologically tolerant to that product
For enzymes, proteins, etc.	
5.	Leukocyte production can be 50–300 g/day
6.	Leukocytes circulate, should release the component or deliver cell-to-cell
7.	Defective tissues should be able to accept the component
8.	The component should find its functional site to a degree adequate to correct the defect.

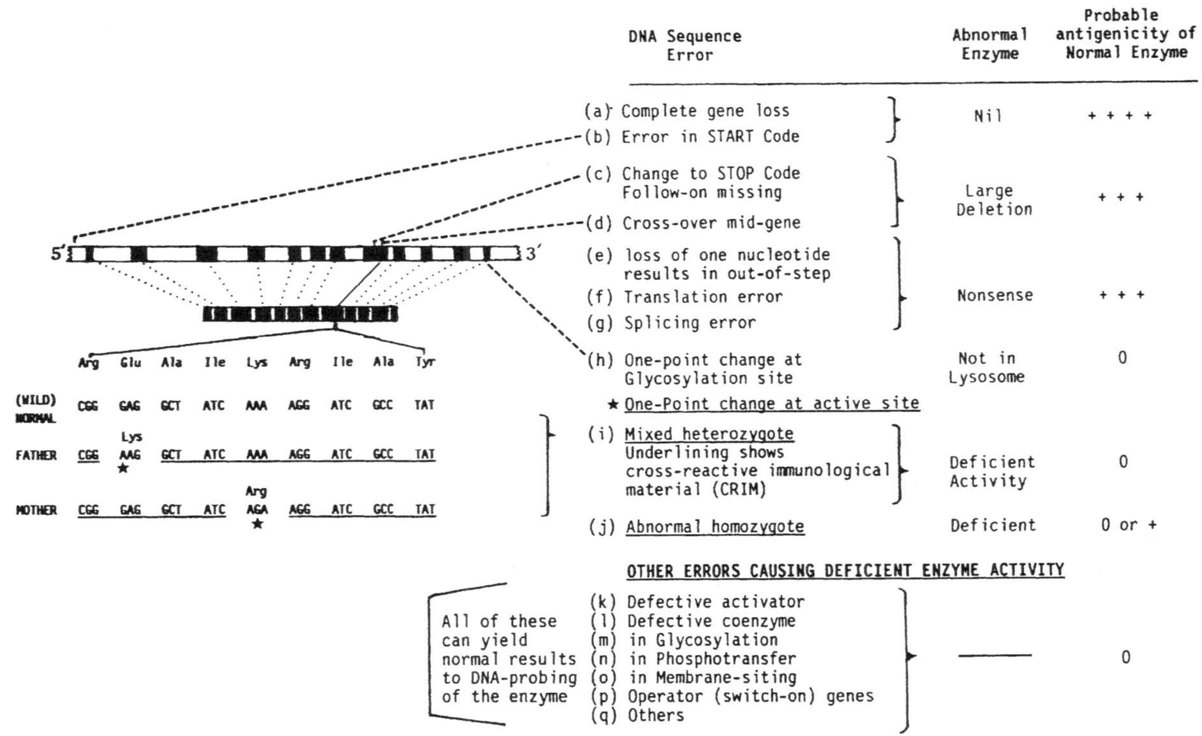

Figure 2 Known errors causing deficient enzyme activity and probable antigenicity in that patient of the normal gene product. The same principles apply to non-enzyme products.

Table 3 Inborn errors where DBMT can provide normal cells

A	*Already successfully corrected*
1.	Reticular dysgenesis (leukocytes)
2.	Sex-linked (helper T $\pm$ B)
3.	Swiss-type autosomal recessive (T + B)
4.	SCID with cartilage-hair dysplasia (T + B)
5.	Late adenosine-deaminase (new T + B)
6.	Late purine nucleoside phosphorylase (new T + B)
7.	Late Di George (new T)
8.	Connatal GVHD (new T)
9.	Wiskott–Aldrich (new T + B + phagocytes)
10.	Autosomal recessive (helper-T)
11.	Bare lymphocyte (new Class II)
12.	Bare lymphocyte (new Class I)
13.	Bare lymphocyte (new Class I + II)
14.	Nezelof/Matsaniotis (T)
15.	Interleukin II receptor (T)
16.	Late onset childhood SCID (T) – not AIDS
17.	Non-functional B (B $\pm$ T)
18.	Adult onset (T + B) – not AIDS
19.	Chronic granulomatous disease (phagocytes)
20.	Chediak–Higashi (phagocytes)
21.	Kostmann, recessive (neutrophils)
22.	Autosomal dominant agranulocytosis (neutrophils)
23.	Lazy phagocyte (phagocytes)
24.	Cyclic neutropenia (phagocytes)
25.	Adhesive proteins (phagocytes)
26.	Diamond–Blackfan (RBC)
27.	Thalassaemia major (RBC)
28.	Sickle cell (RBC)
29.	Spherocytosis (RBC)
30.	Osteopetrosis (osteoclasts)
D	*Possibly correctable*
1.	Severe elliptocytosis (RBC)
2.	Erythropoietic porphyria (RBC)
3.	Severe pyruvate kinase (RBC)
4.	Other severe haemoglobinopathy (RBC)
5.	Homozygous G6PD (phagocytes)
6.	Severe myeloperoxidase (phagocytes)
7.	Lysosome (phagocytes)
8.	Lipochrome histiocytosis (phagocytes)
9.	Lactoferrin (phagocytes)
10.	Strauss defect (phagocytes)
11.	Tubulin (phagocytes)
12.	Severe myosin (phagocytes)
13.	Severe histiocytosis X (phagocytes)
14.	D. Miller's reticuloendotheliosis (phagocytes)
15.	Bruton's (B)
16.	Sporadic hypogammaglobulinaemia (B)
17.	Isolated IgM (B)
18.	Isolated IgG (B)
19.	Severe IgG_2 (B)
20.	Severe isolated IgA (B)
21.	Duncan's X-linked proliferative (T + B)
22.	Severe orotic aciduria (T + B)

Table 4 Inborn errors where DBMT can provide a transferable component

A	*Already successfully corrected*
31.	Chronic mucocutaneous candidiasis (MIF)
32.	Hurlers (α-iduronidase)
33.	Sanfilippo B (acetyl-α-glucosamidase)
34.	Gaucher's type III Norbottnian (cerebroside–β–glucosidase)
35.	Gaucher's, onset < 3 years (cerebroside-β-glucosidase)
36.	Gaucher's, onset 3–16 years (cerebroside-β-glucosidase)
37.	Fabry's (α-galactosidase)
38.	Refsum's (? peroxisomal)
39.	Immunodeficiency (γ-interferon)
40.	Metachromatic leukodystrophy (arylsulphatase-A)
41.	Wolman's (acid esterase)
42.	Fucosidosis (fucosidase)
43.	Omenn's syndrome (biotinidase, holocarboxylase synthetase)
44.	Niemann–Pick B (sphingomyelinase)
45.	Fanconi's (DNA repair enzyme)
B	*Already partially corrected*
46.	Hunter's (iduronidate sulphatase)
47.	Sanfilippo A (heparan sulphatase)
48.	Morquio B (β-galactosidase)
49.	Maroteaux–Lamy (arylsulphatase-β)
50.	Adrenoleukodystrophy (peroxisomal enzyme)
51.	Lesch–Nyhan (hypoxanthine-guanine-phosphoribosyltransferase)
52.	I- cell, mucolipidosis II (mannose processing enzyme)
C	*Known inadequate correction by 100% engraftment*
1.	GM1 gangliosidosis (acid-β-galactosidase)
2.	Pompe's (acid–α-glucosidase)
3.	Niemann–Pick A (sphingomyelinase)
4.	Krabbé's (galactosylceramidase)
5.	Farber's lipogranulomatosis (acid ceramidase)
D	*Possibly correctable*
23.	Scheie's (α-iduronidase)
24.	Hurler–Scheie compound (α-iduronidase)
25.	Sanfilippo C (α-glucosaminide-acetyltransferase)
26.	Sanfilippo D (acetyl-α-glucosaminide-6-sulphatase)
27.	Mannosidosis (α-mannosidase)
28.	Severe sialidosis (sialidase)
29.	Mucolipidosis III (? mannose-phosphorylase)
30.	Niemann–Pick D (?)
31.	Maple syrup urine (leukocyte correctable)
32.	Galactosaemia (galactose-1-phosphate-uridyltransferase)
33.	Ataxia telangiectasia (DNA repair enzyme)
34.	Xeroderma pigmentosa (DNA repair enzyme)
35.	Morquio A (galactosamine-6-sulphate-sulphatase)
36.	Batten's (? peroxisomal enzyme)
37.	Canavan's spongiform leukodystrophy (aspartoacyclase)
38.	Schindler's (α-*N*-acetylgalactosaminidase)
39.	Pseudo-neonatal adrenoleukodystrophy (acyl-CoA-oxidase)
40.	Propionic acidaemia (selected propionyl-CoA-carboxylase deficiency)

Table 5 Optimal conditions when referring patients for elective DBMT

1.	Refer before complications arise (e.g. septic foci, transmitted viral diseases, transfusional sensitization, severe bony deformities, irreparable CNS damage)
2.	If splenectomy is needed, immunization should be planned
3.	If prior enzyme therapy is tried, immunoprophylaxis should have been used
4.	The younger, the better
5.	Use a matched sibling donor or VUD who is a normal homozygote
6.	Refer to a centre with gnotobiotic facilities, especially for transplants from alternative donors

disease as the patient. If a suitable matched healthy sibling is found, then the mixed lymphocyte cultures (MLC) are set up in each direction (donor vs recipient to predict GVHD; recipient vs donor to predict rejection) and nearly always repeated on a second occasion. With our MLC-negative criteria (Hobbs, 1989) over 150 matched transplants have resulted in less than 7% fatal GVHD, even though T-cell depletion is not used. If no suitable sibling donor is available, the search is made among close relatives where, alas, a close match is found for only about 8% of the patients. For Caucasian patients we then turn to the Nolan and allied laboratories with currently a 60% success rate. Any identified prospective donor and the patient are then screened for viral diseases (CMV, HSV, EB, HIV) and where necessary, any other risks (TB, malaria, toxoplasmosis, etc.). Appropriate measures can then be taken for any known risks or blood group differences. At this stage, the parents (and the patient if old enough) are interviewed by a consultant for at least an hour, are given full information (and a booklet), are seen by our experienced psychologists, and given an estimate of the individual risks. They then go away to digest this information and ask any more questions and only at the second interview are they asked to give their final decision as to whether or not to proceed to DBMT. Donors are placed under the care of an independent physician, to assess their fitness; he explains the small risk of having a general anaesthetic and will allow them to change their minds without undue pressure.

When the patient is admitted to hospital, they and the parents are familiarized with the Unit and the staff, and arrangements are made for one parent to be resident; we encourage the parents to alternate sharing the care of their home or the patient and they are trained to be able to enter laminar flow rooms, etc. After initial skin and blood decontamination and further baseline tests, the patient will go to theatre where an autologous bone marrow harvest will be collected to be stored in liquid nitrogen should a rescue be needed; at the same time a triple lumen Hickman line is inserted which avoids excessive needling of the patient. On return from theatre, the patient will enter the laminar flow facility. Our Unit avoids irradiation of children wherever possible and uses the induction outlined in Table 6, for reasons given elsewhere (Hobbs, 1987).

Immunoprophylaxis: We have found that remaining phagocytes function normally after busulphan (or up-front irradiation) and so can process any normal antigens present in the donor buffy coat which can be presented to the recipient's immunocom-

Table 6 Induction for displacement bone marrow transplantation

Day		
-11	To theatre for Hickman line and autologous BM harvest; return to sterile laminar flow room	
-10	Busulphan[a]	4–6 mg/kg
-9	Busulphan	4–6 mg/kg
-8	Busulphan	4–6 mg/kg
-7	Busulphan	4–6 mg/kg
-6	Donor buffy coat	
	Exactly 24 hrs later[b]	
-5	Cyclophosphamide[b,c]	50–75 mg/kg
-4	Cyclophosphamide[b,c]	50–75 mg/kg
-3	Cyclophosphamide[c]	50–75 mg/kg
-2	Cyclophosphamide[c]	50–75 mg/kg
-1	Day of rest	
0	Transplant	

[a]80 mg/m^2 corrected to not < 4 and not > 6 mg/kg
[b]T-helper function is needed here, so cyclosporin A or ATG must not be given before day -3
[c]2 g/m^2 mercapto-ethane sulphonate and diuresis are used daily with the cyclophosphamide

petent lymphocytes. By waiting exactly 24 h, during which time T-helper function must be available (no cyclosporin-A (CsA) or antilymphocyte globulin (ALG)), any immunocompetent lymphocytes which become committed to transform will be eliminated by the cyclophosphamide which follows. This results in deletion of any primary immune responses which might be made by the recipient against the normal components they are about to have engrafted. If a matched sibling DBMT is followed by no GVHD, CsA is abandoned at 3 months but where GVHD above Grade 2 has occurred or in all transplants from any unrelated or MLC-positive family donors, CsA is continued for 1 year at least, if possible.

In principle, we harvest as much marrow as we can and give as large a dose as possible, the primary objective being to achieve 100% donor-type engraftment. Among some 90 patients where this has been achieved for a genetic disease, only once has the graft subsequently been lost; in contrast, mixed chimerism is usually unstable and grafts of up to 88% donor type have eventually been lost up to 1–7 years later. If there is failure of engraftment confirmed by bone marrow biopsy between days + 14 and + 21, our usual procedure is to rescue the patient immediately with autologous marrow and not to attempt to regraft for at least three months after the patient has recovered. Thereafter, a second full induction can be followed by successful engraftment without any serious side effects. In contrast, attempts for early second grafts, even when reserve donors are available, have largely led to complications. In general, donor cells or enzymes are detected by day + 14 and are then monitored. The results of the Westminster group are shown in Table 7. Using MLC-negative family or volunteer unrelated donors, fatal GVHD has been below 8%. Use of MLC-positive donors nearly always causes GVHD, and if not acute, then chronic; measures have to be taken against the competent T-cells of the donor.

Table 7 Results of all BMT for genetic diseases (no exclusions) Westminster Bone Marrow Team 1970–1989

	No. of patients	*Best available donor*	*Survivors of BMT %*	*Long-term survivors*	
				No.	*%*
	51	MLC-neg related (MF)	92	39	76
	11	MLC-neg unrelated	91	8	73
	2	MLC-pos unrelated	0	0	0
	42	MLC-pos related	52	11	26
Total	106		75	58	55
Elective MF	42		98	39	93

At the time of writing, our experience of over 60 such transplants in children has initially achieved over 60% survivors leaving hospital, but later complications and loss of grafts have occurred and the long term results are about 30% surviving with satisfactory outcomes. There is still room for improvement in the selection and use of donors other than a matched family donor, but nevertheless our current success rates seem ethically acceptable, compared to the results of many other kinds of transplantation.

Post-transplant care really amounts to treating the patient rather like a newborn baby for about a year; avoid exposure to virulent infections (chickenpox, etc.), ensure good nutrition, actively rehabilitate to as near a normal lifestyle as possible for age and ensure immediate referral to a centre of excellence if any untoward incident occurs (five of our patients have died of overwhelming septicaemia in outlying districts without such a referral). Where there has been chronic GVHD we advise continuous ampicillin until it resolves, as it can be associated with autosplenectomy (Rogers *et al.*, 1983). When necessary prophylactic IgG can be given; we do not permit live vaccines until immunological recovery has been verified. The majority of our patients are off all treatment within one year of the transplant.

RESULTS FOR SPECIFIC DISEASES

These are numbered as in Tables 3 and 4 and the type of donor is indicated as MF (Matched family MLC-negative), VUD (volunteer matched unrelated donor), or HS (a family donor sharing at least one full genetic haplotype).

A1 Reticular dysgenesis

In a known family the birth was conducted under aseptic conditions and an MF BMT undertaken without any conditioning, to achieve full correction (Levinsky and Tiedman, 1983). If diagnosed after birth, it would be important to eradicate any infection, e.g. using irradiated leukocytes from one parent so that the other could be an HS donor.

A2 Severe combined immune deficiency (SCID)

The first MF BMT without conditioning resulted in a healthy chimera, stable for 21 years, with donor female helper T-cells fortunately co-operating with the recipient's remaining B-cells. After some MF engraftments this has not occurred, so where there is any doubt it would be advisable to use DBMT to achieve all-donor co-operating cells (Hobbs and Hugh-Jones, 1985). T-helper deficiency is the commonest form of SCID, and simple BMT from HS donors, while possible, has mostly failed to achieve complete correction (Fischer *et al.*, 1986).

A3 Non-sex-linked SCID (Swiss type)

BMT without conditioning has been successful (Yamamura *et al.*, 1972) but it is important to treat existing infection with antibiotics, i.v. IgG and even irradiated immune T-cells (e.g. from one parent) to improve the chances of success. Emergency BMT has under 60% good results. Of 12 patients with disseminated BCG, the only two survivors immediately had immune T-cells. Presentation with acute GVHD, transplacental or from non-irradiated blood products, is serious: the graft might be possible after ALG rescue, etc.

A4 SCID with cartilage hair dysplasia

The SCID and hair have been corrected by BMT without conditioning (Fischer *et al.*, 1986). Today it is felt that the cartilage disorder might have responded better to DBMT.

A5–8 T-cell deficiencies diagnosed after the age of 3 months

Today it is important to exclude HIV infection. Serology is unreliable but the HIV genome can be detected within a few hours (Laure *et al.*, 1988). At present there is no justification for the use of BMT to treat HIV as growing T-cells propagate the virus and over 40 failures are known. Deficiencies of adenosine deaminase, purine nucleoside phosphorylase or of the thymus can be corrected by substitution therapy commenced within 6–8 weeks of birth, but after the age of 3 months transient responses are more the rule. One form of adenosine deaminase deficiency arises by deletion of a large part of the genome (Markert *et al.*, 1987) and the normal enzyme will then generate antibody production giving rise to inactivation. DBMT became the treatment of choice, preferably correcting infection, prolonged malnutrition, treatable viral infections (HSV etc.) and even using thymic therapy where indicated, although this can generate GVHD. If enzymes or cells are infused before DBMT it would be important to practise immunoprophylaxis to abrogate a primary immune response.

A9 Wiskott–Aldrich syndrome

The underlying membrane protein defect (Parkman *et al.*, 1981) indicates early DBMT (Hobbs, 1981). Immunostimulation failed to prevent bleeds and malignant transformation.

A10 Autosomal recessive helper T-cell defect

The OKT4 hapten can be absent with completely normal helper function (Amino *et al.*, 1984). Where malfunction is proven, DBMT is essential to achieve co-operating T- and B-cells, unless the donor is perfect MF.

A11–13 Bare lymphocyte syndrome

Defects of class I and class II expression (Touraine *et al.*, 1984) require DBMT for full correction. Donor selection can be complicated by failure of stimulation in the MLC. It is hoped molecular biology methods may be developed to assist matching.

A14–17, 39 Non-functional lymphocytes

Since secondary T-cell deficiency is so common (Hobbs *et al.*, 1984), total absence of the suspected deficient cytokine and failure to induce it with immunomodulators must be shown before undertaking DBMT. The first successfully treated patient who suffered from candidiasis from birth did not produce MIF to all immunogens tested and was not inducible *in vitro* (Valdimarsson *et al.*, 1972): five similar patients not given BMT all died, confirming the seriousness of the condition. Deficiency of gamma interferon can also be so serious that the only treatment seems to be DBMT. More patients with normal numbers of T- and B-subsets are being found with serious malfunction (Fischer *et al.*, 1986). Improving knowledge and assays for cytokines and their receptors may better identify these patients and the best treatments for them. The provision of lymphocytes delivering cytokines at short range seems preferable to the complications of lifelong systemic therapies, where malaise, growth failure and even amyloidogenesis may result. In older patients it is possible that autoimmune mechanisms are active, and where life becomes intolerable, intervention with TBI could eradicate the autoimmune process with an MF BMT establishing normal immune function and good health.

A19–25 Errors intrinsic to phagocytes

BMT intended to replace abnormal by normal phagocytes was first undertaken (Foroozanfar *et al.*, 1977) for chronic granulomatous disease and from it arose the concept of DBMT. The traditional use of TBI in animals by serendipity deleted the abnormal phagocyte stem cells of dogs to correct cyclic neutropenia (Dale and Graw, 1974) and of mice to cure Chediak–Higashi syndrome (Kazmierowski *et al.*, 1976). Kostman's syndrome was corrected by BMT after TBI (Rappeport *et al.*, 1980) but today it and cyclic neutropenia may be corrected by treatment with recombinant human granulocyte colony stimulating factor (Bonilla *et al.*, 1988), avoiding the risks of BMT. Cyclophosphamide induction alone achieved only 30% engraftment in another form of congenital neutropenia (Pahwa *et al.*, 1977), but today a trial of colony stimulating factor should perhaps first be made before proceeding to DBMT. Ordinary BMTs (without displacement) failed for lazy leukocyte syndrome (Camitta *et al.*, 1977), adhesive protein deficiency (Fischer *et al.*, 1983) and human Chediak–Higashi syndrome (Virelizier *et al.*, 1983), although engraftment followed second attempts using TBI, wherafter pneumonitis killed one child. Today our induction protocol (see Table 6) is preferred.

A26–29 Severe genetic anaemia

In discussing previous failures which had occurred in the treatment of genetic anaemias when only cyclophosphamide induction was used, it was predicted that DBMT should be successful (Hobbs, 1981). This prediction was confirmed when thalassaemia major became the first such disorder to be successfully corrected by adding busulphan to the induction (Thomas *et al.*, 1982). DBMT from MF donors has now been used for over 400 children: Class I patients have shown a 93% cure rate, falling to about 50% for Class III patients (older, with serum ferritin above 3000 μg/L with liver damage) (Giardini *et al.*, 1989). The alternative treatment of continuous transfusion with chelates, to reduce iron overload, had had a mortality of 37% within 10 years (Giardina *et al.*, 1987) together with the risks of transmission of cytomegalovirus, hepatitis, and, worst of all, human immunodeficiency and other retroviruses by blood transfusion: 57 children with thalasssaemia have become HIV positive. Tentative dosages of busulphan cyclophosphamide result in unstable chimeras with regression to the disease state (Giardini *et al.*, 1989) so full doses are indicated; the risk of veno-occlusive disease has been overestimated, for it rarely occurs (Hobbs, 1989). The DBMT option seems preferable to conservative management and where parents have to bear the cost it is much more effective. For children in Class III special protocols are being used and are encouraging (Giardini *et al.*, 1989), and pregraft high dose intravenous chelate can remove much iron.

Congenital spherocytosis in animals was corrected because TBI was used (Steinmuller and Motulsky, 1967) and serendipitous displacement cured sickle cell anaemia in a patient who had BMT for leukaemia (Johnson *et al.*, 1984). Current management of spherocytosis and sickle cell disease can result in loss of splenic function, following which septicaemia yearly kills some 3% of patients. Sickle cell disease can be cured by DBMT (Vermylen *et al.*, 1988).

Blackfan–Diamond syndrome has also been completely corrected by DBMT (Iriondo *et al.*, 1984). Improving characterization can now identify severe forms of elliptocytosis, spherocytosis, hexokinase or pyruvate kinase deficiency, etc. For all patients with severe red cell errors, the choice between existing treatments and DBMT is a controversial one, best made on an individual basis (Hobbs, 1989).

A30 Osteopetrosis

In animals four different errors cause this syndrome, but in man two major varieties are known; the infantile form (varying in rate of progress between families) which is due to an unidentified error in osteoclasts, and the late onset or benign form, due to an absence of carbonic anhydrase type II (William *et al.*, 1989). The infantile form justifies DBMT because bone overgrowth crushes the cranial nerves to cause blindness, deafness and other paralyses and eventually obliterates the bone marrow to cause death. Successful parabiosis (Walker, 1975) led to the more practical use of bone marrow, but with the addition of spleen cells, to restore bone resorption in microphthalmic mice. Loutit (1977) showed that simple infusion of bone marrow would do, and in mice displacement was not needed. Unfortunately, in the human situation simple BMT failed (Ballet *et al.*, 1977), as did a heavy induction (Sorell *et al.*, 1978). In 1979 Lamendin recorded success after adding TBI, a practice confirmed by Coccia and colleagues (1980) but today busulphan cyclophosphamide is preferred (Fischer *et al.*, 1986). Mobilization of the bone following the graft demands control of the hypercalcaemia. In some late patients, the bone is so dense that even with DBMT the marrow cannot get established. Ideally, therefore, it should be undertaken as early as possible, even possibly inducing labour at 36 weeks of gestation in order to prevent damage to the cranial nerves. Vitamin D (calcitriol) can delay petrosis during a donor search and brave surgeons can enlarge the optic foramina to buy time. At diagnosis it is important to establish whether the child is blind and/or deaf, so that the parents can be fully informed and may decline a graft option. Chambers (1985) suggested that the osteoclast may have its own precursor in human bone marrow, fortuitously transferred by DBMT. At present there is no way of transferring the osteoblast which, of course, might correct quite a few other diseases.

A32 Hurler's disease

Allotypic variation in the severity of α-iduronidase deficiency has not yet been clarified by molecular biology studies, but all children except those with the rare Scheie variant show mental deterioration for which there has been no satisfactory alternative treatment. Since the first patient was treated by DBMT in 1980 (Hobbs *et al.*, 1981) over 60 others have now received transplants. Of the 24 carried out at the Westminster Hospital, all seven survived the DBMT from MF or VUD, as did nine from 17 HS donors. The seven with the longest follow-up (all over 6 years) showed correction of the hepatosplenomegaly within 6 to 12 months, improvement of visual acuity to 6/12 with glasses, and restoration of normal hearing (sometimes needing grommets). There was normalization of the 24 h output of total urinary glycosaminoglycans, but a continuing excess of dermatan sulphate, presumably derived from those tissues not adequately penetrated by donor enzyme. These include cartilage and the carpal tunnel fibroblasts. Joint mobility and claw-hands improved (with even better results after the carpal tunnel retinaculum was cut) but otherwise dysostosis multiplex was little affected. The lumbar gibbus would increase, but has been halted by posterior spinal fusion. Knock-knees develop, and hip dysplasia can lead to subluxation and flexion deformities. However, the response to surgery in the transplanted patients is good with excellent healing and bone fusion.

With regard to the brain, hydrocephalus improved, NMR imaging showed good myelination and differentiation, and patients are maintaining their British ability scales, especially if engrafted before 2 years of age. Thereafter, patients will probably have lower IQs, consequent to the damage already incurred. It is known that dendrite growth can occur between the ages of 2–3 years and re-establish new connections and, of course, children who get enzyme into their brains before 2 years of age have this benefit. One of our patients died of pneumococcal septicaemia 14 months postgraft, and his brain (after correction for contained blood) had achieved 4% of the normal iduronidase level (Hobbs, 1985), whereas untreated Hurler's children have shown no detectable iduronidase. This has been subsequently confirmed from transplants in Hurler dogs where the brain level reached 7–10% of normal controls (Shull *et al.*, 1987).

As chondrocytes which have collected some donor enzyme migrate deeper from the growing plate, they use up the enzyme and revert to Hurler type; as cartilage gets thicker with age some of the bone problems worsen, but as the bones finally stop growing and revert to membrane type, it is possible that improved enzyme delivery may ameliorate the situation. Certainly the facies of these children have become almost normal apart from the thickened cartilage at the top of the nose, and the parents are very pleased with the results. With five out of the seven long-term survivors at normal schools and with several other teams enjoying similar results, it is still considered that the transplants have been worthwhile, but the bone problems will require careful follow-up.

A33 Sanfilippo B disease

Non-identical twin sisters who had HS DBMT (Hugh-Jones *et al.*, 1982) when just over 2 years of age have not, in the subsequent seven years, followed the disastrous progress of their two elder brothers who were both severely affected by the age of 4. Their donor was heterozygous, and progress was complicated by severe GVHD and leukopenia. One of the girls appears to have recovered almost completely from chronic GVHD but the other is still showing effects. Both have led a reasonably normal life and go to school but require extra assistance in their education. DBMT under the age of 3 still seems justifiable but, of course, follow-up must continue.

A34–36 Gaucher's diseases

In the light of new molecular biology the non-infantile mainly non-neurological forms are preferably classified as 'fast' (symptoms before the age of 3), 'medium' (symptoms at 3–16 years of age), and 'slow' (symptoms only after 16 years of age). Enzyme replacement has had very limited success, and tests for binding antibodies were not done (Brady, 1984). While gene transfer has been accomplished in the test tube (Sorge *et al.*, 1987), there was no test against the mature immune system of a patient. Early attempts at BMT (Hammersmith and Philadelphia) did not use displacement and failed to establish successful grafts. While TBI achieved successful engraftment (Svennerholm *et al.*, 1984), the response seemed slower, with longer persistence of the Gaucher cells than in our patients in whom CAT scans (Starer *et al.*, 1987) showed rapid improvement before all the host monocytes could be replaced, so it is likely that enzyme is actually donated by the engrafted leukocytes to host phagocytes, possibly after apoptosis. Gaucher cells, locked in fibrous cords in the liver, can persist for up to two years, whereas in the bone marrow they clear within six months (Hobbs *et al.*, 1987).

The non-use of immunoprophylaxis could have generated antibodies to explain the high phagocyte enzyme levels in the patients of Svennerholm and colleagues (1984) and of Ginns and colleagues (1984) for some months after the graft. IgG-tagged enzyme would go back into the white cells to be measured by the assay:

delivery elsewhere would be impaired.

Splenectomy under the age of 5 years is followed by many septicaemic deaths (Lowdon *et al.*, 1966) so we initially tried transplants leaving the spleens intact in two children with neutrophil counts above 1000 and platelet counts above 75 000/μL. These patients required up to 356 units of platelets, and one never achieved a neutrophil count above 50/μL and died of aspergillosis. The other recovered completely to normalize spleen, liver and lung function. Three other splenectomized patients had much easier grafts so four subsequent patients had elective splenectomies pregraft. Pre-splenectomy, they can be immunized with pneumococcal, meningococcal and haemophilus vaccines, to set up memory status in B-lymphocytes and antigen-processing cells. Immunizing their donors pre-BMT ensures that immune recipient and donor cells can co-operate postgraft when a booster dose is given to try and obtain good antibody levels. Survivors should take ampicillin for life and while some strains of the offending micro-organisms do become resistant, this does not seem yet to be the case for the DF2-type organisms common in cats and dogs, which are known to be able to kill post-splenectomy patients. A major problem in Gaucher's diseases, found in all our patients in pregraft biopsies, was quite extensive liver fibrosis. The impaired liver function tests and raised IgA have normalized in all our survivors postgraft, but biopsies up to two years later have not shown very much improvement in the degree of fibrosis, although there has been a large amount of clearing of Gaucher cells. Nevertheless, the children have developed a marked increase in wellbeing ('new children' say their parents), and have achieved active lifestyles. A 16-year-old girl abandoned her 2-year-old leg irons at three months, gave up her crutches at four months and now regularly rides a bicycle. Two other girls who had pregraft hip damage now behave as if it did not exist and our orthopaedic surgeon is not going to intervene until there is a better indication than a bad X-ray. This is a most rewarding disease to treat by DBMT, although long-term liver results are awaited.

A37 Fabry's disease

Small increases in serum α-galactosidase-A achieved by fetal liver transplantation benefitted three patients (Touraine, 1982). DBMT could do better and confer tolerance to the enzyme for the lifetime of the patient.

A38 Refsum's disease

Similar benefit followed fetal liver transplantation (Touraine, 1982), so DBMT could work even from a heterozygous donor. Current treatments with aphereses and difficult dietary regimes are not satisfactory for all patients and progress in the knowledge of peroxisomal defects may soon improve patient selection for DBMT.

A40 Metachromatic leukodystrophy

The infantile and juvenile forms are due to a deficiency of arylsulphatase-A, but the heterogeneity of abnormal allomers of this enzyme, including pseudodeficiency, is now being clarified by DNA probes (Stein *et al.*, 1989). With better identification, early DBMT is indicated as soon as the diagnosis is certain. In the first infantile-variety patient treated by DBMT the father's heterozygous enzyme level was achieved, but she died from CMV infection before any benefit occurred (Joss *et al.*, 1982). The second infantile patient continued to progress downhill after an ordinary BMT, but did improve later when a proper DBMT was carried out to achieve full donor engraftment (Bayever *et al.*, 1983). Several other patients have done well after DBMT with measured improvement in CNS function, both of peripheral nerve and brain. Our late-onset-variety (juvenile) patient had full engraftment from an MS with a normal WBC level of arylsulphatase-A, but nevertheless continued to deteriorate and died of respiratory failure: proper immunoprophylaxis was done. It may be that after a certain degree of leukodystrophy is reached (perhaps varying with the genetic variety) it becomes irreversible. It is known that the earlier the patient has DBMT, the better the long term result.

A41 Wolman's disease

The severe form of acid esterase deficiency shows storage visible within leukocytes, and the biochemical liver and gut abnormalities were fully corrected by DBMT, but the infant died on day +80 from aspergillosis (Hobbs *et al.*, 1986).

A42 Fucosidosis

Because affected fibroblasts could be cleared of deposits by adding normal leukocytes to a culture, DBMT was proposed for this disease (Hobbs, 1983). Hopefully, the blood/brain barrier of man can be crossed as easily as in the dog. In dogs, DBMT achieved fucosidase brain levels as high as 48% of normal, with reversal of CNS lesions in dogs given transplants before 4 months of age (Taylor *et al.*, 1986).

A43 Multiple carboxylase deficiency

This apparent deficiency can be due to defects of two known enzymes, biotinidase (the severe homozygous deficiency with a frequency of about 1 : 50 000 births, Dunkel *et al.*, 1989), or holocarboxylase synthetase (Holme *et al.*, 1988), resulting in early onset symptoms subsequent to disorders of all four biotin-dependent carboxylases. In most cases, diagnosed after 3 months of age, replacement biotin treatment does not prevent complications such as deafness (Wilcken and Hammond, 1983). Three patients given biotin from diagnosis at birth had not yet developed any lesions by 1989. A late onset form is described with both these enzymes being present (Holme *et al.*, 1988). Other secondary causes of carboxylase deficiency do occur so it is important that the syndrome is correctly identified (Rosenberg, 1983). Older descriptions such as Omenn's syndrome are now inadequate, but some difficult patients (with SCID also) have been corrected by DBMT (Fischer *et al.*, 1986; Hurvitz *et al.*, 1989).

A44 Niemann–Pick B disease

Our patient continues with good systemic improvement after her DBMT (Vellodi *et al.*, 1987).

A45 Fanconi's syndrome

The underlying defect is a failure to repair DNA (over 30 enzymes are needed) so excess somatic mutations occur throughout life which can end with neoplastic transformation. The tissues are much more susceptible to test doses of irradiation or cyclophosphamide, whereby challenge tests enable early diagnosis before over-transfusion etc. Late patients with aplasia have responded to ordinary BMT, although procarbazine is the preferred induction drug (Auerbach *et al.*, 1983). Fatal GVHD occurred in some 60% of patients over the age of 6 years, but the success rate after Gluckman low-dose induction is now approaching 70% (Ebell *et al.*, 1989). While HS donors have had poor results, two VUD BMT have been successful. In our first patient (Barrett *et al.*, 1977) who had a DBMT, neoplastic epithelia around the eye and in the bladder normalized post-transplant so that the repair enzyme appears to be transferable.

B46 Hunter's disease

There are 'severe' and 'mild' forms of this disease (Orii, 1986). Our two survivors had 'severe' disease and only had their DBMT at 5 years of age, both developing severe chronic GVHD with low levels of leukocyte and enzyme. Although hepatosplenomegaly has gone, neither has shown any evidence of mental improvement and their IQs are falling. It is not known whether a graft from a normal homozygote under the age of 1 year can achieve better results. A boy with a 'mild' variety had a successful DBMT at 7 years of age, appeared to proceed satisfactorily (Warkentin *et al.*, 1986) but then progressed downhill and died. Assuming that random neutralization of the X-chromosome occurs for neurones, the cells with the active X-chromosome of maternal origin which are unable to synthesize enzyme must obtain an adequate supply from their neighbours. It remains to be seen whether an adequate supply can cross the blood/brain barrier after early DBMT.

B47 Sanfilippo A disease

Our patient, grafted at 5.4 years of age, showed marked improvement of the systemic features, but five years postgraft we are disappointed by mental deterioration and would not at present graft any patient over the age of 4. A French child who had DBMT at the age of 2 progressed downhill, whereas some other patients, while not fully corrected, have had pleasing results (Bordignoni *et al.*, 1989).

B48 Morquio's disease

Here again, severe and mild forms exist (Orii, 1986) with at least three distinct enzyme deficiencies. One of our patients with advanced disease did not receive buffy coat immunoprophylaxis and produced postgraft IgG which bound to the normal enzyme and greatly reduced its activity; the child showed improvement only in the liver and spleen (Desai *et al.*, 1983) and finally died after dislocation of her odontoid process. Our second patient had HS DBMT from his father but developed severe chronic GVHD with leukopenia and low enzyme delivery, and again while the liver and spleen has improved, his orthopaedic progress has been disappointing. A recent graft after TBI (no host B-cells) is progressing well (Kato *et al.*, 1989).

B49 Maroteaux–Lamy syndrome

The 13-year-old patient who received DBMT for this disease (McGovern *et al.*, 1986) showed improvement in hepatosplenomegaly, corneal clouding and lung function, but little progress in the joint deformities: her age precluded much new cartilage formation. In a 7-year-old boy, DBMT ensuring immunoprophylaxis not only produced the above improvements but also a clearly improved range of movement within six weeks of the graft. We are still assessing his further progress, but at least can detect no antibodies to arylsulphatase-B.

B50 Adrenoleukodystrophy

This sex-linked disorder (X-linked adrenoleukodystrophy) shows variability in clinical presentation and progress (Moser *et al.*, 1987) and in some families even the female carrier can show neurological disease of the same type later in life. Up to 30% of siblings with the characteristic abnormality of accumulation of long-chain fatty acids similar to their propositi appear to develop no lesions. This heterogeneity is now recognized in the group of peroxisomal disorders (Schutgens *et al.*, 1989) to which X-linked adrenoleukodystrophy belongs with a single enzyme deficiency in peroxisomal very-long-chain acylcoenzyme A synthetase. A distinct neonatal form has loss of peroxisomes and many of their functions. The variation in X-linked adrenoleukodystrophy may yield to future DNA probing. Very-long-chain acylcoenzyme A synthetase must clearly pass from the 'good X-chromosome' neurones of the mothers to the 'bad X-chromosome' neurones (as most are unaffected) and exists in normal WBC. Good engraftment after DBMT from a normal sibling did not benefit one patient who died 145 days postgraft: immunoprophylaxis was not done, so antibodies could have interfered with delivery of very-long-chain acylcoenzyme A synthetase. In a more recent French patient, objective improvement with remyelination detected by nuclear magnetic resonance has followed successful DBMT (Aubourg, personal communication) at a time when only minimal neurological damage had occurred. A similar good result has been obtained in Los Angeles. The only other alternative treatment has been a short-chain fatty acid diet, which to date has not shown significant CNS improvement. It will be important to retain patient (and donor) DNA extracts for future studies of the heterogeneity that exists; perhaps then selection of those varieties responsive to DBMT may be possible. At present well patients with a bad family history or those with measurable but minimal CNS deterioration seem the most suitable candidates.

B51 Lesch–Nyhan syndrome

The original patient received an MS DBMT at 21 years of age and his metabolic disease appears to be completely corrected, but there has been no improvement in his psychosis in the subsequent two years (Nyhan *et al.*, 1986). Two further attempts have been made in children under 1 year of age but, alas, early post-transplant deaths have prevented evaluation.

B52 I-cell disease

Biochemical improvement has followed an MS DBMT from a heterozygote (Kurobane *et al.*, 1986) and the usual downhill course has been prevented. Long-term follow-up is awaited.

C1 GM1 gangliosidosis

By the time the infant is born, there appears to be extensive ganglioside deposition and DBMT at 9 months and even at 3 months of age from a normal homozygote has been unable to reverse the inexorable progression of the disease (Shaw *et al.*, 1986).

C2 Pompe's disease

Three attempts at 5–6 months of age were followed by two deaths from heart failure and one from pneumonia (Harris *et al.*, 1986). Before transplanting our patient, we kept her human voluntary and smooth muscle alive in tissue culture for 24 h, by which time the added donor leukocytes had completely cleared them of glycogen, and that this happened *in vivo* was confirmed at *post mortem* even though the graft had only just taken. We could not test heart tissue *in vitro* and it is not known if there are sufficient coated pits to allow adequate access of donated enzyme.

C3 Niemann–Pick A disease

In a mouse model and in a young infant (Krivit, personal communication) BMT has not been able to reverse the neurological damage present at diagnosis, although it appears that immunoprophylaxis was not practised in either case. Clearly, any antibodies that bound to donor enzyme would almost certainly prevent its entry into the CNS but their postgraft presence has not been sought.

C4 Krabbé's disease

In the Twitcher mouse model, BMT, which must be before the age of 11 days, greatly improves the prognosis (Hoogerbrugge *et al.*, 1988). As this simulates the human disease, two patients have been treated, but with very disappointing results despite full engraftment (Krivit, personal communication).

C5 Farber's lipogranulomatsis

A boy with a severe deficiency of acid ceramidase and brain lesions had a DBMT 18 months ago from his compatible sister who had a normal homozygous level of enzyme. The transplant achieved 100% donor type engraftment with only GVH grade II. The patient nevertheless showed no improvement in the progress of his disease (Souillet *et al.*, 1989).

FUTURE DEVELOPMENTS

While a majority of the original diseases proposed (Hobbs, 1981) have been corrected by a properly undertaken DBMT, Tables 3B and 4D list other diseases which might be correctable through the same principles. While a bad family history guides judgement to the seriousness, it is in those very situations that future births would best be prevented if at all possible by studies of chorionic villus biopsies, or indeed amniotic biopsies. In Britain, some 80% of these diseases tend to be sporadic, with no known family history, and are not preventable. For some, prenatal diagnosis is not yet possible. Diseases 3B 15–21 seem intrinsic to the B-lymphocyte, and indeed absence of IgA has been both conferred upon a BMT recipient (Hammarstrom *et al.*, 1985) and corrected by one of our DBMTs, just as is recorded for the atopic state (Walker *et al.*, 1986). The severe diseases indicated can render a patient's life quite miserable, and intravenous IgG has not prevented acquisition of serious viral infection and other complications. It is possible that cytokine deficiencies may underly some of the diseases (e.g. IL4 or 6 for B21) and that recombinant peptide therapy may become the future choice, as for 3A 21. On the other hand, in some centres, the success rate of over 90% for elective MF DBMT before complications occur may provide a better choice to the parents than more expensive alternatives. It is to be hoped that DNA probes and monoclonal antibodies will better identify those severe forms justifying DBMT, and for many of the currently suggested diseases it is possible to set up fibroblast cultures from affected patients in media without corrective factors (e.g. avoid fetal calf serum), to compare these with what happens after the addition of prospective donor leukocytes or plasma, and to extend this to more relevant tissues such as brain or heart when this becomes feasible.

The difficult area has been those inborn deficiencies causing damage to the brain; *in vitro* tests are not yet available which can predict whether or not adequate correction is possible. In young animals new bone marrow precursors can populate the brain with the cells of the macrophage line (Perry and Gordon, 1989) to become a local source of enzyme. However, just as for gene replacement therapy, DBMT must be tested in an intact animal with all its physiological barriers and a normal immune system. In about half of the diseases so far studied or treated, adequate results are obtained (*Lancet* leader, 1986). It should also be remembered that some animal successes (simple BMT in micro-ophthalmic mice, correction in Twitcher mice) have not been transferable to the human situation.

Cost efficiency of current DBMT is excellent; updating old estimates (Hobbs, 1981) some 100 children born each year in England and Wales could have DBMT for £1.8 million, achieving lifelong correction for over 60 of them, as against £8 million being expended before most of them die from a miserable existence afflicting them and their families.

Currently, most attempts at gene therapy have only been successful in the test tube, but have failed in whole animals. It seems initially that many will be based on harvesting autologous bone marrow from an affected animal, transfecting it with the gene, and restoring it to the host; this is doomed to failure unless DBMT is undertaken, for it is very important to remove the competition from the remaining host stem cells. There is also the problem that the primordial stem cells seem to be turning over in such a way that only 1 out of 8 is ever being used at any given time; this makes them harder to eradicate. Nevertheless, methods are being developed for the positive selection of the earliest bone marrow stem cells which might be totally transfectable without impairing their power to displace those of the host and avoid the risks of allogeneic BMT. The real danger is that the host's remaining B-cells will mount an immune rejection of the new gene product. If total displacement requires an unopposed new start, there may be a return to a TBI induction with its risks and, of course, the ever present risk of infection. Such gene transfers would have to be undertaken with exactly the same facilities and experience which exist in those teams undertaking DBMT, and initially for many of the same diseases. Clearly, there are many factors which will influence the final decision for any given patient; that will have to be made by the parents whom we must advise as best we can, emphasizing that total cure is exceptional but that worthwhile correction may be achievable.

ACKNOWLEDGEMENTS

Much of this review has arisen from the work of the Westminster Children's Bone Marrow Transplant Team (many of whom are named elsewhere; Hobbs, 1983) who are grateful to the Bostic and Dobson Funds of the Westminster Medical School Research Trust and the Riverside Health Authority for their generous support. I personally thank Mrs Rosemary Jenkinson for her excellent secretarial assistance.

REFERENCES

Amino, N., Aozasa, M., Iwatani, Y., Tamakim, H., Miyaim, K., Sato, H. and Gunji, T. Familial OKT4 lymphocyte deficiency. *Lancet* 2 (1984) 94–95

Aubourg, P., Blanche, S., Rocchiccoli, F., Saudreau, C., Roland, M. O. and Fischer, A. Bone marrow transplant in adrenoleukodystrophy. *SSIEM Munich Meeting* (1989) Abstr. 0 11

Auerbach, A. D., Adler, B., O'Reilly, R. J., Kirkpatrick, D. and Chaganti, R. S. Effect of procarbazine and cyclophosphamide on chromosome breakage in Fanconi anaemia cells: Relevance to bone marrow transplantation. *Cancer Genet. and Cytogenet.* 9 (1983) 25–36

Ballet, J. J., Griscelli, C., Coutris, C., Milhaud, G. and Maroteaux, P. Bone marrow transplantation in osteopetrosis. *Lancet* 2 (1977) 1137

Barrett, A. J., Brigden, W. D., Hobbs, J. R., Hugh-Jones, K., Humble, J. G., James, D. C. O., Retsas, S., Rogers, T. R. F., Selwyn, S., Sneath, P. and Watson, J. G. Successful bone marrow transplant for Fanconi's anaemia. *Br. Med. J.* 1 (1977) 420–422

Bayever, E., Feigm, S. A., Philippart, M. and Brill, N. Bone marrow transplantation in the treatment of metachromatic leukodystrophy. *Clin. Res.* 31 (1983) 107a

Bonilla, M. A., Gillio, A. P., Roggiero, M., Kernan, N. A., Brochstein, J. A., Fumagatti, L., Bordignon, C., Vincent, M., Welte, A., Souza, L. M. and O'Reilly, R. J. Correction of neutropenia in patients with congenital agranulocytosis with recombinant human granulocyte colony stimulating factor *in vivo*. *Exp. Hematol.* 16 (1988) 520

Bordigoni, P., Vidailhet, M., Lena, M., Maire, I. and Gelot, S. Bone marrow transplantation for Sanfilipo syndrome. In Hobbs, J. R. (ed.) *Correction of Certain Genetic Diseases by Transplantation, 1989*, COGENT Press, Westminster, 1989, pp. 114–119

Brady, R. O. Enzyme replacement in the sphingolipidoses. In Barranger, J. A. and Brady, R. O. (eds.), *Molecular Basis of Lysosomal Storage Disorders*, Academic Press, New York, 1984, pp. 461–78

Camitta, B. M., Quesenberry, P. J. and Parkmann, R. Bone marrow transplantation for an infant with neutrophil dysfunction. *Exp. Hematol.* 5 (1977) 109–116

Chambers, T. J. The pathology of the osteoclast. *J. Clin. Pathol. (London)* 38 (1985) 241–252

Coccia, P. J., Krivit, W., Cervenka, J., Clawson, C., Kersey, J. H., Kim, T. H., Nesbit, M. E., Ramsay, N. K. C., Warkentin, P. I., Teitelbaum, S. L., Kahn, A. J. and Brown, D. M. Successful bone marrow transplantation for infantile malignant osteopetrosis. *N. Engl. J.*

Med. 302 (1980) 701–708

Dale, D. C. and Graw, R. G. Transplantation of allogeneic bone marrow in canine cyclic neutropenia. *Science* 181 (1974) 83–84

Desai, S., Hobbs, J. R., Hugh-Jones, K., Williamson, S., Barnes, I., Kendra, J. and White, S., Morquio's disease (mucopolysaccharidosis type IV) treated by bone marrow transplant. *Exp. Hematol.* 11 Suppl. 13, (1983) 98–100

Dunkel, G., Clow, C. L., Scriver, C. R. Prospective ascertainment of complete and partial serum biotinidase deficiency in the newborn. *J. Inher. Metab. Dis.* 12 (1989) 131–138

Ebell, W., Friedrich, W. and Kohne, E. Therapeutic aspects of Fanconi anaemia. In Schroeder-Kuth, T. M., Auerbach, A. D. and Obe, G. (eds.), *Fanconi Anaemia: Clinical, Cytogenetic and Experimental Aspects*, Springer-Verlag, Berlin, 1989, pp. 47–59

Fischer, A., Pham Huu, T., Durandy, A., Descamps, B., Grospierre, B., Gerota, I., Gerota, E., Schenmetzler, C. and Griscelli, C. Bone marrow transplantation in two patients with granulocytopathies. *Exp. Hematol.* 11 Suppl. 13, (1983) 93–94

Fischer, A., Friedrich, W., Griscelli, C., Kubanek, B., Landais, P., Levinsky, R., Morgan, G., Vossen, J. and Wagemaker, G. Bone marrow transplantation for immunodeficiencies and osteopetrosis: European survey 1968–1985. *Lancet* 2 (1986) 1080–1083

Foroozanfar, N., Hobbs, J. R., Hugh-Jones, K., Humble, J. G., James, D. C. O., Selwyn, S., Watson, J. G. and Yamamura, M. Bone marrow transplantation from an unrelated donor for chronic granulomatous disease. *Lancet* 1 (1977) 210–213

Gatti, R. A., Allen, H. D., Meuwissen, H. J., Allen, H. D., Hong, R. and Good, R. A. Immunological reconstitution of sex-linked lymphopenic immunological deficiency. *Lancet* 2 (1968) 1366–1369

Giardina, P. J., Ehlers, K., Lesser, M. *et al.* Improved survival in Beta thalassemia major. *Pediatr. Res.* 21 (1987) 229A

Giardini, G., Lucarelli, C., Angelucci, E., Baronciani, D. and Durazzi, S. M. T. Bone marrow transplantation for thalassaemia. The experience of Pesaro. In Hobbs, J. R. (ed.) *Correction of Certain Genetic Diseases by Transplantation*, COGENT Press, Westminster, 1989, pp. 76–77

Ginns, E. I., Caplan, D. B., Rappeport, J. M. and Barranger, J. A. Bone marrow transplantation in severe Gaucher's disease: rapid correction of enzyme deficiency accompanied by continued long term survival of storage cells. In Barranger, J. A. and Brady, R. O. (eds.), *Molecular Basis of Lysosomal Storage Disorders*, Academic Pres, New York, 1984, pp. 429–40

Hammarstrom, L., Lonnquist, B., Ringden, O., Edvard Smith, C. I. and Wiebe, T. Transfer of IgA deficiency to a bone-marrow-grafted patient with aplastic anaemia. *Lancet* 1 (1985) 778–781

Harris, R. E., Hannon, D., Vogler, C. and Hug, G. Bone marrow transplantation in type IIa glycogen storage disease. *Birth Defects* 22 (1) (1986) 119–132

Hobbs, J. R., Humble, J. G., Anderson, I. M. and James, D. C. O. The elective treatment of graft-versus-host disease following a bone marrow graft from a father to a son with severe combined immunodeficiency. *Postgrad. Med. J.* 52 Suppl. 5 (1976) 91–95

Hobbs, J. R. Bone marrow transplantation for inborn errors. *Lancet* 2 (1981) 735–739

Hobbs, J. R. The scope of allogeneic bone marrow transplantation. In Losowsky, M. and Bolton, R. (eds.), *Advanced Medicine Leeds*, Pitman, Bath, 1983, pp. 378–391

Hobbs, J. R. Correction of 34 genetic diseases by displacement bone marrow transplantation. *Plasma Ther. Transpl. Tech.* 6 (1985) 221–246

Hobbs, J. R. Displacement bone marrow transplantation and immunoprophylaxis for genetic diseases. *Adv. Intern. Med.* 33 (1987) 81–118

Hobbs, J. R. (ed.) *The Correction of Certain Genetic Diseases by Transplantation*, 1989, COGENT Press, Westminster, 1989, pp. 147–159*

Hobbs, J. R. and Hugh-Jones, K. Immunodeficiencies better treated by transplantation. *Tokai J. Exp. Clin. Med.* 10 (1985) 85–97

*If sterling £22 is received by Westminster Medical School Research Trust, 17 Horseferry Road, London SW1P 2AR, UK, a copy can be mailed to your address.

Hobbs J. R., Barrett, A. J., Chambers, J. D., James, D. C. O., Hugh-Jones, K., Byrom, N., Henry, K. and Lucas, C. F. Reversal of clinical features of Hurler's disease and biochemical improvement after treatment by bone marrow transplantation. *Lancet* 2 (1981) 709–712

Hobbs, J. R., Byrom, N. A., Chambers, J. D., Williamson, S. A. and Nagvekar, N. Secondary T-lymphocyte deficiencies. In Byrom, N. A. and Hobbs, J. R. (eds.), *Thymic Factor Therapy: Proceedings of the Serono Symposia* 15, Raven Press, New York, 1984, pp. 175–187

Hobbs, J. R., Williamson, S., Chambers, J. D., James, D. C. O., Joshi, R., Shaw, P. and Hugh-Jones, K. Use of donors sharing one genetic haplotype for bone marrow transplantation. *Tokai J. Exp. Clin. Med.* 10 (1985) 207–214

Hobbs, J. R., Hugh-Jones, K., Shaw, P. J., Chambers, D., Clemens, M. E., Parsons, P., Patrick, A. D. and Cheetham, C. M. Wolman's disease corrected by displacement bone marrow transplantation with immunoprophylaxis. *Bone Marrow Transplantation* 1, Suppl. 1 (1986) 347

Hobbs, J. R., Hugh-Jones, K., Shaw, P., Lindsay, I. and Hancock, M., Beneficial effect of pre-transplant splenectomy on displacement bone marrow transplantation for Gaucher's syndrome. *Lancet* 1 (1987) 1111–1115

Holme, E., Jacobsen, G. E. and Kristiannson, B. Biotin-responsive multiple carboxylase deficiency in an 8-year-old boy with normal serum biotinidase and fibroblast holocarboxylase-sulphatase activities. *J. Inher. Metab. Dis.* 1a, 11 (1988) 270–276

Hoogerbrugge, P. M., Suzuki, Kinuko., Suzuki, Kunihiko, Poorthuis, B. J. H. M., Kobayashi, T., Wagemaker, G. and van Bekkum, D. W. Donor-derived cells in the central nervous system of Twitcher mice after bone marrow transplantation. *Science* 239 (1988) 1035–1038

Hugh-Jones, K., Kendra, J., James, D. C. O., Rogers, T. R., Williamson, S., Desai, S., Patrick, A. D. and Hobbs, J. R. Treatment of Sanfilippo B disease (MPS IIIB) by bone marrow transplant. *Exp. Hematol* 10 Suppl. 10 (1982) 50–51

Hurvitz, H., Ginat-Israeli, T., Elpeleg, O. N., Klar, A. and Amir, N. Biotinidase deficiency associated with severe combined immunodeficiency. *Lancet* 2 (1989) 228–229

Iriondo, A., Garijo, J., Baro, J., Conde, E., Pastor, J. M., Sabanes, A., Hermosa, V., Sainz, M. C., Perez de la Lastra, L. and Zubizaretta, A. Complete recovery of hemopoiesis following bone marrow transplant in a patient with unresponsive congenital hypoplastic anaemia. (Blackfan-Diamond syndrome). *Blood* 164 (1984) 348–51

Johnson, F. L., Look, A. T., Gockerman, J., Ruggiero, M. R., Dalla-Pozza, L. and Billings, F. T. Bone marrow transplantation in a patient with sickle cell anaemia. *N. Engl. J. Med.* 311 (1984) 780–783

Joss, V., Rogers, T. R., Hugh-Jones, K., Beilby, B., Joshi, R., Williamson, S., Foroozanfar, N., Riches, P., Turner, M., Benson, P. D. and Hobbs, J. R. A bone marrow transplant for metachromatic leucodystrophy. *Exp. Hematol.* 10 Suppl. 10 (1982) 52–53

Kato, S., Kabota, C., Yabe, H., Yamamura, M., Kurobane, I. and Orii, T. Bone marrow transplantation in Morquio's disease. In Hobbs, J. R. (ed.), *Correction of Certain Genetic Diseases by Transplantation 1989*, COGENT Press, Westminster, 1989, pp. 120–126

Kazmierowski, J. A., Elin, R. J., Reynolds, H. Y., Durbin, W. A. and Wolff, S. M. Chediak-Higashi syndrome: reversal of increased susceptibility to infection by bone marrow transplantation. *Blood* 47 (1976) 555–59

Kurobane, I., Inoue, S., Gotoh, Y-I., Kato, S., Tamura, M., Narisawa, K. and Tada, K. Biochemical improvement after treatment by bone marrow transplantation in I-cell disease. *Tohoku J. Exp. Med.* 150 (1986) 63–68

Lamendin, H. First case of bone resorption evoked by bone marrow transplantation in a human patient with osteopetrosis. *Mater. Med. Pol.* 11 (1979) 67–68

Lancet leader: Bone marrow transplantation for neurovisceral storage disorders. *Lancet* 2 (1986) 788–789

Laure, F., Courgnaud, V., Rouzloux, C., Blanche, S., Veber, F., Jacomet, C., Griscelli, G. and Brechot, C. Detection of HIV1 DNA in infants and children by means of the polymerase chain reaction. *Lancet* 2 (1988) 538–540

Levinsky, R. J. and Tiedman, K. Successful bone marrow transplantation for reticular dysgenesis. *Lancet* 1 (1983) 671–73

Loutit, J. F. Bone marrow grafts in mature osteopetrotic mice. *Transplantation* 24 (1977) 299–301

Lowdon, A. G. R., Stewart, R. H. M. and Walker, W. Risk of serious infection following splenectomy. *Br. Med. J.* 1 (1966) 446–450

McGovern, M. M., Ludman, M., Short, M. P., Kattan, M., Raab, E. L., Krivit, W. and Desnick, R. J. Bone marrow transplantation in Maroteaux–Lamy syndrome (MPS type 6): status 40 months after BMT. *Birth Defects* 22 (1986) 41–53

Markert, M. L., Hershfield, M. S., Wiginton, D. A., States, J. C., Ward, F. E., Bigner, S. H., Buckley, R. H., Kaufman, R. E. and Hutton, J. J. Identification of a deletion in the adenosine deaminase gene in a child with severe combined immunodeficiency. *J. Immunol.* 138 (1987) 3203–3206

Moser, H. W., Naidu, S., Kumar, A. J., Rosenbaum, A. E. The adrenoleukodystrophies. *Crit. Rev. Neurobiol.* 5 (1987) 29–88

Nyhan, W. L., Page, T., Gruber, H. and Parkman, R. Bone marrow transplantation in Lesch–Nyhan disease. *Birth Defects* 22 (1) (1986) 113–117

Orii, T. Screening, enzymatic diagnosis and heterozygote identification of genetic mucopolysaccharidoses. *Asian Med. J.* 29 (1986) 89–99

Pahwa, R. N., O'Reilly, R. J., Broxmeyer, H. E., Smithwick, E. M., Pahwa, S. G., Kapadla, A. and Good, R. A. Partial correction of neutrophil deficiency in congenital neutropenia following bone marrow transplantation (BMT) *Exp. Hematol.* 5 (1977) 45

Parkman, R., Remold-O'Donnell, E., Kenney, D. M., Perrine, S. and Rosen, F. S. Surface protein abnormalities in lymphocytes and platelets from patients with Wiskott–Aldrich syndrome. *Lancet* 2 (1981) 1387–1389

Perry, V. H. and Gordon, S. Macrophages of the central nervous system and their possible role in the delivery of lysosomal hydrolases after bone marrow transplantation. In Hobbs, J. R. (ed.) *The Correction of Certain Genetic Diseases By Transplantation*, 1989, COGENT Press, Westminster, 1989, pp. 64–70

Porter, M. T., Fluharty, A. L. and Kihara, H. Correction of abnormal cerebroside sulfate metabolism in cultured metachromatic leukodystrophy fibroblasts. *Science* 172 (1971) 1263–1265

Rappeport, J. M., Parkman, R., Newburger, P., Camitta, B. M. and Chusid, M. J. Correction of infantile agranulocytosis (Kostmann's syndrome) by allogeneic bone marrow transplantation. *Am. J. Med.* 68 (1980) 605–609

Riches, P., Weatherald, L., Walker, S., Hugh-Jones, K. and Hobbs, J. R. Transition to donor-type immunoglobulin synthesis following BMT. *Bone Marrow Transplantation* 1 Suppl. 1 (1986) 244

Rogers, T. R., Joshi, R., White, S., Riches, P., Foroozanfar, N., Ingram, L. and Pallett, A. Severe pneumococcal infection and splenic atrophy occurring as complications of graft-versus-host disease after haplotype mismatched marrow transplants. *Exp. Hematol.* 11, Suppl. 13 (1983) 123–124

Rosenberg, L. E., Disorders of proprionate and methylmalonate metabolism. In Stanbury, J. B.,, Wyngaarden, J. B., Fredrickson, D. S., Goldstein, J. L. and Brown, M. S. (eds.), *The Metabolic Basis of Inherited Disease*, McGraw Hill, New York, 1983, pp. 471–497

Schutgens, R. B. H., Schrakamp, G., Wanders, R. J. A., Heymans, H. S. A., Tager, J. M. and van den Bosch, H. Prenatal and perinatal diagnosis of peroxisomal disorders. *J. Inher. Metab. Dis.* 12, Suppl. 1 (1989) 118–134

Shaw, P. J., Hugh-Jones, K. and Hobbs, J. R. GM1 gangliosidosis: Failure to halt neurological regression by bone marrow transplantation. *Bone Marrow Transplantation* 1, Suppl. 1 (1986) 339

Shull, R. M., Hastings, N. E., Selcer, R. R., Jones, J. B., Smith, J. R., Cullen, W. C. and Constantopoulos, G. Bone marrow transplantation in canine mucopolysaccharidosis 1: effects within the central nervous system. *J. Clin. Invest.* 79 (1987) 435–43

Sorell, M., Rosen, J. F. and Kapoor, N. Bone marrow transplant for osteopetrosis in a 10-year-old boy. *Pediatr. Res.* 13 (1978) 481

Sorge, J., Kuhl, W., West, C. and Beutler, E. Complete correction of the enzymatic defect of type I Gaucher disease fibroblasts by retroviral-mediated gene transfer. *Proc. Natl. Acad. Sci. USA* 84 (1987) 906–909

Souillet, G., Guibaud, P., Fensom, A. H., Maire, I. and Zabet, M. T. Outcome of displacement bone marrow transplantation in Farber's disease. In Hobbs, J.R. (ed.) *The Correction of Certain Genetic Diseases by Transplantation, 1989*, COGENT Press, Westminster, 1989, pp. 137–141

Starer, F., Sargent, J. D. and Hobbs, J. R. Regression of the radiological changes of Gaucher's disease following bone marrow transplantation. *Br. J. Radiol.* 60 (1987) 1189–1195

Stein, C., Gieselmann, V. and Kreysing, J. Cloning and expression of human arylsulfatase A. *J. Biol. Chem.* 261 (1989) 1252–1259

Steinmuller, D. and Motulsky, A. G. Treatment of hereditary spherocytosis in Peromyscus by radiation and allogeneic bone marrow transplantation. *Blood* 29 (1967) 320

Svennerholm, L., Mansson, J-E., Nilsson, O. and Tibblin, E. Bone marrow transplantation in the Norrbottnian form of Gaucher disease. In Barranger, J. A. and Brady, R. O. (eds.), *Molecular Basis of Lysosomal Storage Disorders*, Academic Press, New York, 1984, pp. 441–459

Taylor, R. M., Farrow, B. R. H., Stewart, G. J. and Healy, P. J. Enzyme replacement in nervous tissue after allogeneic bone marrow transplantation for fucosidosis. *Lancet* 2 (1986) 772–774

Thomas, E. D., Sanders, J.E., Borgna-Pignatti, C., Stefano, P.D., Clift, R.A., Buckner, C.D., Papyannopoulou, T., Sullivan, K. M. and Storb, R. Marrow transplantation for thalassaemia. *Lancet* 2 (1982) 227–229

Touraine, J-L. Fetal liver transplantation in congenital enzyme deficiencies in man. *Exp. Haematol.* 10 Suppl 10 (1982) 46

Touraine, J-L., Betuel, H. and Touraine, F. The bare lymphocyte syndrome. In Griscelli, C. and Vossen, J. (eds.), *Progress in Immunodeficiency Research and Therapy*, Excerpta Medica, Amsterdam, 1984, pp. 27–34

Tutschka, P. J. and Santos, G. W. Bone marrow transplantation in the busulfan-treated rat. *Transplantation* 24 (1977) 52–62

Valdimarsson, H., Holt, P. J. L., Moss, P. D. and Hobbs, J. R. Treatment of chronic mucocutaneous candidiasis with leucocytes from HL-A compatible sibling. *Lancet* 1 (1972) 469–71

Vellodi, A., Hobbs, J. R., O'Donnell, N. M., Coulter, B. S. and Hugh-Jones, K. Treatment of Niemann–Pick disease type B by allogeneic bone marrow transplantation. *Br. Med. J.* 295 (1987) 1375–1376

Vermylen, C., Fernandez Robles, E. Ninane, J. and Cornu, G. Bone marrow transplantation in five children with sickle cell anaemia. *Lancet* 1 (1988) 1427–1428

Virelizier, J. L., Durandy, A., Lagrue, A., Fischer, A. and Griscelli, C. Successful bone marrow transplantation in a patient with Chediak–Higashi syndrome. *Exp. Hematol.* 11 Suppl. 13 (1983) 91–92

Walker, D. G. Bone resorption restored in osteopetrotic mice by transplants of normal bone marrow and spleen cells. *Science* 190 (1975) 784–85

Walker, S. A., Riches, P. G., Wild, G., Ward, A. M., Shaw, P. J., Desai, S. and Hobbs, J. R. Total and allergen-specific IgE in relation to allergic response pattern following bone marrow transplantation. *Clin. Exp. Immunol.* 66 (1986) 633–639

Warkentin, P. I., Dixon Jr., M. S., Schafer, I., Strandjord, S. E. and Coccia, P. F. Bone marrow transplantation in Hunter syndrome: a preliminary report. *Birth Defects* 22 No 1. (1986) 31–39

Wilcken, B. and Hammond, J. Hearing loss in biotinidase deficiency. *Lancet* 2 (1983) 1366

William, S., Hewett-Emmett, D., Whyte, M. P., Yu, Y-SL. and Tashian, R. E. Carbonic anhydrase II deficiency identified as the primary defect in the autosomal recessive syndrome of osteopetrosis with renal tubular acidosis and cerebral calcification. *Proc. Natl. Acad. Sci. USA* 80 (1983) 2752–2756

Yamamura, M., Newton, R. C. F., James, D. C .O., Humble, J. G., Butler, L. J. and Hobbs, J. R. Uncomplicated HL-A matched sibling bone marrow graft for combined immune deficiency. *Br. Med. J.* 2 (1972) 265–69

J. Inher. Metab. Dis. 13 (1990) 597–616

Clinical Application of Somatic Gene Therapy in Inborn Errors of Metabolism

F. D. LEDLEY
Howard Hughes Medical Institute, Departments of Cell Biology and Pediatrics, Baylor College of Medicine, Houston, Texas TX 77030, USA

Summary: Rapid advances in recombinant DNA and gene transfer technologies provide the potential for somatic gene therapy of inborn errors of metabolism in which the genetically defective function will be restored by transfer of a normal gene into somatic cells. The therapeutic potential and safety of gene therapy has been explored in cultured cells and experimental animals, but therapeutic clinical trials have not yet been proposed or performed. The technologies which may make somatic gene replacement therapy feasible need to be considered and criticised from a clinical perspective. Clinical trials will be necessary to determine the efficacy of somatic gene therapy and address concerns about safety.

In 1946 in his inaugural lecture as the Galton Professor of Eugenics at University College London (Penrose, 1946), Sir Lionel Penrose considered the eugenic approach to disease pioneered by his eminent predecessors and concluded that they were wrong. He concluded that they were wrong, not because of their statistical and genetic errors, not because of their inherent racial bias, and not because of the apocalyptic consequences of the eugenic vision: rather, he realized that the genetically determined phenotype of a metabolic disease such as phenylketonuria (PKU) could be amenable to conventional allopathic medical therapy (Ledley, 1987a); he wrote:

> "There may be methods of alleviating the condition, even though it is inborn, in a manner analogous to the way in which a child with club feet may be helped to walk, or a child with congenital cataract to see" (Penrose, 1946).

Within several years, Professor Horst Bickel in Heidelberg and others applied this concept to clinical practice with dietary therapy for PKU. Dietary therapy of PKU is fundamentally palliative; it adapts the patient's input of phenylalanine to match their limited excretory capacity. This therapy does not alter the enzymatic abnormality underlying the disease, but it alters the environment within which these mutations operate and mitigates the phenotypic consequences of the mutation (Scriver *et al.*, 1989). Dietary therapy has proved useful in many inborn errors of metabolism and provides an important paradigm for treating genetic disease (Scriver and Clow, 1980). If we might use Penrose's metaphor, we have provided a crutch and glasses which enable our patients to walk without falling, though the genetic defect remains.

Another approach to the treatment of inborn errors of metabolism is to replace the deficient function. This is the idea behind tissue transplantation in which a genetically defective organ is replaced with a donor organ having normal genetic capacities. Tissue transplantation is useful in treating many metabolic diseases, and with advances in the procurement of organs, techniques for partial or heterotopic transplantation, and management of immunological rejection, these procedures may become a more common therapeutic option.

Recombinant DNA and molecular cloning technologies have introduced a new possibility; that of selectively replacing abnormal genes by somatic gene therapy. This would be a truly therapeutic option in which the fundamental biochemical abnormality would be corrected in a patient's own cells.

The inborn errors of metabolism are ideal candidates for somatic gene therapy for several reasons: the clinical and biochemical courses of many of these diseases are well known; many of the genes involved in inborn errors of metabolism have been cloned; and many experiments have been performed in cultured cells which have established the principle of 'curing' the genetic defect by gene transfer. Within the next 1–2 years, several laboratories will be proposing experiments in somatic gene therapy for inborn errors of metabolism.

Despite the exciting potential of this technology, there is foreboding and mystique about gene therapy outside of the community of molecular geneticists. Gene therapy is portrayed as a creative or even eugenic potential capable of altering the human genome and human inheritance. Its power and applications are often exaggerated and often engender fear. Much of the apprehension about gene therapy arises from the fact that the basic research which will enable somatic gene therapy to be carried out is usually presented in the abstract without reference to the logical and logistical limitations of the clinic. It is important to consider somatic gene therapy within the confines of clinical application, both because the molecular biologist frequently underestimates the complexity of human applications and because there is a wealth of surgical and clinical expertise which may be applied to these problems.

Several extensive reviews have emphasized the technological development of somatic gene therapy (Friedmann and Roblin, 1972; Friedmann, 1983; Anderson, 1984; Office of Technology Assessment, 1984; Williams and Orkin, 1986; Ledley, 1987b, 1989; Nichols, 1988). In this report, I will describe somatic gene therapy in the context of clinical investigation and clinical application. I will consider both the state-of-the-art in gene transfer technology as well as the biochemical and clinical concerns which may affect the design of clinical research protocols.

METHODS FOR SOMATIC GENE THERAPY

Methods for gene transfer

It is a fundamental principle of molecular biology that if a gene is isolated and introduced into a suitable environment it will continue to express its gene product. The transfer of genes among organisms is common in nature. It is best exemplified by viruses whose life cycle involves the transfer of viral genes into infected cells and the subsequent *transformation* of the infected cell to produce a new generation of viruses. The principle of somatic gene therapy is similar to viral infection. In fact, an early, unsuccessful attempt at gene therapy for arginase deficiency (hyperargininaemia, hyperammoniaemia) was made by deliberately infecting patients with the Shope papilloma virus, a virus which expresses a viral form of the enzyme arginase (Rogers *et al.*, 1973; Terhaggen *et al.*, 1975).

There are several ways to transfer a gene into a cell. Purified DNA may be introduced into cells by direct microinjection (Capecchi, 1980), electroporation (in which a powerful electric pulse disrupts the membrane and pushes DNA into a cell; Chu *et al.*, 1987), or transfection (in which particles containing DNA precipitates are taken up by a cell; Graham and Vandereb, 1973). These methods are referred to as *DNA-mediated gene transfer*. Once DNA is in the cell it may become integrated into the host cell's genome by a process resembling DNA repair. This process, called *stable integration*, is inefficient (occurring in < 1 in 10 000 cells) and is frequently associated with damage to the host genome (Scangos and Ruddle, 1981). Thus, DNA mediated gene transfer with contemporary technologies has little application to somatic gene therapy.

Viruses have evolved efficient methods for introducing genes into cells and integrating their genes into the host genome. Research in somatic gene therapy has concentrated in adapting viruses as *vectors* for gene transfer (Reviewed in Ledley, 1989). The use of viral vectors to carry recombinant genes into cells is called *viral-mediated gene transfer*.

RNA viruses such as Moloney murine leukaemia virus (MMLV) are particularly well suited for experiments in gene therapy. MMLV is easily manipulated by recombinant DNA techniques and contains only three viral genes: *gag*, *pol* and *env*. One important property of retroviruses is that the proteins and enzymes required for processing the viral gene are constitutive elements of the virus particle and are carried into the infected cell with the viral gene during infection. It is possible to delete the *gag*, *pol* and *env* genes, package the deleted viral genome into a pre-assembled viral particle, and stably infect cells with the deleted gene (Mann *et al.*, 1983). This so-called *defective retrovirus* encodes no viral proteins and is incapable of further propagation.

Defective retroviruses represent a 'Trojan horse' for gene transfer. Human genes can be recombined with the deleted viral genome, packaged into a viral particle, and introduced into cells by infection. This is done by combining the recombinant human gene with the *long terminal repeat* (LTR) and ψ (packaging) sequences of the viral genome which are necessary and sufficient for packaging a gene into an empty viral particle (Figure 1) (Mann *et al.*, 1983). Empty viral particles can be produced using a *packaging cell line* which contains the *gag*, *pol*, and *env* genes without the LTR and ψ components of the viral genome (Figure 1) (Mann *et al.*, 1983; Markowitz *et al.*, 1988). When a recombinant gene containing the LTR and ψ sequences is introduced into these cells, the recombinant gene is packaged into the viral particles producing a defective retrovirus.

Retroviruses have been used to introduce genes into a variety of cell types including

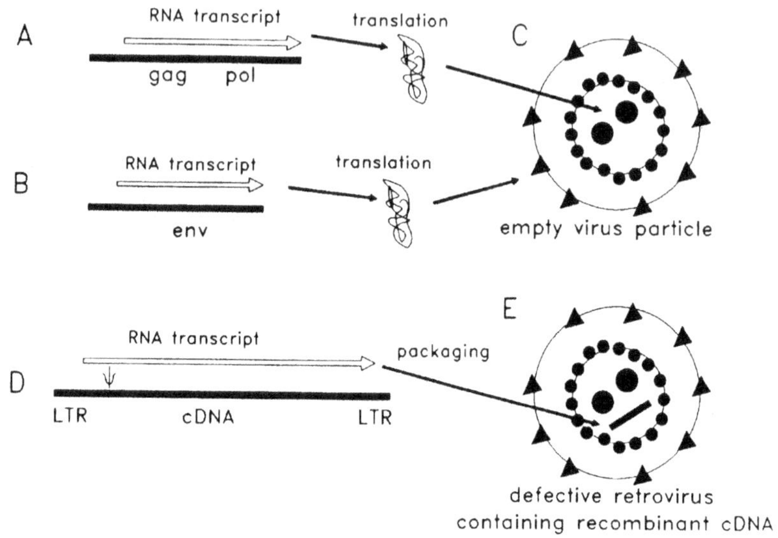

Figure 1 Method for construction of defective recombinant retroviruses. A cell line containing recombinant genes expressing the *gag-pol* polyprotein (A) and the *env* glycoprotein (B) will translate these mRNA on cytoplasmic ribosomes and synthesize empty virus particles (C). If another recombinant gene containing a human cDNA, the ψ sequence, and the LTR sequences (D) is introduced into this cell, the RNA transcript from this recombinant will be packaged into the virus particles produced from recombinants containing only *gag-pol* or *env* giving rise to a defective retrovirus containing the recombinant cDNA (E). This defective retrovirus contains the *gag*, *pol*, and *env* gene products as well as the recombinant cDNA and is capable of infecting host cells and incorporating the recombinant cDNA into the host chromosome. Since this transcript does not carry any viral genes, it is incapable of subsequent viral replication or inducing viral disease.

embryonic cells, hematopoietic stem cells, hepatocytes, endothelial cells, epithelial cells and fibroblasts. *Amphotrophic retroviruses* have been shown to infect human cells (Reviewed in Ledley, 1989).

Methods for expression of a recombinant gene

Introducing a gene into a cell is only the first step in somatic gene replacement therapy. It is essential that this gene be expressed and that the gene product be biologically active. The expression of a recombinant gene requires a *promotor* to direct *transcription* of the integrated DNA into mRNA and the signals for *translation* of the mRNA into protein.

The major problem in the development of somatic gene therapy has been achieving adequate levels of gene expression of recombinant genes in infected cells. Many viral constructions have been reported which directed expression in cultured cells but failed to function *in vivo*. The retroviral LTR sequence contains a promotor capable of directing transcription and recently success has been obtained using simple vectors containing only this LTR promotor (Belmont *et al.*, 1988; Wilson *et al.*, 1988a). Alternatively, the recombinant vector may be designed with a tissue specific or hormonally responsive promotor, and some success has been reported with these constructions (Dzierzak *et al.*, 1988; Peng *et al.*, 1988).

TARGETS FOR SOMATIC GENE THERAPY OF INBORN ERRORS OF METABOLISM

After the recombinant gene is transcribed and translated, the recombinant gene product must be biologically active. This is a particular problem in somatic gene therapy for inborn errors of metabolism since the apoenzyme encoded by the recombinant gene may require cofactors, substrates or regulatory effectors. For example, it is possible to transduce the phenylalanine hydroxylase gene into virtually any cell type, but if the host cell does not provide sufficient reduced biopterin cofactor, the enzyme will be inactive (Ledley et al., 1987a). Similarly, it may be reasoned that ornithine transcarboxylase will be inactive except in cells producing carbamyl phosphate, and enzymes such as hexosaminidase will be biologically useless except in cells which accumulate gangliosides. Moreover, many enzymes are regulated by the concentration of substrate, products, or regulatory enzymes which are expressed in a tissue specific manner. Thus, the target tissue for somatic gene therapy must be carefully selected in order to constitute enzyme function and alter the biochemcial phenotype of the patient.

Gene therapy targeted to bone marrow

Most research in somatic gene therapy has concentrated on introducing genes into the bone marrow. The bone marrow is an ideal target for somatic gene therapy since it is readily accessible for harvest, transplantation, and analysis; because there is extensive clinical and laboratory experience in culturing and transplanting bone marrow; and because bone marrow may be reconstituted from a small number of totipotential stem cells transformed with recombinant vectors. Studies in several laboratories have demonstrated that it is possible to infect a totipotential stem cell with a recombinant retrovirus; to reconstitute murine (Dick *et al.*, 1985; Keller *et al.*, 1985; Belmont *et al.*, 1988; Dzierzak *et al.*, 1988), canine (Stead *et al.*, 1988), or chimpanzee bone marrow (Kantoff *et al.*, 1987) with the transformed cells; and to achieve expression of the recombinant gene in marrow-derived cell lineages.

Many inborn errors of metabolism may be treated by somatic gene therapy targeted to bone marrow (Parkman, 1986; Hobbs, 1990). The best candidates are those diseases currently amenable to heterologous bone marrow transplantation such as Gaucher's disease or adenosine deaminase deficiency. Some inborn errors of metabolism are not amenable to bone marrow transplantation because the affected gene is not expressed in bone marrow-derived cells. Such disorders might be treated by gene therapy targeted to the bone marrow by designing vectors with promoters which will direct *heterotopic* transcription of the gene in marrow-derived cells. *Heterotopic* gene expression could alter a metabolic disease by clearing a toxic metabolite from the blood or by producing a deficient metabolite. This would require the transformed cell to transport the substrate from the plasma and to be able to return the product. Transformed bone marrow cells could alternatively be engineered to secrete an enzyme which could be taken up by other cells as a form of enzyme replacement therapy. Obviously, in considering heterotopic expression as therapy for an inborn error of metabolism, it is essential that the fate of the substrate, product, and the enzyme itself be understood.

Gene therapy targeted to the liver

Not all inborn errors of metabolism will be amenable to somatic gene therapy targeted to the bone marrow. For many inborn errors of metabolism, the obvious target for somatic gene therapy is the liver. Several laboratories have demonstrated that recombinant retroviruses can be used to introduce recombinant genes into hepatocytes in culture and have shown direct expression of the recombinant gene product (Ledley *et al.*, 1987b; Wolff *et al.*, 1987a, 1987b; Peng *et al.*, 1988; Wilson *et al.*, 1988a, 1988b). It has been proposed that gene therapy could be performed by isolating hepatocytes from a partial hepatectomy, infecting these cells with recombinant viruses, and performing autologous transplants back into the patient. Unlike bone marrow transplantation which is in widespread clinical usage, there is no clinical precedent for hepatocellular transplantation in man.

Hepatocellular transplantation techniques have been developed in animals. The most common model is the Gunn rat which is deficient in UDP-glucoronyl transferase and represents an analogue for Crigler–Najjar syndrome. Transplantation of normal (congenic) hepatocytes into the Gunn rat has been shown to lower bilirubin levels. Transplantation techniques have included injection of isolated hepatocytes into the peritoneum (Mukherjee and Krasner, 1973; Matas *et al.*, 1976; Groth *et al.*, 1977; Sutherland *et al.*, 1977; Demetriou *et al.*, 1986a, 1986b, 1986c), portal vein (Matas *et al.*, 1976; Groth *et al.*, 1977), spleen (Mito *et al.*, 1979; Vroemen *et al.*, 1985), or fat pads (Jirtle and Michalopoulous, 1982). Studies in analbuminaemic rats have demonstrated that transplantation of hepatocytes into these animals will increase the amount of circulating albumin (Demetriou, 1986a, 1986b, 1986c). It has also been shown that animals with experimentally induced hepatic failure can be rescued by implantation of hepatocytes (Makowka *et al.*, 1980; Baumgartner *et al.*, 1983; Contini *et al.*, 1983; Minato *et al.*, 1984; tenBerg *et al.*, 1985). Hepatocytes from a transgenic mouse expressing human α-1-antitrypsin (Shen *et al.*, 1987) transplanted into normal mice have led to the stable expression of human α-1-antitrypsin in the mouse serum, demonstrating successful engraftment and function of the transplanted cells (Parker and Woo, unpublished data).

Many studies have demonstrated function of transplanted hepatocytes for short periods of time (weeks or months). One problem is that few of the transplanted cells become vascularized and remain viable. Improved vascularization has been reported using 'gel-foam' soaked with angiogenesis factor (Thompson *et al.*, 1988) or collagen IV coated supports (Anderson *et al.*, 1989). Improved results may also result from injection of cells into the portal or splenic vein rather than into an avascular space.

Even if hepatocellular transplantation protocols prove to be efficacious in rodent models, these methods are unlikely to be in the vanguard of human gene therapy protocols since there is no clinical or surgical precedent for these transplantation procedures. Only the bone marrow has been shown to be amenable to reconstitution by cellular transplant following *in vitro* culture. Extensive research on cellular transplantation for diabetes (Yasumizu *et al.*, 1987) or Parkinson's disease (Madrazo *et al.*, 1987) has not met with unambiguous success. Furthermore, there is a thousand-fold difference in the scale between humans and rodents, and it is difficult to imagine 'scaling-up' *in vitro* culture to this degree.

The lack of clinical precedent for hepatocellular transplantation represents a major impediment to such gene therapy protocols. Hepatocellular transplantation techniques would most likely have to be established in human clinical trials before they could be incorporated into protocols for somatic gene therapy. Such experiments could be done now using normal (living or cadaveric) donor cells, though these experiments have never been attempted. The only advantage to transplanting genetically engineering cells versus heterologous donor cells is that it affords the opportunity to perform autologous transplants without immunosuppression. Indeed, the molecular biologist's interest in cellular transplantation as an adjunct to somatic gene therapy may provide the impetus for such clinical experiments.

There are exciting developments in the field of hepatic transplantation which may be applicable to somatic gene therapy, including the development of methods for transplanting portions or isolated lobes of livers and heterotopic transplantation. It has been suggested by some researchers that familial donation of liver lobes may provide an alternative to cadaveric liver transplantation (Broelsch *et al.*, 1988). Somatic gene therapy for inborn errors of metabolism will have to take advantage of the considerable clinical experience in the harvest, preservation, and transplantation of these organs in developing clinically applicable methods for somatic gene therapy.

Gene therapy targeted to fibroblasts, endothelial cells, and epidermal cells

Other cell types have been proposed as potential targets for gene therapy including epidermal cells (Morgan *et al.*, 1987), fibroblasts (Choudary *et al.*, 1986; Palmer *et al.*, 1987; Sorge *et al.*, 1987), and endothelial cells (Nabel *et al.*, 1989; Wilson *et al.*, 1989). These targets have the advantage that they are easily harvested, cultured and transplanted. It has been proposed that epidermal cells could be reimplanted using established procedures for skin grafting, that endothelial cells could be reimplanted as part of a vascular graft, and that fibroblasts might be injected virtually anywhere. The disadvantage of these cells is that they may not have the accessory functions required for activity of the recombinant gene product, and that only a relatively small number of cells could be transplanted.

Gene therapy targeted to the central nervous system

The central nervous system is an important, though difficult, target for somatic gene therapy for several reasons; the CNS is protected by a blood–brain barrier which prevents infection with most viruses, and integration of retroviruses may require cell division. Thus, the approach to diseases such as Lesch–Nyhan syndrome has been to circumvent the need for transformation of neurons by engrafting non-neuronal cells containing recombinant transgenes (Gage *et al.*, 1987; Rosenberg *et al.*, 1988). The expectation is that the recombinant gene in the graft would provide essential metabolites or eliminate toxic products within the CNS. This expectation was not supported by the experience in a patient with advanced Lesch–Nyhan syndrome treated with a heterologous bone marrow transplantation (Nyhan *et al.*, 1986) who failed to show a clinical response. In one experimental model for gene therapy of the CNS, fibroblasts expressing a recombinant nerve growth factor have been grafted into rat brains following surgical ablation of specific regions and shown to stimulate the growth of neurons into the ablated region (Rosenberg *et al.*, 1988). The absence of any clinical precedent for these procedures in man, however, makes the application of somatic gene therapy to these disorders more distant.

Gene therapy to solid organs

There is little precedent for somatic gene therapy into solid organs such as muscle, heart, kidney or lung. Recent experiments with myoblast injection into the muscles of patients with Duchenne's dystrophy raise the possibility that the introduction of a few transformed cells might alter the phenotype of muscle, perhaps by formation of heterokaryons. Cells with complex architecture such as the kidney will not be amenable to cellular transplantation although they might be infected *in situ* or *ex situ*. The lung may be a particularly important site for experiments in gene therapy because of the prevalence and continuing morbidity of cystic fibrosis.

Somatic gene therapy by *in vivo* infection

The simplest scheme for gene therapy would be to infect a patient with recombinant retroviruses *in vivo*, thus obviating the need for explanation and transplantation of organs or cells. It is likely, however, that initial experiments will require greater control over the target and distribution of the recombinant retroviruses than will be afforded by the current generation of recombinant vectors. It is considered essential that somatic gene therapy avoids even accidental contamination of the germline which would result in vertical transmission of the recombinant gene to future generations (see below). Several laboratories are addressing the possibility of designing vectors with particular tissue specific trophism which might enable *in vivo* infection to take place.

Somatic cells vs germ cells

One of the most important issues in gene therapy is the distinction between the introduction of genes into *germ cells*, where the recombinant gene may become part of the human germline and be passed on to future generations, and the introduction of genes into *somatic cells*, where the recombinant gene will only alter the phenotype of the individual. The germline would appear to be an obvious target for gene replacement therapy, since this would lead to replacement of the gene function in all cells. Moreover, repair of mutations in the germline could prevent the inheritance of the genetic disease by subsequent generations. For technical and ethical reasons, the consideration of gene therapy is restricted to somatic cells. There is serious concern that engineering of the human germline could lead to eugenic interventions or unacceptable interference in human variability or evolution. Germline interventions, however, may be inappropriate and impractical for logistical as well as ethical reasons. Studies with transgenic mice (in which gene transfer vectors are introduced into the mouse germline) demonstrate that germline manipulations are associated with a high frequency of insertional mutagenesis and the genesis of new genetic diseases (Palmiter and Brinster, 1985). Also, germline gene therapy would require prior identification of germ cells containing mutant genes. While it is technically possible using the polymerase chain reaction to perform genetic diagnosis on embryos fertilized *in vitro* (Handysmith *et al.*, 1989), such diagnosis would necessarily reveal that genetic disease was transmitted to only a fraction of the embryos. Since gene transfer into germ cells is known to be associated with significant risk, it would obviously be inappropriate to chance damage to the majority of germ cells carrying the normal allele. The profound risk of gene transfer into an embryo would have to be compared with the cost of selectively reimplanting the non-affected embryos (generally only a fraction of fertilized embryos are implanted).

ALTERNATIVE STRATEGIES FOR SOMATIC GENE THERAPY OF INBORN ERRORS OF METABOLISM

Somatic gene therapy as gene addition

Somatic gene therapy, as generally conceived, will constitute a metabolic function adding a normal gene to somatic cells which are genetically deficient in that gene product. The inborn errors of metabolism are well suited to this approach since they are single gene disorders, are commonly recessive (autosomal or X-linked), and even one normal gene would be expected to prevent the pathological phenotype. Moreover, in many inborn errors of metabolism even small amounts of residual function (5–10% of normal) may prevent the clinical pathology associated with complete deficiency of the gene product. Thus, even low level expression of the recombinant gene could ameliorate many inborn errors of metabolism.

The potential for replacement of a mutant gene

There are other approaches to somatic gene therapy. One approach is *gene replacement* in which a normal gene would be integrated in place of the defective gene. Gene replacement is practical in cultured cells using techniques of homologous recombination. When a recombinant gene is introduced into a cell, there is a relatively high probability (1:100–1:1000 integrants) that it will integrate into the genome in its proper (homologous) position (Smithies *et al.*, 1985; Doetschman *et al.*, 1987; Thomas and Capecchi, 1987). (This is a high probability considering that there are 3×10^9 bases in the human genome which represent potential non-homologous recombination sites.) This process of *homologous recombination* is thought to involve matching between the recombinant gene sequence and the (homologous) gene present in the genome.

Homologous recombination has been used to repair a mutation in the germline of a mouse with hypoxanthine phosphoribosyltransferase deficiency (Thompson *et al.*, 1989). Gene repair by homologous recombination has little application to gene therapy in man at the present time because it remains relatively inefficient. It may be imagined that homologous recombinaion can be used to correct a gene defect in a haemotopoietic stem cell. Even this procedure would require significant advances in the frequency of homologous recombination and methods for culturing stem cells.

Somatic gene therapy by constitution of novel pathways

Another approach is to circumvent a defective pathway by constitution of alternative pathways. Conventional therapy for the inborn errors of metabolism offers important precedents for this approach. For example, the administration of pharmacological doses of sodium benzoate in disorders of the urea cycle stimulates activity of a normally minor alternative pathway for ammonia fixation (Brusilow *et al.*, 1984); the administration of pharmacological doses of betaine in homocystinuria stimulates a minor pathway for homocysteine metabolism (Wilcken *et al.*, 1983); and the administration of phenylalanine ammonia lyase in phenylketonuria would provide a mechanism for metabolizing phenylalanine (Ambrus *et al.*, 1987). Genetic constitution of alternative pathways could similarly prevent the pathological consequences of a genetic deficiency without restoring the deficient enzyme activity. This could provide a means of treating diseases in which the deficient gene product is difficult to transfer, requires critical regulation, or requires expression in an inaccessible site. For example, it has been suggested that the presence of urate oxidase protects the HPRT deficient mouse from the pathological consequence of Lesch–Nyhan syndrome in humans (this enzyme is not present in humans) (Lee *et al.*, 1988). Constitution of urate oxidase in human cells might present an alternative to the introduction of HPRT into neurons.

Somatic gene therapy altering metabolite regulation

Another strategy is to use gene transfer to alter the regulation of a gene. There is a precedent for this approach in the use of Mevinolin to treat hypercholesterolaemia associated with LDL receptor deficiency. Mevinolin inhibits HMG-CoA reductase and leads indirectly to increased expression of the normal LDL receptor gene (Ma *et al.*, 1986). Another precedent is the attempt to treat thalassaemia by activation of fetal haemoglobin genes. Somatic gene therapy could similarly be used to alter the production of substrates or abnormal metabolites and thus alter the pathophysiological consequences of the enzyme deficiency. This approach to gene therapy may have increasing significance in the future as the factors involved in gene regulation are themselves cloned and become available for gene therapy.

Somatic gene therapy directed at pathophysiological mechanisms

The pathological phenotype of an inborn error of metabolism frequently involves the epigenetic action of a metabolite on pathways or processes unrelated to the mutant gene locus. For example, mental retardation in phenylketonuria is due to the action of phenylalanine (or abnormal metabolites of phenylalanine) on processes regulating amino acid levels or myelin formation in the brain where there is no phenylalanine hydroxylase. It may be anticipated that as such epigenetic processes come to be understood, somatic gene therapy may be used to alter the pathophysiology of many inborn errors of metabolism without restoring the deficient enzyme.

SAFETY OF SOMATIC GENE THERAPY

There are legitimate concerns about the safety of somatic gene therapy. Extensive studies in cells and animals will be performed prior to human investigations to minimize the potential for adverse effects. There is particular concern about the efficacy of using vectors based on MMLV for gene transfer in humans. There are two theoretical problems with MMLV based vectors: the first is concern that introduction of the recombinant gene into a cell may cause mutations by interruption (*insertional mutagenesis*) of an essential gene or that the promotor elements in the LTR may activate a normally silent gene. The possibility of activating *proto-oncogenes* is of particular concern since this is one mechanism by which retroviruses may cause tumorigenesis. In order to prevent activation of cellular proto-oncogenes, crippled retroviruses have been designed in which the enhancer and promotor functions of the LTR have been deleted (Yu *et al.*, 1986; Yee *et al.*, 1987). Such viruses are less likely to cause activation of oncogenes, but to date have also been inherently less efficient in producing sufficient virus particles for gene therapy experiments. The potential for insertional mutagenesis may theoretically be circumvented by using vectors which do not integrate into the host chromosome, but rather are replicated as 'mini-chromosomes' or *episomes*. Viruses such as papilloma virus and SV40 naturally replicate as episomes; however, it has been difficult to separate mechanisms for episomal replication from the malignant transforming potential of these viruses. The second concern is that replication of a defective retrovirus may spontaneously *recombine* with retroviruses in the environment giving rise to new, infectious viruses with unknown pathological potential. There is little data in experimental animals (and no data in man) to calculate the potential for such an event. It should be noted, however, that extensive research was performed in the 1960s and 1970s seeking to find naturally occurring human viruses related to murine retroviruses. These studies were uniformly unsuccessful in identifying endogenous or 'wild type' recombinants between human sequences and common murine retroviruses.

Experiments currently underway at the National Institutes of Health are using recombinant retroviral vectors as genetic markers as part of a bone marrow transplantation protocol in patients with multiply relapsed malignancies. While these experiments are not intended to evaluate the therapeutic potential of gene transfer, they will provide important data about the safety of these agents in humans and the applicability of animal experiments to predicting the efficacy and safety of these agents in man.

THE ETHICS OF SOMATIC GENE THERAPY

There has been extensive debate about the ethics of gene transfer in man (Friedman, 1983; Anderson, 1985; Fletcher, 1985; Ledley, 1987a; Nichols, 1988). Most authors agree that there is an essential difference between '*somatic gene therapy*' which involves only differentiated somatic cells and '*germline manipulations*' which effect the sperm and egg and thus potentially human progeny. Somatic gene therapy is fundamentally allopathic in nature (Ledley, 1987a). In principle, it is no different from the replacement of a failing organ, limb, or function with a heterologous or artificial graft.

There is also concern that the technologies developed to treat human disease could be abused to 'enhance' or alter normal human capacities (Anderson and Fletcher, 1980) or that the application of gene therapy to human diseases could lead down a 'slippery slope' of applications for cosmetic or social purposes. While the issue of potential abuse is legitimate, it is not unique to gene therapy and it does not warrant limiting the development or application of potentially life-saving medical therapies.

WHEN WILL CLINICAL RESEARCH IN SOMATIC GENE THERAPY FOR INBORN ERRORS OF METABOLISM BEGIN?

The development of methods for somatic gene transfer in cultured cells and experimental animals represents the first step in the development of this technology for clinical application. Ultimately, somatic gene therapy, like any other new therapeutic technique, will also have to be evaluated in clinical trials to determine the safety, complications and efficacy of this approach to human disease as well as of the specific agents which will be employed. It is naive to think that the results of these clinical experiments can be inferred from animal models of genetic disease. It is also naive to think that somatic gene therapy will provide an entirely safe and uncomplicated method for treating genetic disease. In the history of medical innovation, the best considered ideas of medical science can prove to be great advances and can prove to have undesirable consequences or inadequate therapeutic effects. The first attempts to treat PKU by dietary therapy did not prevent mental retardation, but may have exacerbated the pathology by inadvertent protein deprivation. Many productive careers have been spent translating Penrose's concept of treating inborn errors of metabolism into effective clinical practice. The application of somatic gene therapy will similarly require careers of clinical investigation and innovation.

It is true that there is more societal concern and public interest surrounding somatic gene therapy experiments than most other clinical research protocols. The first experiments in somatic gene therapy will certainly take place under intense public scrutiny. It has been argued that science as a discipline cannot afford failure or unanticipated complications in a public exercise. It has also been argued that society has an interest in limiting technologies whose ramifications may be incompletely understood and delimited. Despite the social implications of experimental success or failure, the tangible interest of individuals with a genetic disease must be considered in league with society's abstract and sometimes ephemeral concern about the propriety or potential of genetic engineering. A recent *Lancet* editorial made this point, arguing that 'the individual's responsibility and choice, provided it harms no-one else, is fundamental to a democratic society' (Anon, 1989). The recent trend towards allowing AIDS patients premature access to untested therapeutic agents affirms the principle that the individual's right to a potentially life-saving technology supercedes concerns about public policy. In fact, the physician's responsibility to patients with inborn errors of metabolism may require active advocation of the patients' rights to such technologies.

It is appropriate at the present time to consider in detail how clinical trials for somatic gene therapy will be designed and performed. The Recombinant Advisory Committee of the National Institutes of Health, anticipating the development of proposals for gene therapy, has promulgated a document entititled: *Points to Consider in the Design and Submission of Human Somatic-Cell Gene Therapy Protocols* detailing questions posed by the scientific and lay community about somatic gene therapy.

While there is considerable interest in the molecular biology behind human gene therapy experiments, there are also important clinical issues which must be considered in the design of gene therapy experiments. These include:

i) Selection of an inborn error of metabolism with unacceptable mortality or morbidity which is not effectively palliated by conventional therapy. The potential benefits of somatic gene therapy must be weighed against the morbidity or mortality of the disease as well as the efficacy and availability of other therapeutic approaches. The balance of risk vs. benefit may weigh more heavily in favour of experiments involving untreatable and lethal childhood diseases than those associated with qualitative defects such as mental retardation, growth retardation, moderate handicap, or cosmetic impairment. The balance is also altered by the development of competing technologies in pharmacology, transplantation and clinical management.

Many previous reviews on human gene therapy have emphasized the selection of diseases which might serve as models for human experimentation (Friedmann and Roblin, 1972; Friedmann, 1983; Anderson, 1984; Office of Technology Assessment, 1984; Ledley, 1987b; Ledley, 1989). The earlier works considered the availability of cloned genetic material and the development of vector systems as limiting factors. In recent years, the cloning of genes for many common inborn errors of metabolism and the development of general principles of vector design have made many inborn errors of metabolism potential candidates for somatic gene therapy. Human experiments will not only be performed for 'ideal' model diseases. It is likely that progress towards gene therapy for any particular disease will depend upon the specific assessment of risk vs. benefit, the availability of patients, and the interests of individual investigators in developing the methods, preliminary data, and protocols for human experiments.

ii) Demonstration that the disease can be reversed by transplantation of cells with normal genetic function. Experience with conventional transplantation is extremely important in demonstrating whether a pathological phenotype can be reversed by implantation of a particular pool of cells. Thus, it is likely that somatic gene therapy will be attempted first for diseases which are known to be amenable to conventional transplantation rather than diseases in which somatic gene therapy involves the use of cells whose capacity to reverse the pathological phenotype is unproven.

Ideally, it would be advantageous to have an animal model in which to study somatic gene therapy of a homologous human disease and demonstrate the efficacy of the genetic intervention. Unfortunately, few animal models of inborn errors of metabolism exist, and the phenotypes of these diseases are often dramatically different from that seen in man. For example, genetically engineered deficiency of hypoxanthine phosphoribosyltransferase in mice does not cause the clinical or biochemical abnormalities characteristic of Lesch–Nyhan syndrome (Finger *et al.*, 1988). Thus, it is likely that most experiments in somatic gene therapy for inborn errors of metabolism will be performed without the benefit of specific animal models of the genotype or phenotype.

iii) Demonstration that recombinant vectors are capable of stably transforming cells in a rodent or large animal model and directing adequate expression of the recombinant gene for prolonged periods of time. One of the contentious and unresolved issues is whether gene transfer experiments must be performed on non-human primates prior to humans. It has not been established whether data describing expression and stability of recombinant vectors in animals is a reliable indicator of their function in man. It is impractical (and in itself perhaps unethical) to demand that all gene therapy vectors be tested in non-human primates. Moreover, the unequivocal determination of whether the rodents, large non-primates, or non-human primates are appropriate models for vector function in man will ultimately require data from human trials. Thus, initial human experiments may have to be performed in conjunction with experiments in large animals or non-human primates in order to determine the design of subsequent experimental protocols.

iv) Demonstration that the infectability and expression of the recombinant gene is similar in human cells and that of the animal model. *In vitro* studies with human cells will be essential to substantiate quantitatively the applicability of animal data to predicting the consequences of gene therapy in man. Thus, vectors and methods must be shown to work in human cells before clinical experiments can begin. It is important also to remember that humans are three orders of magnitude (1000 ×) larger than rodents. In designing a clinical protocol, it is essential to demonstrate the ability to manipulate organs or cells of equivalent magnitude to human subjects.

v) Application of clinically accepted surgical techniques for cellular manipulations and transplantation. It is essential that protocols for somatic gene therapy be based on state-of-the-art surgical and medical procedures and do not require radical departures from accepted medical practice or materials. As described above, techniques such as hepatocellular, fibroblast or endothelial cell transplant or selection of haematopoietic stem cells need to be evaluated independently from protocols involving somatic gene therapy.

vi) Evaluation of safety of recombinant agents in experimental animals. Extensive work remains to be done in experimental animals to evaluate the safety of recombinant retroviral vectors. Of particular importance is the need to assess the potential of vertical or horizontal transmission of viral agents or recombination to 'wild type' infectious viruses. It should be remembered that naturally occurring retroviruses (and even naturally occurring 'recombinant' retroviruses) are ubiquitous in our environment. In fact, nature may have already done this experiment; the absence of murine retroviral-like elements in the human genome and the absence of such agents contributing to human disease may be significant evidence that these agents are not capable of vertical or horizontal transmission in man.

vii) Informed consent and institutional review. Clinical research represents an honourable tradition. It is safeguarded by the sometimes coincident and sometimes conflicting interests of the physician concerned with the advance of medical science and the patients' concern with their own well-being. Ultimately, it will be necessary to approach our colleagues who serve on Human Investigation Committees (Institutional Review Boards) and the patients themselves with our proposals for clinical research involving somatic gene therapy. We will have to describe the potentials and the pitfalls, the reasons and the risks. There are ample precedents for clinical investigation of procedures and protocols which are unproven or even untested in animal models, and ample clinical precedents for trials of therapies which are potentially life-threatening or oncogenic.

Those of us who have watched the course of genetic disease devastate individuals and their families know the confluence of hope, concern, and despair that attends genetic disease. We also know that these individuals can make informed decisions to participate as subjects in clinical research. Our responsibility is thus to inform. We must inform our colleagues who will evaluate our protocols, the lay public who are concerned about untoward consequences of our work, and most importantly our patients. Our research must be directed not only at developing scientific models for gene therapy and satisfying scientific and philosophical concerns about their efficacy, but at answering the questions which the patients will ask about themselves, their children, and their families. When we have answered our patients' questions to the best of our ability, then it will be time to begin clinical investigations of somatic gene therapy. It is only clinical investigation which can ultimately determine the efficacy of this approach to human disease.

ACKNOWLEDGEMENTS

Original research described in this report was performed in the laboratory of Dr Savio Woo. This work was supported in part by NIH grant HD-24186 to Fred D. Ledley, grants HD-21452 and HL-40162 to Savio L. C. Woo, and the ACTA foundation. Fred D. Ledley is an Assistant Investigator in the Howard Hughes Medical Institute.

REFERENCES

Ambrus, C. M., Anthone, S., Horvath, C., Kalghatgi, K., Lele, A. S., Eapen, G., Ambrus, J. L., Ryan, A. J. and Li, P. Extracorporeal enzyme reactors for depletion of phenylalanine in phenylketonuria. *Ann. Intern. Med.* 106 (1987) 531–537

Anderson, K. D., Thompson, J. A., DiPietro, J. M., Montgeomery, K. T., Reid, L. M. and Anderson, W. F. Gene expression in implanted rat hepatocytes following retroviral-mediated gene transfer. *Somat. Cell. Mol. Genet.* 15 (1989) 215–227.

Anderson, W. F. Prospects for human gene therapy. *Science* 226 (1984) 401–409

Anderson, W. F. Human gene therapy: scientific and ethical considerations. *J. Med. Philos.* 10 (1985) 275–291

Anderson, W. F. and Fletcher, J. C. Sounding boards. Gene therapy in human beings: when is it ethical to begin? *N. Engl. J. Med.* 303 (1980) 1293–1297

Anon. Gene therapy (editorial). *Lancet* 1 (1989) 193

Baumgartner, D., LaPlante-ONeill, P. M., Sutherland, D. E. and Najarian, J. S. Effects of intrasplenic injection of hepatocytes, hepatocyte fragments and hepatocyte culture supernatants on D-galactosamine-induced liver failure in rats. *Eur. Surg. Res.* 15 (1983) 129–135

Belmont, J. W., MacGregor, C. R., Wager-Smith, K., Fletcher, F. A., Moore, K. A., Hawkins, D., Villalon, D., Change, S. M. and Caskey, C. T. Expression of human adenosine deaminase in murine hematopoietic cells. *Mol. Cell. Biol.* 8 (1988) 5116–5125

Broelsch, C. S., Emond, J. C., Thistlethwaite, J. R., Whitington, P. F., Zucke, A. R., Baker, A. L., Aran, P. F., Rouch, D. A. and Lichtor, J. L. Liver transplantation, including the concept of reduced-size liver transplants in children. *Ann. Surg.* 208 (1988) 410–420

Brusilow, S. W., Danney, M., Waber, L. J., Batshaw, M., Burton, B., Levitsky, L., Roth, K., McKeethren, C. and Ward, J. Treatment of episodic hyperammonemia in children with inborn errors of urea synthesis. *N. Engl. J. Med.* 310 (1984) 1630–1634

Capecchi, M. R. High efficiency transformation by direct microinjection of DNA into cultured mammalian cells. *Cell* 22 (1980) 479–488

Choudary, P. V., Barranger, J. A., Tsuji, S., Mayor, J., LaMarca, M. E., Cepko, C. L., Mulligan, R. C. and Ginns, E. I. Retrovirus-mediated transfer of the human glycocerebrosidase gene to Gaucher fibroblasts. *Mol. Biol. Med.* 3 (1986) 293–299

Chu, G., Hayakawa, H., and Berg, P. Electroporation for the efficient transfection of mammalian cells with DNA. *Nucleic Acids Res.* 15 (1987) 1311–1326

Contini, S., Pezzarossa, A., Sansoni, P., Mazzoni, M. P. and Botta, G. C. Hepatocellular transplantation in rats with toxic induced liver failure: results of iso-, allo- and xenografts. *Ital. J. Surg. Sci.* 13 (1983) 25–30

Demetriou, A. A., Levenson, S. M., Novikoff, P. M., Novikoff, A. B., Chowdhury, N. R., Whiting, J., Reisner, A. and Chowdhury, J. R. Survival, organization, and function of microcarrier-attached hepatocytes transplanted in rats. *Proc. Natl. Acad. Sci. USA* 83 (1986a) 7475–7479

Demetriou, A. A., Whiting, J., Levenson, S. M., Chowdhury, N. R., Schechner, R., Michalski, S., Feldman, D. and Chowdhury, J. R. New method of hepatocyte transplantation and extracorporeal liver support. *Ann. Surg.* 204 (1986b) 259–271

Demetriou, A. A., Whiting, J. F., Feldman, D., Levenson, S. M., Chowdhury, N. R., Moscioni, A. D., Kram, M. and Chowdhury, J. R. Replacement of liver function in rats by transplantation of microcarrier-attached hepatocytes. *Science* 233 (1986c) 1190–1192

Dick, J. E., Magli, M. C., Huszar, D., Phillips, R. A. and Bernstein, A. Introduction of a selectable gene into primitive stem cells capable of long-term reconstitution of the hemopoietic system of W/Wv mice. *Cell* 42 (1985) 71–79

Doetscham, T., Gregg, R. G., Maeda, N., Hooper, M. L., Melton, D. W., Thompson, S. and Smithies, O. Targetted correction of a mutant HPRT gene in mouse embryonic stem cells. *Nature* 330 (1987) 576–578

Dzierzak, E. A., Papayannopoulou, T. and Mulligan, R. C. Lineage-specific expression of a human beta-globin gene in murine bone marrow transplant recipients reconstituted with retrovirus-transduced stem cells. *Nature* 331 (1988) 35–41

Finger, S., Heavens, R. P., Sirinathsinghji, D. J., Kuehn, M. R. and Dunnett, S. B. Behavioral and neurochemical evaluation of a transgenic mouse model of Lesch–Nyhan syndrome. *J. Neurol. Sci.* 86 (1988) 203–213

Fletcher, J. C. Ethical issues in and beyond prospective clinical trials of human gene therapy. *J. Med. Philos.* 10 (1985) 293–309

Friedmann, T. *Gene Therapy, Fact and Fiction in Biology's New Approaches to Disease*, Cold Spring Harbor Laboratory, Cold Spring Harbor, New York, 1983

Friedmann, T. and Roblin, R. Gene therapy for human genetic disease? *Science* 175 (1972) 949–955

Gage, F. H., Wolff, J. A., Rosenberg, M. B., Zu, L., Yee, J. K., Shults, C. and Friedmann, T. Grafting genetically modified cells to the brain: possibilities for the future. *Neuroscience* 23 (1987) 795–807

Graham, F. L. and VanderEb, A. J., A new technique for the assay of infectivity of human adenovirus 5 DNA. *Virology* 52 (1973) 456–467

Groth, C. G., Arborgh, B., Bjorken, C., Sundberg, B. and Lundgren, G. Correction of hyperbilirubinemia in the glucuronyltransferase-deficient rat by intraportal hepatocyte transplantation. *Transplant Proc.* 9 (1977) 313–316

Handysmith, A. H., Penketh, R. J. A., Pattinson, J. K., Delhanty, J. D. A., Winston, R. M. L. and Tuddenham, E. G. D. Biopsy of human preimplantation embryos and sexing by DNA amplification. *Lancet* 1 (1989) 347

Hobbs, J. Displacement bone marrow transplantation for some inborn errors *J. Inher Metab. Dis.* 13 (1990) 572–596

Jirtle, R. L. and Michalopoulos, G. Effects of partial hepatectomy on transplanted hepatocytes. *Cancer Res.* 42 (1982) 3000–3004

Kantoff, P. W., Gillio, A. P., McLachlin, J. R., Bordignon, C., Eglitis, M. A., Kernan, N. A., Moen, R. C., Kohn, D. B., Yu, S. F., Karson, E., Karlsson, S., Zweibel, J. A., Gilboa, E., Blaese, R. M., Neinhuis, A., O'Reilly, R. J. and Anderson, W. F. Expression of human adenosine deaminase in non-human primates after retrovirus-mediated gene transfer. *J. Exp. Med.* 166 (1987) 219–234

Keller, G., Paige, C., Gilboa, E. and Wagner, E. F. Expression of a foreign gene in myeloid and lymphoid cells derived from multipotent hematopoietic precursors. *Nature* 318 (1985) 149–154

Ledley, F. D. Somatic gene therapy for human disease: a problem of eugenics? *Trends in Genetics* 3 (1987a) 112–115

Ledley, F. D. Somatic gene therapy for human disease: background and prospects. *J. Pediatr.* 110 (1987b) (Part I) 1–8 (Part II) *ibid* 167–174

Ledley, F. D. Human gene therapy In: Jacobson, G. (ed.), Biotechnology. *VCH Verlagsgesellschaft* (1989) 401–457

Ledley, F. D., Hahn, T. and Woo, S. L. C. Selection for phenylalanine hydroxylase activity in cells transformed with recombinant retroviruses. *Somat. Cell Mol. Genet.* 13 (1987a) 145–154

Ledley, F. D., Darlington, G., Hahn, T. and Woo, S. L. C. Retroviral gene transfer into primary hepatocytes. Implications for genetic therapy of liver specific functions. *Proc. Natal. Acad. Sci. USA* 84 (1987b) 5335–5339

Lee, C. C., Wu, X. W., Gibbs, R. A., Cook, R. G., Muzny, D. M. and Caskey, C. T., Generation of cDNA probes directed by amino acid sequence: cloning of urate oxidase. *Science* 239 (1988) 1288–1291

Ma, P. T., Gil, G., Sudhof, T. C., Bilheimer, D. W., Goldstein, J. L. and Brown, M. S. Mevinolin, an inhibitor of cholesterol synthesis, induces mRNA for low density lipoprotein receptor in livers of hamsters and rabbits. *Proc. Natl. Acad. Sci. USA* 83 (1986) 8370–8374

Madrazo, I., Drucker-Colin, R., Diaz, V., Martinez-Mata, J., Torres, C., and Becerril, J. J. Open microsurgical autograft of adrenal medulla to the right caudate nucleus in two patients with intractable Parkinson's disease. *N. Engl. J. Med.* 316 (1987) 831–834

Madowka, L., Falk, R. E., Rostein, L. E., Falk, J. A., Nossal, N., Langer, B., Blendis, L. M. and Phillips, M. J. Cellular transplantation in the treatment of experimental hepatic failure. *Science* 210 (1980) 901–903

Mann, R., Mulligan, R. C. and Baltimore, D. Construction of a retrovirus packaging mutant and its use to produce helper-free defective retrovirus. *Cell* 33 (1983) 153–159

Markowitz, D., Geoff, S. and Bank, A. A safe packaging line for gene transfer: separating viral genes on two different plasmids. *J. Virol.* 62 (1988) 1120–1124

Matas, A. J., Sutherland, D. E., Steffes, M. W., Mauer, S. M., Sowe, A., Simmons, R. L. and Najarian, J. S. Hepatocellular transplantation for metabolic deficiencies: decrease of plasma bilirubin in Gunn rats. *Science* 192 (1976) 892–894

Minato, M., Houssin, D., Demma, I., Morin, J., Gigou, M., Szekely, A. M. and Bismuth, J. Transplantation of hepatocytes for treatment of surgically induced acute hepatic failure in the rat. *Eur. Surg. Res.* 16 (1984) 162–169

Mito, M., Ebata, H., Kusano, M., Onishi, T., Hiratsuka, M. and Saito, T. Studies on ectopic liver utilizing hepatocyte transplantation into the rat spleen. *Transplant Proc.* 11 (1979) 585–591

Morgan, J. R., Barrandon, Y., Green, H. and Mulligan, R. C. Expression of an exogenous growth hormone gene by transplantable human epidermal cells. *Science* 237 (1987) 1476–1479

Mukherjee, A. B. and Krasner, J. Induction of an enzyme in genetically deficient rats after grafting of normal liver. *Science* 182 (1973) 68–70

Nabel, E. G., Plautz, G., Boyce, F. M., Stanley, J. C. and Nabel, G. J. Recombinant gene expression *in vivo* within endothelial cells of the arterial wall. *Science* 244 (1989) 1342–1344

Nichls, E. K. *Human Gene Therapy*, Harvard University Press, Cambridge, MA, 1988

Nyhan, W. L., Parkman, R., Page, T., Gruber, H. E., Pyati, J., Jolly, D. and Friedmann, T. Bone marrow transplantation in Lesch–Nyhan disease. *Adv. Exp. Med. Biol.* 195 (1986) 167–170

Office of Technology Assessment. *Human Gene Therapy*, background paper, US Government Printing Office, Washington, DC, 1984

Palmer, T. D., Hock, R. A., Osborne, W. R. and Miller, A. D. Efficient retrovirus-mediated transfer and expression of a human adenosine deaminase gene in diploid skin fibroblasts from an adenosine deaminase-deficient human. *Proc. Natl. Acad. Sci. USA* 84 (1987) 1055–1059

Palmiter, R. D., and Brinster, R. L. Transgenic mice. *Cell* 41 (1985) 343–345

Parkman, R. The application of bone marrow transplantation to the treatment of genetic diseases. *Science* 232 (1986) 1373–1378

Peng, H., Armentano, D., Graham, L., Ledley, F. D., and Woo, S. L. C. Tissue specific expression of human phenylalanine hydroxylase in mouse hepatocytes following retroviral mediated gene transfer. *Proc. Natl. Acad. Sci. USA* 85 (1988) 8146–8150

Penrose, L. S. Phenylketonuria: a problem of eugenics. *Lancet* 1 (1946) 949–954

Rogers, S., Lowenthal, A., Tereggen, H. G. and Columbo, J. P. Induction of arginase activity with the Shoppe papilloma virus in tissue culture cells from an argininemic patient. *J. Exp. Med.* 137 (1973) 1091–1096

Rosenberg, M. B., Friedmann, T., Robertson, R. C., Tuszynski, M., Wolff, J. A., Breakefield, X. O. and Gage, F. H. Grafting genetically modified cells to the damaged brain: restorative effects of NGF expression. *Science* 242 (1988) 1575–1578

Scangos, G. and Ruddle, F. H. Mechanisms and applications of DNA-mediated gene transfer in mammalian cells – a review. *Gene* 14 (1981) 1–10

Scriver, C. R. and Clow, C. L. Phenylketonuria: epitome of human biochemical genetics. *N. Engl. J. Med.* 303 (1980) 1336–1342 (part I) 1394–1400 (part II)

Scriver, C. R., Kaufman, S. and Woo, S. L. C. The hyperphenylalaninemias. In Scriver, C. R., Beaudet, A. L., Sly, W. S., and Valle, D. (eds.), *The Metabolic Basis of Inheritied Disease*, McGraw-Hill, New York, 1989, pp. 495–546

Shen, R. F., Li, Y, Sifers, R. N., Wang, H., Hardick, C., Tsai, S. Y. and Woo, S. L. C. Tissue-specific expression of the human alpha-1-antitrypsin gene is controlled by multiple cis-regulatory elements. *Nucleic Acids Res.* 15 (1987) 8399–8415

Smithies, O., Gregg, R. G., Boggs, S. S., Koralewski, M. A. and Kucherlapati, R. S. Insertion of DNA sequences into the human chromosomal beta-globin locus by homologous recombination. *Nature* 317 (1985) 230–234

Sorge, J., Kuhl, W., West, C. and Beutler, E. Complete correction of the enzymatic defect of type I Gaucher disease fibroblasts by retroviral-mediated gene transfer. *Proc. Natl. Acad. Sci. USA* 84 (1987) 906–909

Stead, R. B., Kwok, W. W., Storb, R., and Miller, A. D. Canine model for gene therapy: inefficient gene expression in dogs reconstituted with autologous marrow infected with retroviral vectors. *Blood* 71 (1988) 742–747

Sutherland, D. E., Numata, M., Matas, A. J., Simmons, R. L. and Najarian, J. S. Hepatocellular transplantation in acute liver failure. *Surgery* 82 (1977) 124–132

tenBerg, R. G., Ernst, P., vanMaldegen-Dronkers, C., Marquet, R. and Westbroek, D. L. Effect of viable isolated hepatocytes or hepatocyte fractions on survival rate following galactosamine-induced acute liver failure. *Eur. Surg. Res.* 17 (1985) 109–118

Terhegen, H. G., Lowenthal, A., Lavinha, F., Colombo, J. P., and Rogers, S. Unsuccessful trial of gene replacement in arginase deficiency. *Z. Kinderheilkd* 119 (1975) 1–3

Thomas, K. R. and Capacchi, M. R. Site-directed mutagenesis by gene targeting in mouse embryo-derived stem cells. *Cell* 51 (1987) 503–512

Thomspon, J. A., Anderson, K. D., DiPietro, J. M., Zwiebel, J. A., Zametta, M., Anderson, W. F. and Maciag, T. Site-directed neovessel formation *in vivo*. *Science* 241 (1988) 1349–1352

Thompson, S., Clarke, A. R., Pow, A. M., Hooper, M. L. and Melton, D. W. Germ line transmission and expression of a corrected HPRT gene produced by gene targeting in embryonic stem cells. *Cell* 56 (1989) 313–321

Vroemen, J. P., Blanckaert, N., Buurman, W. A., Heirwegh, K. P. and Kootstra, G. Treatment of enzyme deficiency by hepatocyte transplantation in rats. *J. Surg. Res.* 39 (1985) 267–275

Wilcken, D. E., Wilcken, B., Dudman, N. P. and Tyrrell, P. A. Homocystinuria – the effects of betaine in the treatment of patients not responsive to pyridoxine. *N. Engl. J. Med.* 309 (1983) 448–453

Williams, D. A. and Orkin, S. H., Somatic gene therapy. Current status and future prospects. *J. Clin. Invest.* 77 (1986) 1053–1056

Wilson, J. M., Jefferson, D. M., Chowdhury, J. R., Novikoff, P. M., Johnston, D. E. and Mulligan, R. C. Retrovirus-mediated transduction of adult hepatocytes. *Proc. Natl. Acad. Sci. USA* 85 (1988a) 3014–3018

Wilson, J. M., Johnston, D. E., Jefferson, D. M. and Mulligan, R. C. Correction of the genetic defect in hepatocytes from the Watanabe heritable hyperlipidemic rabbit. *Proc. Natl. Acad. Sci. USA* 85 (1988b) 4421–4425

Wilson, J. M., Birinyi, L. K., Salomon, R. N., Libby, P., Callow, A. D. and Mulligan, R. C. Implantation of vascular grafts lined with genetically modified endothelial cells. *Science* 244 (1989) 1344–1346

Wolff, J. A., Yee, J. K., Skelly, H., Moores, J., Respess, J., Friedmann, T. and Leffert, H. Adult mammalian hepatocyte as target cell for retroviral gene transfer: a model for gene therapy. *Somat. Cell Mol. Genet.* 13 (1987a) 423–428

Wolff, J. A., Yee, J. K., Skelly, H. F., Moores, J. C., Respess, J. G., Friedmann, T. and Leffert, H. Expression of retrovirally transduced genes in primary cultures of adult rat hepatocytes. *Proc. Natl. Acad. Sci. USA* 84 (1987b) 3344–3348

Yasumizu, R., Sugiura, K., Iwai, H., Inaba, M., Makino, S., Ida, T., Imura, H., Hamashimo, Y., Good, R. A. and Ikehara, S. Treatment of type 1 diabetes mellitus in non-obese diabetic mice by transplantation of allogeneic bone marrow and pancreatic tissue. *Proc. Natl. Acad. Sci. USA* 84 (1987) 6555–6557

Yee, J. K., Moores, J. C., Jolly, D. J., Wolff, J. A., Respess, J. G. and Friedmann, T. Gene expression from transcriptionally disabled retroviral vectors. *Proc. Natl. Acad. Sci. USA* 84 (1987) 5197–5201

Yu, S. F., vonRuden, T., Kantoff, P. W., Garber, C., Seiberg, M., Ruther, U., Anderson, W. F., Wagner, E. F., and Gilboa, E. Self-inactivating retroviral vectors designed for transfer of whole genes into mammalian cells. *Proc. Natl. Acad. Sci. USA* 83 (1986) 3194–3198

SOCIETY FOR THE STUDY OF INBORN ERRORS OF METABOLISM

The SSIEM was founded in 1963 by a small group in the North of England but now has more than 70% of its members outside the UK. The aim of the Society is to promote the exchange of ideas between professional workers in different disciplines who are interested in inherited metabolic disorders. This aim is pursued in scientific meetings and publications.

The Society holds an annual symposium concentrating on different topics each year with facilities for poster presentations. There is always a clinical aspect as well as a laboratory component. The meeting is organized so that there is ample time for informal discussion; this feature has allowed the formation of a network of contacts throughout the world. The international and multidisciplinary approach is also reflected in the *Journal of Inherited Metabolic Disease*.

If you are interested in joining the SSIEM then contact the Treasurer: Dr. D. Isherwood, Department of Clinical Biochemistry, Royal Liverpool Children's Hospital, Alder Hey, Liverpool, L12 2AP, UK. The current subscription is £25 per year payable January 1st each year. This subscription includes the 6 issues of the *Journal of Inherited Metabolic Disease* as well as the regular circulation of a newsletter.

J. Inher. Metab. Dis. 13 (1990) 617–626

Maternal PKU Workshop

Transport of Amino Acids by the Human Placenta: Predicted Effects thereon of Maternal Hyperphenylalaninaemia

Y. KUDO and C. A. R. BOYD*
Department of Human Anatomy, Oxford University, South Parks Road, Oxford, OX1 3QX, UK

Summary: Brush border and basal plasma membrane vesicles prepared from normal term human placental syncytiotrophoblast have been used to study amino acid transport. Such studies are reviewed and novel results presented which confirm that saturation of placental transport by phenylalanine is unlikely to limit delivery of this amino acid to the fetus even with grossly raised maternal concentrations. Such raised maternal levels of phenylalanine are, however, likely to severely embarrass the delivery to the fetus across the placental brush border membrane of L-tyrosine and, to a lesser extent, of L-tryptophan. Reasons for thinking that this may be relevant to the fetal damage found in maternal PKU are discussed.

In the scientific analysis of biological events it is usually essential experimentally to separate the problem under investigation into a number of component parts. Thus for analysis of amino acid transfer across the human placenta, these parts are several, including separation of the events occurring at the plasma membranes facing the maternal and fetal circulations and the study of but one particular amino acid as a transport substrate with analysis of its interactions with other amino acids. When faced with a clinical problem such as that posed by maternal PKU (Levy, 1987), it is worth considering how useful such an analytical approach will be in aiding understanding of the many complex transport interactions which must result from the abnormally high level of phenylalanine in the mother found in this condition. In this brief review we will try to consider this while also discussing both methodology and recent findings, mostly unpublished.

THE PLACENTA

The unit of placental function, analogous to the renal nephron, is the chorionic villus, perfused externally with maternal blood flowing through the intervillous spaces and

*Correspondence

perfused internally with fetal blood flowing through the capillary loops which lie in the loose connective tissue of the stromal core of the villus. Separating the two circulations lies the trophoblast, the placental 'epithelium'. Genetically fetal in origin (unlike some other populations of cells found in the mature shed placenta), the trophoblast consists of an external layer, the multinuclear syncytiotrophoblast, which is derived from the underlying cellular epithelium, the cytotrophoblast. In early gestation the trophoblast is composed of both layers with the cytotrophoblast acting as the stem cell for the syncytium; however, as gestation proceeds the syncytiotrophoblast outgrows the cytotrophoblast (Langhans cells) and at term the trophoblast is composed very largely of a single rather thin layer of syncytiotrophoblast. There are no experiments of which we are aware relating to human cytotrophoblast transport of amino acids, although it is likely that at the stage at which the embryo is damaged in maternal PKU (see below) the trophoblast is completely stratified with both syncytium and cytotrophoblast separating maternal from fetal compartments.

THE SYNCYTIOTROPHOBLAST

Since this is the cellular element across which all placental exchange between mother and fetus must occur, it is worth considering some aspects of syncytiotrophoblast design. This is a terminally differentiated epithelium, with marked structural polarity: the maternal-facing 'apical' surface is covered with a lawn of stubby microvilli which lie in direct contact with maternal blood. The fetal-facing 'basal' membrane lies upon the basal lamina itself in direct contact with the fetal core of the villus. From the transport physiologist's perspective the most remarkable feature of this tissue is that it is a genuine syncytium, a multinucleate structure lacking any lateral cell membranes. The anatomical route for a paracellular pathway across the epithelium is thus lacking. (Stulc (1989) has recently reviewed the evidence that a physiological route may be present.) Although in places the syncytium is markedly attenuated, an adaptation for gas exchange particularly clearly seen in association with fetal capillaries (the histologist's 'vasculo-syncytial membrane'), the syncytiotrophoblast forms a complete cellular epithelium separating maternal from fetal compartments. It is therefore reasonable that this paper should focus upon the apical and basal surfaces of this structure when considering the processes involved in maternal–fetal exchange. It is also worth bearing in mind that the placenta functions not only as a gastrointestinal tract, as a kidney and as a lung for the fetus, but also possesses an array of metabolic, endocrine and immunological functions which enable it normally to cherish the fetus during its separate intrauterine life. These other separate physiological functions may clearly also be relevant to the topic of placental transport of amino acids including their metabolic interconversions and biosynthesis.

METHODS USED TO STUDY AMINO ACID TRANSPORT

In the human two very different approaches have been adopted to study amino acid transfer by the placenta. Perfused preparations have been used both in the analysis of steady state rates of amino acid removal from and delivery to the maternal and fetal blood supply; additionally, such preparations have been studied by single pass indicator dilution analysis (a nice example in the guinea pig is given by the work of Eaton *et al.*, 1982). The second method, which will be considered particularly in this review, is the study of placental transport by means of isolated plasma membrane vesicles prepared respectively from the maternal-facing brush border and fetal-facing basal surfaces of the syncytiotrophoblast.

Transport experiments using brush border membrane vesicles have been used extensively over the last decade (Boyd and Lund, 1981; Ganapathy *et al.*, 1986; Kudo *et al.*, 1987; Karl *et al.*, 1989) but only very recently have studies been undertaken on amino acid transport across the basal plasma membrane (Hoeltzli and Smith, 1989; Kudo and Boyd, 1990). Earlier work on amino acid transport has been reviewed by Yudilevich and Sweiry (1985).

EXPERIMENTAL FINDINGS

Classification of transport systems

Table 1 shows the results from experiments by Kudo *et al.* (1987) and by Kudo and Boyd (1990) on the brush border and basal surfaces of human placenta respectively. In this classification the sodium dependence of transport has been used as an initial discriminant between different categories of transport protein; subsequent further separation has been based on competitive interactions between different groups of inhibitor amino acids. The table shows some similarity with the orthodox classification of amino acid transport systems originally proposed by Christensen (1975) (see Yudilevich and Boyd, 1987); however, there are some transport systems apparent in the placenta which have not as yet been found in other tissues. In particular there is evidence that there may be 'fetal' isoforms of some of the amino acid transporters (e.g. for alanine).

Energetics of amino acid transport

Many of the amino acid transporters are energized by secondary active transport coupled to the electrochemical gradient of sodium ions between the external and internal environment of the trophoblast. This is particularly obvious for A system substrate amino acids. Boyd and Lund (1981) showed that such amino acids (proline) are indeed powered by both the chemical and electrical gradients across the brush border surface of human placental membrane vesicles.

The other important energy supply available to the sodium independent transporters depends upon transacceleration of amino acid; thus amino acids which are substrates for more than a single transporter, and for which one such system is by secondary active sodium coupled transport, may be able to exchange with other amino acids through the sodium independent system and generate 'up hill' transfer of other such substrates. These amino acids themselves, now out of electrochemical equilibrium, may power the movement of yet a third amino acid via transacceleration.

Together such secondary and tertiary active transport systems must underly the observed gradients of amino acid concentration across the placenta, fetal concentrations being consistently higher than maternal (Yudilevich and Sweiry, 1985).

Table 1 **Amino acid transport systems in human placental basal membrane***

System	*Transports*	*Other interacting amino acids*	*Non-interacting amino acids*
Na^+-independent systems			
1.	Methionine Glycine Leucine Lysine Glutamate Proline Methyl-AIB	None	None
2.	Methionine Glycine Leucine Lysine	Glutamate	Proline Methyl-AIB
3.	Lysine	Methionine Glycine Leucine	Glutamate Proline Methyl-AIB
Na^+-dependent systems			
1.	Proline	None	Alanine Glycine Methionine Leucine
2.	Alanine Glycine Proline	None	Methionine Leucine
3.	Alanine Glycine Methionine Proline	Proline	None
4.	Alanine Glycine Methionine Proline	None	Leucine
5.	Methionine Leucine	Alanine Glycine	Proline

*Modified from Kudo and Boyd (1990)

L-phenylalanine transport

We have recently examined phenylalanine transport in isolated membrane vesicles from both faces of the placenta in order to establish, in membranes prepared from the same placenta, whether L-phenylalanine is a substrate for sodium-coupled translocation. Clearly, in neither membrane (Figure 1) is sodium able to alter the rate of amino acid entry: nor is there evidence of anion dependence of amino acid transport. In both membranes the kinetics of L-phenylalanine influx show saturation (Figure 2). The amino acid transport systems for phenylalanine are not identical in brush border and basal membranes since the kinetics of L-phenylalanine influx are different. Other differences between the two preparations with regard to L-phenylalanine transport relate to the pattern of inhibition induced by other amino

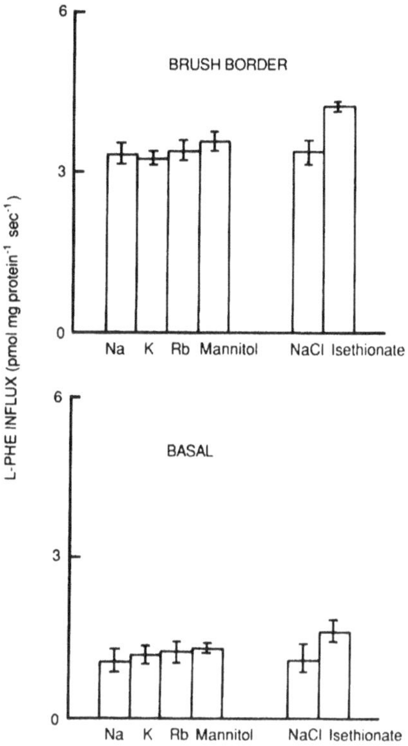

Figure 1 Influence of inwardly-directed cation or anion gradients on initial rates of influx of L-phenylalanine (60 μmol/L) into brush border and basal placental membrane vesicles

acids (Figure 3). The most straightforward interpretation of these findings is that whereas in the basal membrane phenylalanine is transported exclusively via an L-system, in the brush border this amino acid is also a substrate for an additional pathway, possibly system t (Ganapathy *et al.*, 1986 notwithstanding). Figure 4, however, provides evidence that in the brush border there is no extra inhibition of L-phenylalanine influx when maximal inhibitory concentrations of L-tryptophan and of the L-system substrate BCH are combined than when they are applied separately.

Influence of phenylalanine on transport of other amino acids in brush border membrane vesicles

Tyrosine: Figure 5 shows the influence of L-phenylalanine (0–2 mmol/L) on L-tyrosine (50 μmol/L) influx into brush border membrane vesicles prepared from human placenta. Strong inhibition of tyrosine uptake is observed at 1 mmol/L L-phenylalanine; much less inhibition is observed at lower concentrations. Indeed,

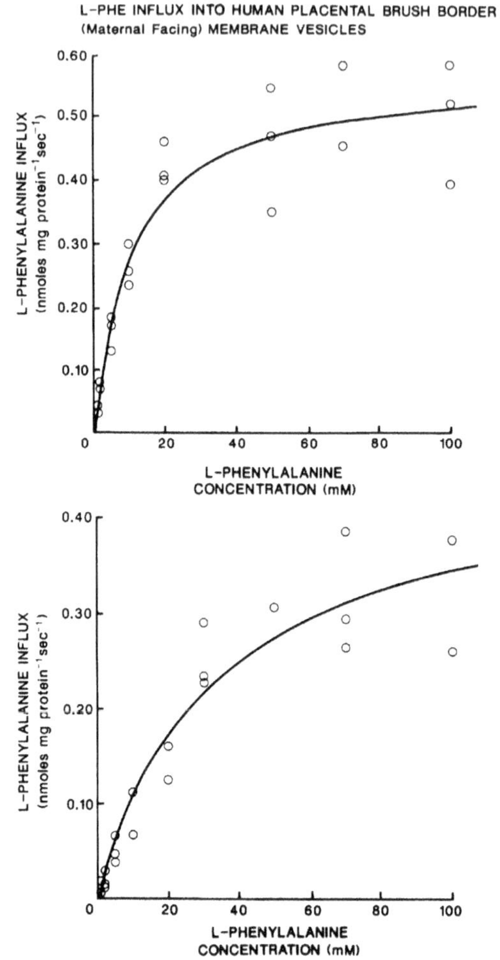

Figure 2 Influx of L-phenylalanine into brush border (upper) and basal (lower) membrane vesicles as a function of substrate concentration

one might predict that the change from a physiological (100 μmol/L) to a pathological (1 mmol/L) level of phenylalanine would alter the inhibition of tyrosine influx from about 20% to 90%. It seems possible that this placental effect of phenylalanine on tyrosine transport may be significant in looking for clues as to the aetiology of fetal damage in maternal PKU.

Tryptophan: Figure 5 also shows the influence of L-phenylalanine on L-tryptophan transport. The concentration of substrate, mimicking that of maternal plasma, was

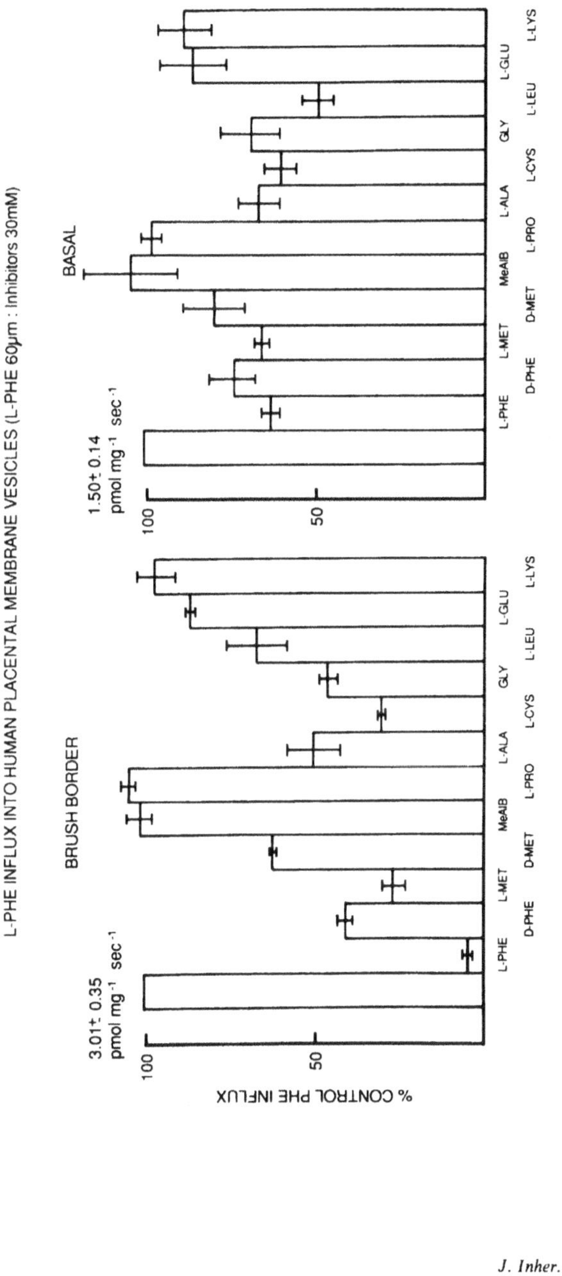

Figure 3 L-Phenylalanine (60 μmol/L) influx into brush border membrane vesicles in the presence of combinations of certain inhibitor amino acids

Taurine: Preliminary experiments using taurine as a transport substrate showed it to be transported very slowly across the brush border membrane, in a fashion which was sodium-independent and quite unaffected by the presence or absence of addition of phenylalanine.

CONCLUSIONS

Because phenylalanine transport has such a very high K_m at both the maternal and fetal sides of the placenta it seems very unlikely that the trophoblast will of itself form any barrier to transplacental phenylalanine transfer from mother to fetus in maternal hyperphenylalaninaemia (Levy, 1987). This theoretical prediction is matched by observations on cord blood obtained at delivery in babies of mothers with maternal PKU (Lenke *et al.*, 1983; Levy *et al.*, 1984). However, this does not mean that the placenta cannot be an important site of phenylalanine action in the pathogenesis of fetal abnormalities associated with maternal PKU. For example, it is at least possible that tyrosine and tryptophan delivery to the fetus is inhibited under these conditions and it will be important to establish the plasma concentration of free tryptophan (the fraction which is not albumin-bound) and tyrosine in the cord blood of such babies at birth. Because of the rôle of these two amino acids in neurotransmitter biosynthesis (Huether, 1986), and because the pattern of abnormalities seen in maternal PKU is characteristic of damage to neural crest derivatives (Kirby *et al.*, 1985; Pratt *et al.*, 1987) it seems at least possible that the pathogenesis of this syndrome may relate to the failure of normal neural crest migration and development associated with insufficient precursor amino acid to meet the particular requirements of this cell lineage. It is worth remembering that neural crest cell formation and migration occurs very early in the developing embryo, at a time when phenylalanine hydroxylase activity will be absent and therefore unable to make up for any deficient delivery of tyrosine and tryptophan to the embryo. The hypothesis that tyrosine/tryptophan deficiency may be responsible for fetal damage in maternal PKU has the merit of being easily tested in animal experiments (Suyama *et al.*, 1989), and moreover raises the possibility that pre-conceptional therapy using dietary addition of tryptophan and tyrosine may mitigate against fetal damage. However, until more is known about the transport kinetics of these two amino acids it would be rash to imply that at the placental level regulation of inhibitor (phenylalanine) concentration may not also be required.

ACKNOWLEDGEMENTS

We are grateful to the MRC for financial support, and to Dr G. M. Morriss-Kay for discussion.

REFERENCES

Boyd, C. A. R. and Lund, E. K. L-proline transport by brush border membrane vesicles prepared from human placenta. *J. Physiol.* 315 (1981) 9–19

Christensen, H. N. *Biological Transport*, 2nd edn., W. A. Benjamin, Reading, Mass., 1975

Eaton, B. M., Mann, G. E. and Yudilevich, D. L. Transport specificity for neutral and basic amino acids at maternal and fetal interfaces of the guinea-pig placenta. *J. Physiol.* 328 (1982) 245–258

Ganapathy, M. E., Leibach, F. H., Mahesh, V. B., Howard, J. C., Devoe, L. D. and Ganapathy, V. Characterization of tryptophan transport in human placental brush-border membrane vesicles. *Biochem. J.* 238 (1986) 201–208

Hoeltzli, S. D. and Smith, C. H. Alanine transport systems in isolated basal plasma membrane of human placenta. *Am. J. Physiol.* 256 (1989) C630–C637

Huether, G. The depletion of tryptophan and serotonin in the brain of developing hyperphenylalaninemic rats is abolished by the additional administration of lysine. *Neurochem. Res.* 11 (1986) 1663–1668

Karl, P. I., Tkaczevski, H. and Fisher, S. E. Characteristics of histidine uptake by human placental microvillous membrane vesicles. *Pediatr. Res.* 25 (1989) 19–26

Kirby, M. L., Turnage, K. L. and Hays, B. M. Characterization of conotruncal malformations following abalation of 'cardiac' neural crest. *Anat. Rec.* 213 (1985) 87–93

Kudo, Y. and Boyd, C. A. R. Characterization of amino acid transport systems in human placental basal membrane vesicles. *Biochim. Biophys. Acta* 1021 (1990) 169–174

Kudo, Y., Yamada, K., Fujiwara, A. and Kawasaki, T. Characterization of amino acid transport systems in human placental brush-border membrane vesicles. *Biochim. Biophys. Acta* 904 (1987) 309–318

Lenke, R. R., Koch, R., Fishler, K. and Platt, L. D. Tyrosine supplementation during pregnancy in a woman with classical phenylketonuria. *J. Reprod. Med.* 28 (1983) 411–141

Levy, H. Maternal phenylketonuria. *Enzyme* 38 (1987) 312–320

Levy, H. L., Lenke, R. R. and Koch, R. Lack of fetal effect on blood phenylalanine concentration in maternal phenylketonuria. *J. Pediatr.* 104 (1984) 245–247

Pratt, R. M., Goulding, E. H. and Abbott, B. D. Retinoic acid inhibits migration of cranial neural crest cells in the cultured mouse embryo. *J. Craniofacial Gen. Dev. Biol.* 7 (1987) 205–217

Stulc, J. C. Placental paracellular transport. *Placenta* 10 (1989) 113–119

Suyama, I., Tani, M., Matsumura, M., Isshiki, G., Okano, Y., Oura, T. and Nishimura, K. Fetal heart malformations in experimental hyperphenylalaninemia in pregnant rats. *Congen. Anom.* 29 (1989) 15–29

Yudilevich, D. L. and Boyd, C. A. R. *Amino Acid Transport in Animal Cells*, Manchester University Press, Manchester, 1987

Yudilevich, D. L. and Sweiry, J. H. Transport of amino acids in the placenta. *Biochim. Biophys. Acta* 822 (1985) 169–201

J. Inher. Metab. Dis. 13 (1990) 627–633

Maternal PKU Workshop

Transport of Amino Acids across the Blood–Brain Barrier: Implications for Treatment of Maternal Phenylketonuria

R. M. GARDINER
Departments of Paediatrics and Human Metabolism, University College London, The Rayne Institute, University Street, London WC1E 6AU, UK;
Present address: Department of Paediatrics, John Radcliffe Hospital, Headington, Oxford OX3 9DU, UK

Summary: Amino acid transport at the mammalian blood–brain barrier has been extensively characterized. Transport of L-phenylalanine and related neutral amino acids is known to be mediated by a stereospecific, sodium independent, saturable carrier. The affinity of this carrier is much higher than that of comparable systems in other tissues. This feature renders it susceptible to inhibition. It has been suggested that inhibition of neutral amino acid influx into the brain by hyperphenylalaninaemia contributes to the pathophysiology of brain damage in this condition.

Methods for investigation of amino acid transport at the blood–brain barrier are discussed, and current knowledge of blood–brain barrier amino acid transport at the blood–brain barrier is reviewed. Developmental changes are delineated, with particular reference to recent work on the ovine blood–brain barrier.

There is insufficient information concerning blood–brain barrier transport of amino acids in the fetal brain to allow firm conclusions to be drawn concerning implications for treatment of maternal PKU. Reasonable extrapolation from animal data suggests that transport inhibition may contribute to impaired fetal brain growth in maternal PKU, and can be minimized by attempts to maintain a normal milieu from the time of conception.

The precise mechanisms by which raised circulating phenylalanine levels exert a deleterious effect on the developing brain, either *in utero* or postnatally, remain uncertain. It has been suggested that the special properties of the transport mechanisms which mediate transfer of amino acids from the circulation to their site of metabolism within neurones may be relevant to the pathophysiology of cerebral damage in hyperphenylalaninaemia. In particular, it has been proposed that inhibition of blood–

brain barrier transport of related neutral amino acids by a high concentration of phenylalanine may be an important pathogenetic mechanism (Pratt, 1982).

Information necessary to evaluate fully the rôle of amino acid transport at the blood–brain barrier in the pathophysiology of hyperphenylalaninaemia *in utero* remains incomplete. Amino acid transport at the blood–brain barrier has been extensively characterized in a variety of animal species, but there is limited information on changes occurring during development. However, a non-invasive approach to quantifying blood–brain barrier transport in human patients, let alone the fetus, is not available, and interspecies extrapolation in this area is notoriously difficult.

This paper reviews the methods available for the study of blood–brain barrier amino acid transport, and summarizes current knowledge of these transport systems in the mammalian brain. Developmental changes are considered, with particular reference to changes at the ovine blood–brain barrier. The possible rôle in pathophysiology of transport at this interface is discussed, with special emphasis on maternal PKU, and gaps in our present knowledge are identified.

TRANSPORT AT THE BLOOD–BRAIN BARRIER

It is now generally accepted that the anatomical basis of the blood–brain barrier lies in the characteristic structure of cerebral capillaries (Bradbury, 1979). In particular, the tight-junctions between capillary endothelial cells create a vascular barrier impermeable to water soluble substrates (such as amino acids) in the absence of a specific transport mechanism.

The plasma membrane of brain capillary endothelial cells is the site of several specific transport mechanisms including those for glucose, monocarboxylic acids, and amino acids. There is evidence for polarity: different systems may be present at the luminal and abluminal interfaces.

Maturation of barrier function has been studied in several species (Bradbury, 1979). The old idea that the blood–brain barrier in the 'newborn' is 'open', is now known to be false and represents a gross oversimplification of the complex anatomical and functional changes which have been documented in a variety of species at various periods of gestation.

METHODS FOR INVESTIGATING AMINO ACID TRANSPORT AT THE BLOOD–BRAIN BARRIER

During the last two decades both *in vivo* and *in vitro* techniques have been developed, but none are applicable in man. Quantitative information is obtained, including values for the kinetic parameters of transport, but the particular method employed has an important bearing on the interpretation of the results. Measurement of net uptake into the brain is extremely difficult as A-V concentration differences are small.

In vivo methods:

Single-pass	– tissue sampling (Oldendorf, 1971)
Single-pass	– indicator-dilution (Yudilevich *et al.*, 1972)
Variable-infusion	– tissue sampling (Pratt, 1976)
In situ brain perfusion	– tissue sampling (Takasato *et al.*, 1984)

In vitro methods:
Observations on isolated brain capillaries (Joo, 1985).

Sampling of brain tissue (following decapitation) after intracarotid injection of the test amino acid and a highly diffusible reference tracer was originally employed by Oldendorf (1971). Results are expressed as a brain uptake index. Although kinetic parameters may be estimated, quantitation of influx and permeability is not possible, and the degree of mixing of bolus and circulating blood is poorly defined.

A recent modification of this approach, the *in situ* brain perfusion technique (Takasato *et al.*, 1984) has several advantages. In particular, permeability can be estimated and the composition of the perfusion fluid is not changed appreciably by mixing with blood (Momma *et al.*, 1987).

The single-pass indicator dilution technique was first applied to the study of transcapillary exchange in the cerebrovascular bed by Crone (1965) and Yudilevich *et al.* (1972). If combined with measurements of flow and arterial concentration, quantitative values can be obtained (see below). It represents the obverse of the tissue sampling approach, the reference tracer being completely unextracted rather than freely diffusible.

The variable intravenous infusion technique has been used extensively by Banos *et al.* (1975) and is particularly suited for detailed analysis of regional uptake.

Studies on isolated brain capillaries (Joo, 1985) provide information *in vitro*, and allow the antiluminal side of the capillary to be examined. Interpretation difficulties arise concerning the structural and functional state of the capillaries following the isolation procedure, and the problem of distinguishing 'transport' from 'uptake'.

The most important methodological considerations include the following:

(i) A non-invasive method applicable to man is not available. Developments in NMR spectroscopy may provide a new approach.
(ii) In general, influx rather than 'net uptake' is measured.
(iii) Kinetic parameters obtained differ depending on whether transport of the amino acid is measured in isolation or in the presence of competing amino acids.

AMINO ACID TRANSPORT AT THE BLOOD–BRAIN BARRIER

Transport of amino acids in the mammalian cerebral nervous system has been extensively investigated (Yudilevich *et al.*, 1988). The existence of separate transport systems at the blood–brain barrier and in brain cells is well established, and the anatomical site of blood–brain barrier transport is now recognized to be the plasma membrane of the brain capillary endothelial cells (Bradbury, 1979).

Amino acid transport at the blood–brain barrier has been investigated using the methods described above in several animal species. Available evidence indicates the existence at the luminal interface of a stereospecific, saturable transport system mediating transport of large neutral amino acids. Fourteen neutral amino acids have been shown to demonstrate measurable affinity for this system (Smith *et al.*, 1987). The order of affinity is similar to that of the L-system of Christensen (1973), but the measured K_m values are both lower and extend over a wider range.

Tryptophan is the only neutral amino acid showing significant binding to plasma proteins. The contribution of albumin-bound tryptophan to influx of this amino acid remains uncertain (Sarna *et al.*, 1985). Transport of basic amino acids, arginine and lysine, has been documented in the rat and sheep but was not observed in the dog (Yudilevich *et al.*, 1972). Transport of small neutral amino acids (glycine, serine, alanine) appears to be limited. Betz and Goldstein (1978) proposed from their observations on isolated brain capillaries that there may be a system-A carrier located at the abluminal side of the brain capillary.

Transport of acidic amino acids, glutamate and aspartate, is not measurable by most methods although small, saturable extractions of these amino acids have been demonstrated by the Oldendorf technique.

KINETIC PARAMETERS OF NEUTRAL AMINO ACID TRANSPORT INCLUDING PHENYLALANINE

Neutral amino acids are transported across the blood–brain barrier by a single facilitated system which is stereospecific and follows Michaelis-Menten saturation kinetics. Amino acid side chain hydrophobicity appears to be a critical determinant of transport affinity. The order of affinity is similar to that of the L-system of Christensen (1973), but the K_m values are mostly between 1–10% of values found in other tissues. At normal plasma concentrations the transporter is therefore nearly saturated and uniquely susceptible to competitive inhibition.

Recent measurements using the *in situ* brain perfusion technique indicate that the true K_m values are even lower than previous measurements suggested (Smith *et al.*, 1987). Measurements made in the presence of competing neutral amino acids (K_m apparent) are elevated by competition effects. For example, the K_m (app) for phenylalanine during plasma perfusion is approximately 20 times greater than the K_m during saline perfusion.

DEVELOPMENTAL CHANGES

Available evidence suggests that blood–brain barrier transport systems are functional in the newborn of several species, including the rabbit (Braun *et al.*, 1980), rat (Cremer *et al.*, 1976; Sershen and Lajtha, 1976) and mouse (Seta *et al.*, 1972). Fetal measurements are not available. Brain uptake indices have been measured for various amino acids during postnatal development in the rat: no difference was found for lysine, valine or glycine between 19–23-day-old and adult rats (Cremer *et al.*, 1976).

Kinetics of L-phenylalanine transport at the blood–brain barrier have been determined in the newborn rabbit (Pardridge and Mietus, 1982). J_{max} and K_m values were both higher than the corresponding values in the adult rat.

TRANSPORT OF L-PHENYLALANINE AND RELATED AMINO ACIDS AT THE OVINE BLOOD–BRAIN BARRIER

The aim of these experiments was to determine the kinetic parameters of blood–brain transport of L-phenylalanine in the lamb and sheep in order to identify any postnatal developmental changes occurring in this species, and to quantify cross-inhibition between L-phenylalanine and several other amino acids (Brenton and Gardiner, 1988).

Observations were made on 30 lambs and five adult sheep under sodium pentobarbitone anaesthesia. Extraction of amino acids was determined using a single-pass venous sampling technique. Venous sampling was from the sagittal sinus. Simultaneous measurements of cerebral blood flow were made using hydrogen clearance and influx calculated from the equation

$$J_{in} = \text{cerebral blood flow} \times \text{fractional extraction} \times \text{arterial blood concentration}$$

Kinetic parameters of transport were determined from measurements of influx made over a range of arterial blood concentrations.

In the lamb, influx of both L-phenylalanine ($14 \pm 1\,\text{nmol}\,\text{g}^{-1}\,\text{min}^{-1}$) and L-alanine ($12 \pm 2\,\text{nmol}\,\text{g}^{-1}\,\text{min}^{-1}$) was greater than in the sheep (L-phenylalanine influx $9 \pm 1\,\text{nmol}\,\text{g}^{-1}\,\text{min}^{-1}$; L-alanine influx, $5 \pm 1\,\text{nmol}\,\text{g}^{-1}\,\text{min}^{-1}$, $p < 0.01$). This difference reflected higher blood concentrations of these amino acids in the younger animal.

Concentration dependence of L-phenylalanine influx was best described by a model with a saturable and non-saturable component. Maximum influx (J_{max}) was higher and the apparent affinity constant (K_m app) lower in the lamb. Values obtained (mean $\pm$ SEM) were: lamb, J_{max} $138 \pm 6\,\text{nmol}\,\text{g}^{-1}\,\text{min}^{-1}$; K_m app $0.85 \pm 0.10\,\text{nmol}\,\text{L}^{-1}$; sheep, J_{max} $107 \pm 7\,\text{nmol}\,\text{g}^{-1}\,\text{min}^{-1}$; K_m app, $2.25 \pm 0.25\,\text{nmol}\,\text{L}^{-1}$.

L-Phenylalanine inhibited influx of L-leucine, L-tyrosine, L-valine and L-glutamine, but not L-arginine and L-lysine. In the lamb, L-phenylalanine inhibited L-histidine influx with an apparent inhibitor constant (K_n) of $139\,\mu\text{mol}\,\text{L}^{-1}$, and maximum inhibition of 92%. In the sheep, L-phenylalanine inhibited L-methionine influx with an apparent K_n of $33\,\mu\text{mol}\,\text{L}^{-1}$ and a maximum inhibitor of 82%.

Evidence was therefore obtained for developmental changes in the kinetic parameters of L-phenylalanine transport at the ovine blood–brain barrier, and significant inhibition of influx of related neutral amino acids by hyperphenylalaninaemia.

DISCUSSION

Implications for treatment of maternal PKU

Although definitive evidence is lacking, current knowledge of transport of phenylalanine and related neutral amino acids at the blood–brain barrier suggests a plausible mechanism by which pathogenetic effects may arise from specific features of this transport system.

In those species studied, it is known that several neutral amino acids share a single carrier and that their affinity constants for this system are within the range of plasma concentrations. The transporter is therefore nearly saturated with neutral amino acids at normal plasma concentrations, and an increase in concentration of one amino acid, such as phenylalanine, will inhibit influx of the others. If net uptake is thereby reduced, cerebral metabolic pathways may be deranged by impairment of substrate supply.

Does such a mechanism represent one way in which the developing CNS is damaged in the fetus of a mother with PKU? It is certainly possible, but the information necessary to examine the question rigorously is not available. The plasma neutral amino acid concentrations in the unstressed human fetus at 18 weeks gestation are very similar to those found in the adult rat. The changes which occur in response to maternal hyperphenylalaninaemia during the first trimester are of critical importance, but uncertain. It is possible that inhibition effects at the placental interface generate further distortions in the fetal plasma amino acid profile which could exacerbate inhibition by further reducing the concentration of vulnerable amino acids.

Obviously there is no information concerning the kinetic parameters of neutral amino acid transport at the blood–brain barrier in the developing fetus, nor can there be certainty concerning the blood–brain barrier function in the human fetus during those early stages of gestation when maternal hyperphenylalaninaemia is known to be most deleterious.

If influx of neutral amino acids into the brain is indeed inhibited, this may not be sufficient to reduce net uptake. A reduction in net uptake will not necessarily impair metabolic pathways such as those involved in protein synthesis, although this is clearly more likely in the rapidly growing brain.

If transport inhibition is an important component of the pathophysiology of the microcephaly found in infants of mothers with PKU, the described correlation with the degree of maternal hyperphenylalaninaemia could be anticipated (Levyjy*et al.*, 1983; Drogari *et al.*, 1987). Our present knowledge does not allow specific recommendations to be made concerning the management of this condition. Strenuous efforts to ensure a normal maternal amino acid profile from before conception would certainly minimize any deleterious effects mediated by inhibition of amino acid influx into the brain. In addition, if hyperphenylalaninaemia of some degree is present, attempts to ensure normal or raised concentrations of neutral amino acids known to share the same carrier (in other mammalian species) should tend to maintain a normal spectrum of amino acid influx into the brain.

REFERENCES

Banos, G., Daniel, P. M., Moorhouse, S. R. and Pratt, O. E. The requirements of the brain for some amino acids. *J. Physiol.* 246 (1975) 539–548

Betz, A. L. and Goldstein, G. W. Polarity of the blood–brain barrier: neutral amino acid transport into isolated brain capillaries. *Science* 202 (1978) 225–227

Bradbury, M. W. B. *The Concept of a Blood–Brain Barrier*, John Wiley, Chichester and New York, 1979

Braun, L. D., Cornford, E. M. and Oldendorf, W.H. Newborn rabbit blood–brain barrier is selectively permeable and differs substantially from the adult. *J. Neurochem.* 34 (1980) 147–152

Brenton, D. P. and Gardiner, R. M. Transport of L-phenylalanine and related amino acids at the ovine blood–brain barrier. *J. Physiol.* 402 (1988) 497–514

Christensen, H. N. On the development of amino acid transport systems. *Fed. Proc.* 32 (1973) 19–28

Cremer, J. E., Braun, L. D. and Oldendorf, W. H. Changes during development in transport processes of the blood–brain barrier. *Biochim. Biophys. Acta* 448 (1976) 633–637

Crone, C. Facilitated transfer of glucose from blood into brain tissue. *J. Physiol.* 181 (1965) 103–113

Drogani, E., Bearley, M., Smith, I. and Lloyd, J. K. Timing of strict diet in relation to fetal damage in maternal phenylketonuria. *Lancet* 2 (1987) 927–930

Joo, F. The blood–brain barrier *in vitro*: ten years of research on microvessels isolated from the brain. *Neurochem. Int.* 7(1) (1985) 1–25

Levy, H. L. and Waisbren, S. E. Effects of untreated maternal phenylketonuria and hyperphenylalaninaemia on the fetus. *N. Engl. J. Med.* 309 (1983) 1269–1274

Momma, S., Aoyagi, M., Rapoport, S. I. and Smith, Q. R. Phenylalanine transport across the blood–brain barrier as studied with the *in situ* brain perfusion technique. *J. Neurochem.* 48 (1987) 1291–1300

Oldendorf, W. H. Brain uptake of radiolabelled amino acid, amines and hexoses after arterial injection. *Am. J. Physiol.* 221 (1971) 1629–1639

Pardridge, W. M. and Mietus, L. J. Kinetics of neutral amino acid transport through the blood–brain barrier of the newborn rabbit. *J. Neurochem.* 38 (1982) 955–962

Pratt, O. E. The transport of metabolisable substances into the living brain. *Adv. Exp. Med. Biol.* 69 (1976) 55–75

Pratt, O. E. Transport inhibition in the pathology of phenylketonuria and other inherited metabolic diseases. *J. Inher. Metab. Dis.* 5 Suppl. 2 (1982) 75–81

Sarna, G. S., Kantamareni, B. D. and Curzon, G. Variables influencing the effect of a meal on brain tryptophan. *J. Neurochem.* 44 (1985) 1575–1580

Sershen, H. and Lajtha, A. Capillary transport of amino acids in the developing brain. *Exp. Neurol.* 53 (1976) 465–474

Seta, K., Sershen, H. and Lajtha, A. Cerebral amino acid uptake *in vivo* in newborn mice. *Brain Res.* 47 (1972) 415–425

Smith, Q. R., Momma, S., Aoyagi, M. and Rapoport, S. I. Kinetics of neutral amino acid transport across the blood–brain barrier. *J. Neurochem.* 49 (1987) 1651–1658

Takasato, Y., Rapoport, S. I. and Smith, Q. R. An *in situ* brain perfusion technique to study cerebrovascular transport in rat. *Am. J. Physiol.* 247 (1984) H484–H493

Yudilevich, D. L., De Rose, N. and Sepulveda, F. V. Facilitated transport of amino acids through the blood brain barrier of the dog. Studies in a single capillary circulation. *Brain Res.* 44 (1972) 569–578

Yudilevich, D. L., Wheeler, C. P. D. and Bustamante, J. C. A comparative view of amino acid transport across the blood–brain barrier (endothelium) and the placenta (trophoblast). In: *Proceedings of Symposium on Peptide and Amino Acid Transport Mechanisms in the Central Nervous System*, (In press)

J. Inher. Metab. Dis. 13 (1990) 634–640

Maternal PKU Workshop

The Effects of High Phenylalanine Concentration on Chick Embryonic Development

M. L. Kirby and S. T. Miyagawa
Department of Anatomy, Medical College of Georgia, Augusta, Georgia 30912-2000, USA

Summary: Cells from a particular portion of the cranial neural crest (cardiac neural crest) migrate from the neural fold into pharyngeal arches 3, 4 and 6, where they provide the support for the endothelium of the aortic arch arteries, and by migration into the outflow tract become involved in septation of the truncus arteriosus. Ablation of the premigratory cardiac neural crest results in persistent truncus arteriosus and other defects reminiscent of the DiGeorge syndrome in man. Removal of a small area of the cardiac neural crest causes a spectrum of heart defects classified together as dextraposed aorta including changes like that of Fallot's tetralogy in man. Some inflow tract anomalies have also been found. Pilot studies injecting phenylalanine into developing chick embryos at a very early stage had little effect on embryo viability or on the incidence of congenital heart defects. However, sham-treated animals produced predominantly small simple ventricular septal defects but phenylalanine-treated embryos had more serious and complex heart anomalies. It is not possible to say yet that congenital heart disease in the offspring of mothers with untreated phenylketonuria is due to phenylalanine-induced damage to the neural crest, but the pilot studies in chick suggest that this idea is worth pursuing.

Uncontrolled maternal phenylketonuria is associated with a variety of congenital defects. Among untreated pregnancies, the frequency of intrauterine growth retardation, mental retardation, microcephaly, congenital heart disease and various other congenital malformations is significantly increased compared with the normal population (Lenke and Levy, 1980; Levy and Waisbren, 1983; Fisch *et al.*, 1986; Hanley *et al.*, 1987). The increase in occurrence of these defects is directly correlated with the mother's blood levels of phenylalanine. All of the defects can be prevented by strict dietary control beginning shortly before and extending throughout the pregnancy (Drogari *et al.*, 1987).

Although the most common abnormalities in these offspring are growth inhibition, microcephaly and mental retardation (40–90%), the most recognized congenital malformations occur in the heart (Fisch *et al.*, 1986; Hanley *et al.*, 1987). The incidence of malformation of the cardiovascular system is 13–17% depending on the concentration of maternal blood phenylalanine over 11 mg/dl (Fisch *et al.*, 1986). By contrast, the incidence of congenital heart disease in the normal population is less than 1%.

Many different anomalies of the cardiovascular system have been reported, but the majority of defects are ventricular septal defect, tetralogy of Fallot, coarctation of the aorta or other anomalies of the aortic arch derivatives and patent ductus arteriosus (Fisch *et al.*, 1986).

Peculiar facial features are also typical of children of mothers with phenylketonuria. In one study of 22 children, 21 had a peculiar facial appearance including long, undeveloped philtrum, thin upper lip, flattened nasal bridge, epicanthic folds, small upturned nose, maxillary hypoplasia and micrognathia (Lipson *et al.*, 1984).

A new model of cardiac dysmorphogenesis has recently been developed which may be of help in understanding the pathogenesis of the defects in maternal phenylketonuria. This model involves removing various amounts of the premigratory neural crest in very early chick embryos. The neural crest contributes to the development of many organs including the heart, aortic arch derivatives and face, all of which are affected in maternal phenylketonuria.

THE NEURAL CREST

The neural crest arises from the neural folds which develop bilaterally from the lateralmost extent of the neural plate (Horstadius, 1950; Weston, 1970; Le Douarin, 1982). The neural crest cells migrate away from the vicinity of the neural folds as the neural plate closes to form the neural tube (Tosney, 1982). The neural crest is divided into two regions (Figure 1): the cranial neural crest extends from the mid-diencephalon to the caudal limit of somite 5 and the trunk neural crest extends caudally from somite 5 (Noden, 1983). Cells of the cranial neural crest can seed mesenchyme to the face, pharyngeal apparatus, glands of the neck and outflow region of the heart (Le Lièvre and Le Douarin, 1975; Kirby *et al.*, 1983; Noden, 1983; Bockman and Kirby, 1984; Bockman *et al.*, 1989). These mesenchymal cells are referred to as ectomesenchymal because of their unique origin from ectoderm. In addition to their ectomesenchymal potential, cranial neural crest cells differentiate into neurons and supporting cells of the peripheral nervous system and melanocytes (Horstadius, 1950; Weston, 1970; Le Douarin, 1982).

The cranial neural crest participating directly in heart development has been mapped to the region extending caudally from the mid-otic placode to the cranial limit of somite 4 (Phillips *et al.*, 1987). This neural crest, called the cardiac neural crest, migrates from the neural folds into pharyngeal arches 3, 4 and 6 (Figure 2). In the pharyngeal region the crest cells provide the support for the endothelium of the aortic arch arteries (Bockman *et al.*, 1989). Some cells migrate from the pharyngeal arches into the outflow tract where they form the outflow septation (Phillips *et al.*, 1987). The ectomesenchymal cells form distinctive whorls in the truncal folds and

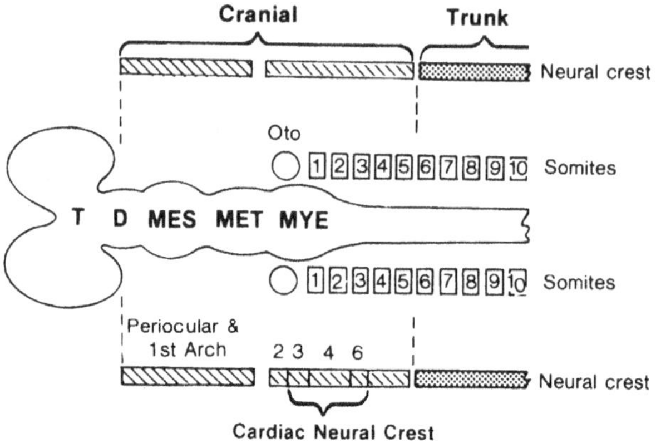

Figure 1 A diagram illustrating the location of various parts of the neural crest and areas of the neural crest which seed the pharyngeal arches. The division of neural crest into cranial and trunk regions is at somite 5. The cranial neural crest seeds structures in the face, pharyngeal apparatus and heart. The part of the cranial neural crest seeding the heart is located between the mid-otic placode and the caudal limit of somite 3. Key: T, telencephalon; D, diencephalon; MES, mesencephalon; MET, metencephalon; MYE, myelencephalon; Oto, otic placode.

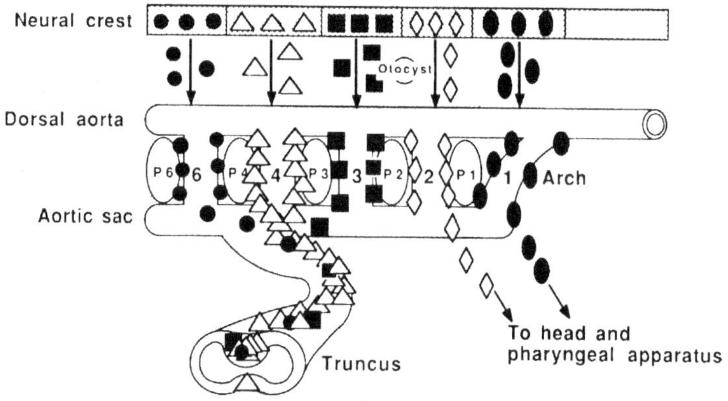

Figure 2 A diagram illustrating the neural crest seeding the pharyngeal arches and heart. Neural crest cells which have previously seeded arches 3–6 migrate into the outflow region of the heart where they participate in outflow septation.

these whorls seem to be the active factor in closure of the outflow septum (Kirby *et al.*, 1983).

REMOVAL OF THE NEURAL CREST

Ablation of the premigratory cardiac neural crest results in persistent truncus arteriosus (Nishibatake *et al.*, 1987). The single vessel usually originates from the right ventricle but has also been found to straddle the ventricular septum or originate from the left ventricle. The conditions which determine the placement of the vessel have not been elucidated (Figure 3). The persistent truncus arteriosus is accompanied by aplasia or hypoplasia of the thymus, parathyroids and thyroid gland as well as interruption of the aortic arch (Bockman and Kirby, 1984). This constellation of defects mimics the DiGeorge syndrome seen in humans and it has been speculated that the DiGeorge syndrome results from some basic defect of the neural crest (Van Mierop and Kusche, 1985).

Removal of a small area of the cardiac neural crest results in a spectrum of heart defects which have been classified together as dextraposed aorta (Figure 3; Nishibatake *et al.*, 1987). Subtypes of this malformation include double outlet right ventricle, tetralogy of Fallot and Eisenmenger's complex. Rare cases of transposition of the great vessels have been found.

Neural crest ablation has also been shown to cause changes in atrioventricular alignment (Figure 3; Nishibatake *et al.*, 1987). The inflow tract anomalies noted include tricuspid atresia, tricuspid stenosis, straddling of the tricuspid valve with or without tricuspid atresia, and double inlet left ventricle. A few atrioventricular canals have been found following neural crest ablation, but these are rare. All of the inflow tract anomalies occur with outflow anomalies although a single case of anomalous

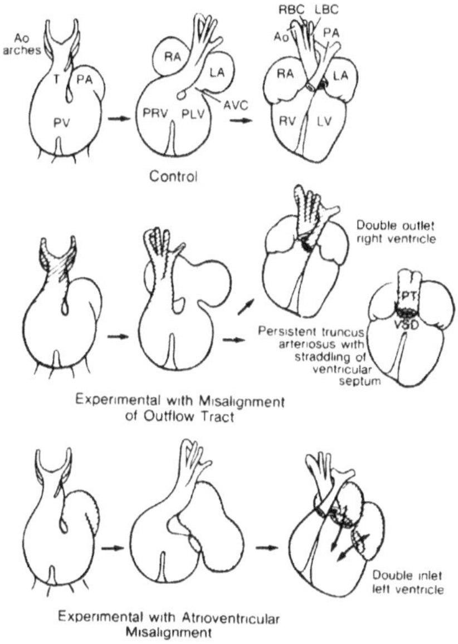

Figure 3 Malalignment of the inflow and outflow portions of the heart are common in neural crest-related heart defects. It is currently thought that partial non-looping of the heart is caused by dilatation of the ventricle during early development. This may account for the origin of the outflow vessel(s) from the right ventricle as well as atrioventricular malalignment.

inflow tract was found in a heart with infundibular ventricular septal defect with right fourth aortic arch hypoplasia.

Even though the heart and great arteries are severely affected by neural crest ablation, neither the systemic nor pulmonary veins are affected, even in hearts with severe outflow tract anomalies (Phillips *et al.*, 1988). This indicates that the neural crest does not influence venous development.

It should be obvious from the foregoing discussion that removal of premigratory cardiac neural crest is not an appropriate model of maternal phenylketonuria. However, development of a model of hyperphenylalaninaemia in the chick embryo would provide the setting in which to determine whether neural crest is directly affected.

EXPERIMENTAL HYPERPHENYLALANINAEMIA STUDIES IN THE CHICK

Only two studies have been published of hyperphenylalaninaemia in chick embryos (Alejandre *et al.*, 1984, Marco *et al.*, 1984). In both of these experiments the chick embryos were injected with either L-phenylalanine and/or α-methyl-DL-phenylalanine beginning on day 10 or 11 of incubation. Brain and liver weights were decreased accompanied by a 14-fold increase in the brain phenylalanine/tyrosine ratio and this was accompanied by some changes in the lipid composition of myelin after 9 days of treatment. This model of hyperphenylalaninaemia involving the second half of the developmental period is not useful for studying neural crest-related defects because the neural crest is only present in the first few days of development.

We have recently carried out a series of pilot studies to determine the effects of hyperphenylalaninaemia on chick embryos at early periods in incubation when the cardiac neural crest is most susceptible to injury. Three treatment regimens were used (Table 1) which included a single dose, two doses per day, and three doses per day with three different concentrations of L-phenylalanine. Sham-injected controls were treated with a similar volume of vehicle at comparable times. The embryos were allowed to develop to day 11 of incubation. The viability in the treatment group was 53% as compared to 63% in the shams (Table 2). The occurrence of heart defects was 43% in experimental embryos as compared with 39% in the shams (Table 2). Significantly, the majority of the heart defects in the shams were small simple ventricular septal defects while the heart defects in the embryos treated with phenylalanine comprised more serious defects such as large ventricular septal defect, double outlet right ventricle, and in one embryo an aortic arch anomaly (Tables 3 and 4).

Table 1 Phenylalanine treatment regimens

1.	1 dose (500 μl of 6, 12, 24, 48 mmol/L solution) at stages 15–18
2.	2 doses/day for 3 days (100 μl of 2, 4 or 6 mmol/L solution) at stages 17–20
3.	3 doses/day for 3 days (100 μl of 2, 4 or 6 mmol/L solution) at stages 10–14

Table 2 Viability and incidence of heart defects in phenylalanine-treated chick embryos (regardless of dose)

Treatment	*No. of embryos*
L-Phenylalanine	216
Viable (11–12 days)	114
Heart defects	46
Saline	65
Viable (11–12 days)	41
Heart defects	16

Table 3 Type and incidence of cardiovascular anomalies induced by L-phenylalanine

	Treatment	*Control*
VSD	45	16
DORV	4	0
Arch anomaly	1	0
Total	50	16

VSD = ventricular septal defect
DORV = double outlet right ventricle

Table 4 Characterization of ventricular septal defects in L-phenylalanine-treated and control embryos

A. Position (%)

	Proximal	*Midconal*	*Distal*	*Total*
Treatment	7 (16)	24 (54)	13 (30)	44*
Control	1 (6)	11 (69)	4 (5)	16

*One heart was not available for analysis

B. Size (%)

	Small	*Moderate*	*Large*	*Total*
Treatment	26 (58)	12 (27)	7 (15)	45
Control	10 (62)	3 (19)	3 (19)	16

CONCLUSIONS

Although it is still not possible to determine directly whether the neural crest is damaged in maternal phenylketonuria, indirect evidence suggests that this might be the case. Continued development of the hyperphenylalaninaemia model in early chick embryos may provide the setting for testing whether or not the neural crest is directly affected.

ACKNOWLEDGEMENTS

The authors wish to thank Dr Harvey Levy for suggesting the possibility that neural crest might be involved in maternal phenylketonuria and continuing discussions on the subject. This work was supported by PHS grant HL36059.

REFERENCES

Alejandre, M. J., Marco, C., Ramirez, H., Segovia, J. L. and Garcia-Peregrin, E. Lipid composition of brain myelin from normal and hyperphenylalaninemic chick embryos. *Comp. Biochem. Physiol.* 77B (1984) 329–332

Bockman, D. E. and Kirby, M. L. Dependence of thymus development on derivatives of the neural crest. *Science* 223 (1984) 498–500

Bockman, D. E., Redmond, M. E. and Kirby, M. L. Alteration of early vascular development after ablation of cranial neural crest. *Anat. Rec.* 225 (1989) 209–217

Drogari, E., Smith, I., Beasley, M. and Lloyd, J. K. Timing of strict diet in relation to fetal damage in maternal phenylketonuria. An international collaborative study by the MRC/DHSS phenylketonuria register. *Lancet* 2 (1987) 927–930

Fisch, R. O., Burke, B., Bass, J., Ferrara, T. B. and Mastri, A. Maternal phenylketonuria-chronology of the detrimental effects on embryogenesis and fetal development: pathological report, survey, clinical application. *Pediatr. Pathol.*, 5 (1986) 449–461

Hanley, W. B., Clarke, J. T. R. and Schoonheyt, W. Maternal phenylketonuria (PKU) – A review. *Clin. Biochem.* 20 (1987) 149–156

Horstadius, S. *The Neural Crest: Its Properties and Derivatives in the Light of Experimental Research*, Oxford University Press, London, 1950

Kirby, M. L., Gale, T. F. and Stewart, D. E. Neural crest cells contribute to normal aorticopulmonary septation. *Science* 220 (1983) 1059–1061

Le Douarin, N. M. *The Neural Crest*, Cambridge University Press, London, 1982

Le Lièvre, C. S. and Le Douarin, N.M. Mesenchymal derivatives of the neural crest: Analysis of chimeric quail and chick embryos. *J. Embryol. Exp. Morphol.* 34 (1975) 125–154

Lenke, R. R. and Levy, H. L. Maternal phenylketonuria and hyperphenylalaninemia. An international survey of the outcome of untreated and treated pregnancies. *N. Engl. J. Med.* 303 (1980) 1202–1208

Levy, H. L. and Waisbren, S. E. Effects of untreated maternal phenylketonuria and hyperphenylalaninemia on the fetus. *N. Engl. J. Med.* 309 (1983) 1269–1274

Lipson, A., Beuhler, B., Bartley, J., Walsh, D., Yu, J., O'Halloran, M. and Webster, W. Maternal hyperphenylalaninemia fetal effects. *J. Pediatr.* 104 (1984) 216–220

Marco, C., Alejandre, J., Zafre, M. F., Segovia, L. and Garcia-Peregrin, E. Induction of experimental phenylketonuria-like conditions in chick embryo. Effect on amino acid concentration in brain, liver and plasma. *Neurochem. Int.* 6 (1984) 485–489

Nishibatake, M., Kirby, M. L. and Van Mierop, L. H. S. Pathogenesis of persistent truncus arteriosus and dextroposed aorta in the chick embryo after neural crest ablation. *Circulation* 75 (1987) 255–264

Noden, D. M. The role of the neural crest in patterning of avian cranial skeletal, connective, and muscle tissues. *Dev. Biol.* 96 (1983) 144–165

Phillips, M. T., Kirby, M. L. and Forbes, G. Analysis of cranial neural crest distribution in the developing heart using quail-chick chimeras. *Circ. Res.* 60 (1987) 27–30

Phillips, M. T., Waldo, K. L. and Kirby, M. L. Neural crest ablation does not alter pulmonary vein development in the chick embryo. *Anat. Rec.* (1988) 292–298

Tosney, K. W. The segregation and early migration of cranial neural crest cells in the avian embryo. *Dev. Biol.* 89 (1982) 13–24

Van Mierop, L. H. S. and Kutsche, L.M. Cardiovascular anomalies in DiGeorge syndrome and importance of neural crest as a possible pathogenetic factor. *Am. J. Cardiol.*, 58 (1986) 133–137

Weston, J. A. The migration and differentiation of neural crest cells. *Adv. Morphol.* 8 (1970) 41–117

J. Inher. Metab. Dis. 13 (1990) 641–650

Maternal PKU Workshop

A Preliminary Report of the Collaborative Study of Maternal Phenylketonuria in the United States and Canada

R. Koch[1], W. Hanley[2], H. Levy[3], R. Matalon[4], B. Rouse[5], F. Dela Cruz[6], C. Azen[1] and E. Gross Friedman[1]
[1]*PKU Program, Division of Medical Genetics, Children's Hospital of Los Angeles, 4650 Sunset Boulevard, Los Angeles, CA 90027, USA*
[2]*PKU Programme, Hospital for Sick Children, 555 University Avenue, Toronto, Ontario, Canada M5G 1X8*
[3]*Biochemical Genetics, Children's Hospital Medical Center, 300 Longwood Avenue, Gardner 648, Boston, MA 02115, USA*
[4]*Division of Genetics and Metabolism, University of Illinois Hospital, 840 S. Wood St., Chicago, IL 60612, USA*
[5]*Child Development Division, University of Texas Medical Branch, 301 University Blvd., Galveston, TX 77550, USA*
[6]*Mental Retardation and Developmental Disabilities Branch, 6130 Executive Blvd. North, Rockville, MD 20892, USA*

Summary: The Maternal Phenylketonuria Collaborative Study (MPKUCS), encompassing all the United States and provinces of Canada, is a prospective, longitudinal investigation designed to ascertain the efficacy of phenylalanine-restricted therapy in protecting the fetus from high maternal phenylalanine concentrations in women with hyperphenylalaninaemia.

Preliminary findings are reported for 147 pregnancies for whom the recommended therapeutic range of blood phenylalanine was 120–360 μmol/L. Sixty-three pregnancies had complete data for analysis. Dietary control was attempted prior to conception in 10 out of 63 women. Significant negative correlations were noted in length, weight and head circumference and blood phenylalanine concentrations during pregnancy. Average reported phenylalanine levels by trimester for 63 hyperphenylalaninaemic pregnancies resulting in live births revealed that no group requiring treatment achieved levels below 360 μmol/L until the third trimester. Median birth measurement percentiles revealed that all groups studied generally had smaller head size compared with birth length and weight. Those started on diet after the first trimester achieved a head circumference below the 10th percentile.

The implication of small head circumference for subsequent intellectual development is unclear at this time. Furthermore, the study must evaluate more offspring of women having optimal preconception and pregnancy restriction of phenylalanine.

The Maternal Phenylketonuria Collaborative Study has been previously described (Koch *et al.*, 1986, 1987). It is an ongoing longitudinal prospective study of pregnant women with hyperphenylalaninaemia and their offspring. The risk to these offspring of classical phenylketonuria (PKU) (McKusick 26160) and its milder forms has been well documented (Table 1) (Lenke and Levy, 1980, 1982; Lipson *et al.*, 1984; Drogari *et al.*, 1987; Koch *et al.*, 1988). The objective of this investigation is to determine how best to reduce the morbidity associated with maternal hyperphenylalaninaemia. The study has completed its fourth year and is in the process of collecting data on the 147 pregnancies followed to date. Study design includes outcome data on the medical, nutritional and biochemical parameters gathered prospectively during the pregnancy and developmental course of the offspring (Table 2). All PKU centres in the United States and Canada are included in this study which is supported by the National Institute of Child Health and Human Development (USA) and the National Health Research and Development Programme (Canada). The study organization is outlined in Table 3 and Figure 1, with one Coordinating and four Contributing Centers

Table 1 Effects of maternal phenylketonuria or hyperphenylalaninaemia on pregnancy outcome[a]

	Maternal phenylalanine levels (μmol/L)			
	≥ 1200	960–1140	660–900	180–600
	Percentage affected in each group			
Mental retardation	92	73	22	21
Microcephaly	73	68	35	24
Congenital heart disease	12	15	6	0
Birth weight ≤ 2500 g	40	52	56	13
Spontaneous abortion	24	30	0	8

Adopted from Lenke and Levy (1980)
[a]Offspring with PKU or hyperphenylalaninaemia are excluded

Table 2 Maternal Phenylketonuria Collaborative Study outcome measures

Rate of spontaneous abortion
Rates of major complications of pregnancy and delivery on offspring:
Growth retardation
Intrauterine growth by ultrasound
Birth length, weight and head circumference
Pediatric evaluation of gestational age
Congenital heart defect
Microcephaly
Congenital malformations
Cognitive/behavioural development

Table 3 Maternal PKU Collaborative Study Centers

COORDINATING CENTER
Principal Investigator:
Richard Koch, MD
Associate Director:
Eva Gross Friedman
Coordinator, Biostatistics:
Colleen Azen, MS

Maternal PKU Collaborative Study
Children's Hospital of Los Angeles,
4650 Sunset Blvd.,
Los Angeles, CA 90027
Telephone: 213-669-2152

NICHD Project Officer:
Felix de la Cruz, MD, MPH
Chief, Mental Retardation and
Developmental Disabilities
Branch, NICHD, NIH
Executive Plaza North, Rm 631,
6130 Executive Blvd. North,
Rockville, MD 20892
Telephone: 301-496-1383

NICHD Contracting Officer:
Harvey Shifrin
Contracts Management Section,
NICHD, NIH
Executive Plaza North, Rm 515,
6130 Executive Blvd. North,
Rockville, MD 20892
Telephone: 301-496-4611

CONTRIBUTING CENTERS

NORTHEAST REGION: Connecticut, Delaware, Maine, Maryland, Massachusetts, New Hampshire, New Jersey, New York, Vermont, Pennsylvania, Rhode Island, Virginia, West Virginia, District of Columbia

Principal Investigator:
Harvey Levy, MD
Project Coordinator:
Deborah Lobbregt
Biochemical Genetics
Children's Hospital Medical Center
300 Longwood Ave., Gardner 648,
Boston, MA 02115
Telephone: 617-735-7945

SOUTHEAST REGION: Alabama, Arkansas, Georgia, Florida, Texas, Mississippi, North Carolina, Louisiana, South Carolina, Tennessee, Puerto Rico

Principal Investigator:
Bobbye Rouse, MD
Project Coordinator:
Lois Castiglioni, MS, RD
Department of Pediatrics, C19
University of Texas Medical Branch,
301 University Blvd.,
Galveston, TX 77550
Telephone: 409-761-2355

MIDWEST REGION: Illinois, Iowa, Ohio, Kentucky, Michigan, Kansas, Wisconsin, Missouri, Nebraska, North Dakota, South Dakota, Indiana, Minnesota, Oklahoma

Principal Investigator:
Reuben Matalon, MD, PhD
Project Coordinator:
Barbara Swift, RDMS
Department of Pediatrics,
RM 1311-N-CSB,
University of Illinois Hospital,
840 S. Wood St.,
Chicago, IL 60612
Telephone: 312-996-5326

WESTERN REGION: Alaska, Utah, Idaho, Arizona, California, Montana, Nevada, Colorado, Hawaii, New Mexico, Oregon, Washington, Wyoming

Principal Investigator:
Richard Koch, MD
Project Coordinator:
Cindy Bauman, MPH
Maternal PKU Collaborative Study,
Children's Hospital of Los Angeles,
4650 Sunset Blvd.,
Los Angeles, CA 90027
Telephone: 213-669-2152

CANADA
Principal Investigator
William B. Hanley, MD
Project Coordinator:
Wanda Schoonheyt, RN

The Hospital for Sick Children,
555 University Ave.,
Toronto, Ontario,
Canada M5G 1X8
Telephone: 416-597-1500

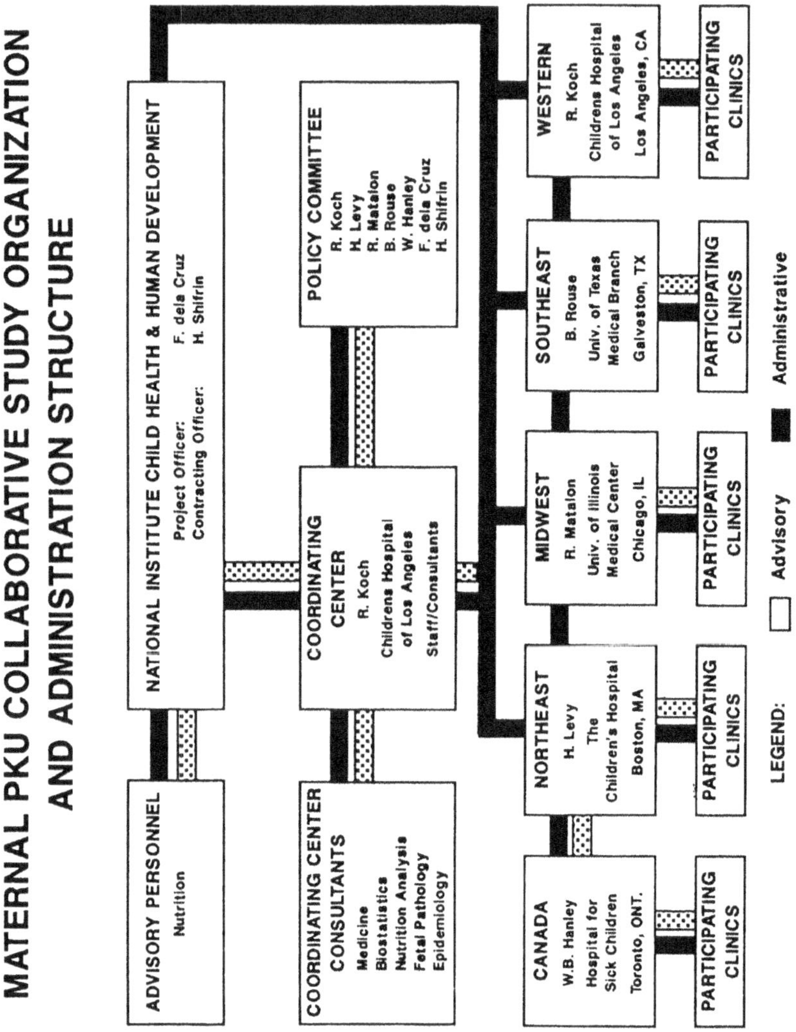

Figure 1 Organization of the Maternal PKU Collaborative Study

located in different geographic regions across the continent. The purpose of this report is to provide a preliminary summary of the data collected as of January 1989.

THE SAMPLE

Approximately 1500 women with hyperphenylalaninaemia have been identified by the project (Table 4). They range in age from 12 to over 35 years, but the majority are in the peak reproductive years of 18 to 30 years of age. An additional 206 are actively enrolled in the study at various participating clinics (Table 5). Fifty-nine percent were identified by newborn screening and are within the normal range of intelligence. Another 20% were identified by family screening and 13% by abnormal phenotype. Forty-eight percent of the pregnant women with hyperphenylalaninaemia were between 21 and 25 years of age at the time of conception; 36% were from 15 to 20 years of age at conception; and 16% were between 26 and 35 years of age.

By 31 January 1989, 147 pregnancies had been followed, of which 20 were currently ongoing. Unfortunately, 80% of the pregnant women with hyperphenylalaninaemia in the study were enrolled with significantly elevated blood phenylalanine concentrations due to an unrestricted diet around the time of conception. Thus, only 20% of the pregnancies studied were planned with average blood phenylalanine concentrations within or close to the recommended therapeutic range of 120–360 μmol/L (2–6 mg/dl).

Table 4 Hyperphenylalaninaemic individuals identified in the United States and Canada[a]

Age (yrs)	*Female*	*Male*	*Total*
12–14	223	155	378
15–17	309	160	469
18–20	269	148	417
21–25	324	140	464
26–30	199	84	283
31–35	88	32	120
> 35	66	26	92
Unknown	22	4	26
Subtotal	1500	749	2249

[a]Excludes enrollees

Table 5 Present age of 206 enrolled hyperphenylalaninaemic females

Age (yrs)	*Number*	*Percentage*
15–17	6	3
18–20	44	21
21–25	99	48
26–30	43	21
31–35	13	6
> 35	1	< 1
Total	206	100

It should be noted that the initial research protocol recommended dietary therapy in women whose natural blood phenylalanine concentrations were above 600 μmol/L (10 mg/dl). By 1988 the Study Policy Committee had revised the upper limit to 360 μmol/L. Of the 127 completed pregnancies, 86 resulted in live births, 19 in spontaneous abortions, 20 in therapeutic abortions, and 2 in stillbirths (Table 6).

For the purposes of this report, complete data were available for analysis on 63 pregnancies resulting in live births, including one set of twins. In addition to the pregnancies in women with hyperphenylalaninaemia, 27 control pregnancies have been completed, all of which resulted in live births.

DIETARY CONTROL DURING PREGNANCY

Dietary control was monitored by evaluating blood phenylalanine levels monthly prior to conception and weekly during pregnancy. For the purposes of statistical analysis, mean phenylalanine levels were calculated for each woman during specific time periods: preconception and the first, second and third trimesters. Table 7 summarizes reported blood phenylalanine concentrations before and during pregnancy for 63 pregnancies resulting in live births, grouped by time, relative to the pregnancy, when diet was initiated.

Mean blood phenylalanine concentrations for mildly hyperphenylalaninaemic women who did not require treatment were 298 μmol/L in the first trimester, decreasing to 210 μmol/L in the third trimester. Women on dietary restriction of phenylalanine prior to pregnancy had average reported phenylalanine concentrations by trimester of 500, 438 and 342 μmol/L, respectively. Average reported phenylalanine concentrations for women who started diet during the first trimester were 641 μmol/L initially, and 400 and 328 μmol/L during the second and third trimesters. Sixteen women were started on dietary restriction during their second or third trimester, and their group mean concentrations ranged from 432 to 1140 μmol/L. The one untreated woman's mean concentrations were above 1200 μmol/L during each trimester.

BIOCHEMICAL PARAMETERS DURING PREGNANCY

Plasma amino acids, trace metals (serum zinc, copper, selenium and blood chromium and manganese), serum ferritin, serum total protein, albumin and cholesterol, red

Table 6 Pregnancy status and outcome of 147 hyperphenylalaninaemic pregnancies

Termination status	*Number of women*	*Percentage*
Currently pregnant	20	
Completed pregnancies		
Liveborn	86	68
Stillborn	2	1
Spontaneous abortion	19	15
Therapeutic abortion	20	16
Total	127	100

Table 7 Average reported blood phenylalanine levels by trimester for 63 pregnancies in women with hyperphenylalaninaemia resulting in live births

		Average phenylalanine by trimester (μmol/L)		
Diet group	n^a	*1st*	*2nd*	*3rd*
Hyperphenylalaninaemia: not treated	6	298 (1)	234 (5)	210 (5)
PKU (preconception)	10	500 (9)	438 (8)	342 (8)
PKU (1st trimester)	30	641 (27)	400 (26)	328 (24)
PKU (2nd trimester)	15	–	780 (15)	432 (14)
PKU (3rd trimester)	1	–	–	1140 (1)
PKU (refused therapy)	1	1296 (1)	1326 (1)	1242 (1)

[a]n = Number of pregnancies in this category of diet group. The numbers of subjects for whom phenylalanine levels were available are specified in parentheses.

blood cell folate, serum vitamin B-12, haemoglobin and haematocrit and plasma carnitine were monitored regularly throughout the pregnancy. In addition, urinary pterin studies were conducted prior to and once during pregnancy. In general, the patterns of these various biochemical markers were within normal limits, although variations did occur. For example, serum zinc concentrations were reduced in the third trimester, as were carnitine values, while copper and cholesterol concentrations increased gradually throughout pregnancy. Haemoglobin concentrations stayed above 11 g/dl during pregnancy with a slight rise near the time of delivery, a pattern comparable between women with hyperphenylalaninaemia and controls, while ferritin concentrations were higher in the women with hyperphenylalaninaemia than in controls, possibly due to dietary supplementation. However, at this time, few clinical signs could be related to these selected findings. Notably, plasma tyrosine levels were consistent with observations in control women.

BIRTH DATA

The average gestational age at delivery was 39 weeks in 63 women with hyperphenylalaninaemia and 40 weeks in 27 control pregnancies. Although the percentage of preterm deliveries in the former was not significantly different from controls, the gestational age at termination was negatively correlated with the time of diet initiation ($r = -0.32$, $p = 0.016$) and also with phenylalanine concentrations during pregnancy ($r = -0.43$, $p = 0.001$).

In order to adjust for differences in gestational age at delivery, birth measurement percentiles were calculated, using as standards the data reported by Lubchenco and colleagues (1963, 1977). Table 8 presents median birth measurements and percentiles for offspring of controls and women with hyperphenylalaninaemia, grouped by time of initiation of diet. Medians for control offspring were above the 80th percentile for

Table 8 Median birth measurements and birth measurement percentiles for completed pregnancies in women with hyperphenylalaninaemia by study group

Study group	*n*	*Weeks gestation*	*Length (cm)*	*(%)*	*Weight (g)*	*(%)*	*Head circumference (cm)*	*(%)*
Control	27	40	51.5	86	3610	88	35.5	83
HPA – diet not indicated	5	40	50.8	78	3150	62	33.5	38
PKU/HPA – diet initiated								
Preconception	10	39	48.9	44	3151	47	32.9	28
Trimester 1	27[a]	39	48.5	61	2926	44	33.0	31
Trimester 2	15	38	47.0	24	2880	41	31.0	< 10
Trimester 3	1	39	44.5	< 10	2211	< 10	28.0	< 10
Refused treatment	1	36	39.0	< 10	1705	< 10	26.5	< 10

[a]Excluding one set of twins

length, weight and head circumference. Median birth length percentile in the offspring of pregnancies in 16 women with hyperphenylalaninaemia ranged from 78 for women not requiring treatment to less than the tenth percentile for women not treated until after the second trimester. Median birth weight percentile was 62 for offspring of women with hyperphenylalaninaemia not requiring treatment, and below the 50th percentile for all other groups. Median head circumference percentiles were well below the 50th percentile for offspring of all groups of women with hyperphenylalaninaemia.

When birth data for offspring of women with hyperphenylalaninaemia were evaluated in relation to actual blood phenylalanine concentrations during pregnancy, significant negative correlations were noted for length ($r = -0.49$, $p = 0.005$), weight ($r = 0.35$, $p < 0.05$) and head circumference ($r = -0.61$, $p < 0.005$).

FETAL OUTCOME

In addition to the higher frequency of relatively small head circumference at birth, there were six infants with congenital heart disease, two of which died before 2 weeks of age. Only one child of all the 64 offspring studied (which included the offspring from one twin pregnancy) was diagnosed as having PKU. At this point, no pattern of major malformations has been observed in the treated offspring.

DEVELOPMENTAL FOLLOW-UP

Developmental assessment with the Bayley Scales of Infant Development at 1 and 2 years of age and the McCarthy Scales of Children's Abilities at 3 years of age are part of the protocol for monitoring offspring. At the age of 6 years, the Revised Wechsler Intelligence Scale for Children will be administered. Bayley scores at or near 12 months are available at present for 24 offspring for the motor portion and for 30 individuals for the mental portion. These show a mean score of 90 on the motor and 95 on the mental development indices respectively. Due to the insufficient amount of data available, no conclusions are possible until the cohort becomes older.

DISCUSSION

The data in this report are disappointing since so few PKU women are planning their pregnancies carefully to commence dietary therapy prior to conception. When one considers that the occurrence of teenage pregnancy is of epidemic proportions worldwide, these results are probably consistent with the lack of reproductive planning generally present today. Thus, it may be too optimistic to hope that the occurrence of preconceptual dietary restriction of phenylalanine will increase. If this is true, then many of the benefits associated with newborn screening will be negated. To date, the participating clinics have not made extensive use of resources such as public health departments, schools and antenatal clinics to help in early identification of PKU women at risk for pregnancy. It is already apparent that far greater efforts to do so are required.

Another important general conclusion, however, is apparent. Dietary restriction of phenylalanine is beneficial, and it is obvious that the occurrence of congenital anomalies in our sample is significantly below that reported by Lenke and Levy in their international survey published in 1980 (see Table 1). The protocol recommends enrolling women at the age of 18 years, independent of pregnancy plans, to encourage conception while on a well controlled dietary regimen, in order to evaluate fetal outcome under more optimal conditions.

More time is needed to assess the value of dietary phenylalanine restriction with respect to cognitive and behavioural outcome, and to determine whether a relationship exists with various biochemical parameters which are being documented in this project.

CONCLUSION

Preliminary data suggest that the head circumference at birth, even in generally well treated PKU pregnancies, is small relative to birth length and weight. More cases are needed to be certain of this, since the percentage of PKU women restricting their diet prior to conception is limited. The relationship between small head circumference at birth and subsequent intelligence is unclear at this time.

No biopterin metabolic defects were identified in the first 147 pregnancies observed to date. While some biochemical parameters are abnormal, their significance remains to be elucidated.

ACKNOWLEDGEMENTS

This work was supported by the National Institute of Child Health and Human Development under Contract No. NO1-HD-4-3807, National Institutes of Health, Bethesda, Maryland and the National Health Research and Development Programme, Health and Welfare Canada, Project No. 6606-3265.

REFERENCES

Drogari, E., Beasley, M., Smith, I. and Lloyd, J. Timing of strict diet in relation to fetal damage in maternal phenylketonuria. *Lancet* 2 (1987) 927–930

Koch, R., Gross Friedman, E., Wenz, E., Jew, K., Crowley, C. and Donnell, G. Maternal phenylketonuria. *J. Inher. Metab. Dis.* 9 suppl. 2 (1986) 159–168

Koch, R., Gross Friedman, E., Azen, C., Wenz. E. and Andre, C. The maternal PKU collaborative study. In Therrell, B. J. (ed.), *Advances in Neonatal Screening*, Elsevier Science Publishers BV (Biomedical Division), New York, 1987, pp. 169–174

Koch, R., Wenz, E., Bauman, C., Friedman, E., Azen, C., Fishler, K. and Heiter, B. Treatment outcome of maternal phenylketonuria. *Acta Pediatr. Jpn.* 30 (1988) 410–416

Lenke, R. R. and Levy, H. L. Maternal phenylketonuria and hyperphenylalaninaemia. *N. Engl. J. Med.* 303 (1980) 1202–1208

Lenke, R. R. and Levy, H. L. Maternal phenylketonuria – results of dietary therapy. *Am. J. Obstet. Gynecol.* 142 no. 5 (1982) 548–553

Lipson, A., Beuhler, B., Bartley, J., Walsh, D., Yu, J., O'Halloran, M. and Webster, W. Maternal hyperphenylalaninaemia fetal effects. *J. Pediatr.* 104 (1984) 216–220

Lubchenco, L. O., Hansman, C., Dressler, M. and Boyd, E. Intrauterine growth as estimated from birth-weight data at 24 to 42 weeks of gestation. *Pediatrics* 32 (1963) 793–800

Lubchenco, L. O., Hansman, C. and Boyd, E. Intrauterine growth in length and head circumference as estimated from live births at gestational ages from 26 to 42 weeks. *Pediatrics* 37 (1977) 403–408

J. Inher. Metab. Dis. 13 (1990) 651–657

Maternal PKU Workshop

Fetal Damage due to Maternal Phenylketonuria: Effects of Dietary Treatment and Maternal Phenylalanine Concentrations around the Time of Conception

(An interim report from the UK Phenylketonuria Register)

I. SMITH, J. GLOSSOP and M. BEASLEY
Department of Child Health, Institute of Child Health, 30 Guilford Street, London WC1N 4NP, UK

Summary: In 94 infants born to women with PKU, birth weight and head circumference were inversely and linearly related to the mothers' phenylalanine concentrations close to conception; with each 200 μmol/L rise in phenylalanine concentrations, birth weight fell by 98 g and head circumference by 0.46 cm. This relationship was highly significant and appeared to be the same whether or not the mother received a low phenylalanine diet. Even in the 28 infants whose mothers conceived on a strict low phenylalanine diet, birth weights and head circumferences, corrected for sex and gestation, were a little below the population norms (3421 g and 34.7 cm compared with 3600 g and 35.2 cm respectively) although the differences were not statistically significant. Optimal fetal growth occurred only in infants whose mothers had phenylalanine concentrations close to the normal range at conception. Dietary treatment started after conception did not appear to confer any benefit.

Infants born to women with phenylketonuria (PKU) are often mentally retarded, microcephalic and of low birth weight (Fisch *et al.*, 1969; Lenke and Levy, 1980); they may also have malformations, notably of the cardiovascular system. Case reports on the offspring of women who have received a strict low pheylalanine diet from before conception suggest that such infants are usually healthy (Nielson *et al.*, 1979; Soeters *et al.*, 1986; Rohr *et al.*, 1987). However, there is a problem in defining 'normality' in individuals as opposed to populations. There is also an inherent bias in the selection of infants born to untreated women (usually because they have abnormalities), and an unknown proportion of women who start treatment after conception, or who receive no treatment, may give birth to apparently healthy infants (Davidson *et al.*, 1981; Levy and Waisbren, 1983). It has therefore been difficult to assess the true influence of dietary treatment on the outcome of pregnancy.

As the evidence linking better outcome with dietary treatment from before conception is already quite convincing, a randomized trial to assess the relationship between outcome and the timing of treatment would not be ethically acceptable and it will be necessary to rely on within-group studies. One such study was set up in 1978 by the Phenylketonuria Register (MRC Steering Committee 1981) which lists virtually all known female subjects with PKU born in the UK since 1964 and a high proportion of those born earlier. A few subjects continue to be notified for the first time when they are discovered as a result of abnormalities in their offspring. The aim of the study is to alert the patient's medical advisors to the risks of maternal PKU, to provide an overall view of the problem in the UK and to collect data which will allow us to compare the outcome of pregnancy in women receiving dietary intervention at different stages in pregnancy. Outcome will be assessed on the basis of infant size at birth, the frequency of malformations, and postnatal growth and intellectual progress. Factors such as maternal phenylalanine concentrations before, during and after pregnancy will be incorporated into the analysis.

Because of the urgent need for more information on the management of pregnancy in young women with PKU, details of the first 37 live births documented by the Register were presented in 1986 (Drogari *et al.*, 1987a) and later published in combination with similar data from another 27 pregnancies occurring in seven other countries (Czechoslovakia, Poland, Switzerland, Australia, Denmark, Holland and Italy) (Drogari *et al.*, 1987b). The present report adds another 30 live births which have been documented in the UK since 1986, providing 94 subjects in all. As before, birth weight and head circumference have been used as measures of outcome. We have examined the relationship between outcome and both the stage of pregnancy when diet was started, and the maternal phenylalanine concentrations around the time of conception.

METHODS

The Register has followed up 341 women aged 14 to 43 years. Between 1978 and the end of 1988 32 women were sterilized, 18 of whom had no children. Over the same period there were 143 pregnancies, including 70 live births. Of the 73 pregnancies which failed to go to term, all but seven were terminated because the mother had conceived on a normal diet. The additional 27 pregnancies from outside the UK have been included in the present report.

As described previously (Drogari *et al.*, 1987b), pregnancies have been grouped according to the mother's dietary treatment during pregnancy (group I = strict diet preconception, phenylalanine concentration $<601\,\mu$mol/L, group II = relaxed diet preconception, phenylalanine concentration $>600\,\mu$mol/L, group III = diet from 1st trimester, group IV = diet from 2nd or 3rd trimester, group V = no diet). Women were only considered to be 'on diet' if they were receiving regular supplements of a phenylalanine-low protein substitute. The phenylalanine concentrations best representing concentrations around the time of conception were defined for each pregnancy (in groups I and II the value closest to the conception date, in group III the phenylalanine value immediately preceding the introduction of diet and in groups

IV and V the value on a normal diet, closest in time to conception).

In the 30 new subjects birth weights and head circumferences were plotted on boys' centile charts allowing for gestational age (girls were placed in their proportionate centile positions). As the distributions were very similar to those observed previously, the data on the 94 subjects was combined. The growth measurements were corrected for sex and gestational age as described previously (Drogari *et al.*, 1987b), and means and standard deviations were calculated for each diet group. The frequencies of malformations in each diet group were also documented. Corrected birth weights and head circumferences were plotted against maternal phenylalanine concentrations around the time of conception; the relationships were examined using linear regression.

RESULTS

In the 30 new infants, birth weights and head circumferences in infants born to mothers who had received a strict diet from before conception were distributed between the 97th and 3rd centiles whereas an excess of values in the remaining subjects fell below the 3rd centiles (particularly head circumferences); the distributions were very similar to those observed previously. The combined data from all 94 subjects is shown in Figures 1a and 1b (group I represented as open circles). Subjects in group I, although significantly ($p < 0.01$) larger for gestational age and sex than subjects in other diet groups, nevertheless included more with measurements below than above the 50th centiles (20 out of 28 for birth weight, 16 out of 27 for head circumference) and mean values were below the norms (although not significantly so) (Table 1). Infants in group II were somewhat larger than those in groups III, IV and V (in whom birth weights and head circumferences were similar) but in all four groups the mean values were significantly below ($p < 0.001$) the norms.

Table 1 Birth weight, head circumference and frequency of malformations in different diet groups (I = strict diet preconception, II = relaxed diet preconception, III = diet 1st trimester, IV = diet 2nd or 3rd trimester, V = no diet)

Group	*Birth weight*			*Head circumference*			*Malformations*	
	No.	*Mean*	*SD*	*No.*	*Mean*	*SD*	*No.*	*%*
I	28	3421	375	27[a]	34.7	1.28	0	0
II	17	3178	526	17	33.7	1.45	1	0.6
III	11	2865	354	11	32.8	1.43	4	19
IV	10	2790	480	10	32.9	1.31	0	0
V	28	2816	437	27[a]	31.5	1.78	8	29
Norms		3600			35.2			<2

[a]missing value
*50th centiles for males

When birth weights and head circumferences were plotted against maternal phenylalanine concentrations around the time of conception (Figures 2a and 2b) there was an obvious and linear trend downwards as maternal phenylalanine concentrations rose. The values in the 30 new cases fitted remarkably closely into the distributions recorded previously. Estimates of the trend based on regression analysis in 94 infants showed that with each 200 μmol/L rise in blood phenylalanine concentrations above the normal range, birth weight fell by 98 g and head circumference by 0.46 cm.

Amongst the 30 new cases no recognized malformations occurred in infants whose mothers had started the diet preconception but 3 subjects born to untreated mothers had malformations. The malformation rate based upon the total series of 94 children is shown in Table 1. The higher rate in group V (29%) compared with groups III, IV and V combined (19%) is likely to be due to the bias involved in the selection of untreated mothers because of abnormalities in their infants rather than any real difference due to treatment. Almost half the malformations occurred in women with plasma phenylalanine concentrations below 1200 μmol/L when receiving a normal diet. The types of malformation varied widely (Table 2) although, as reported previously, cardiac lesions predominated.

Table 2 Character of malformations in 13 infants with mothers' phenylalanine concentrations (μmol/L) at conception

Malformation	*Phenylalanine concentration* (μmol/L)
Cardiac:	
Mitral/aortic stenosis	1411
Mitral/aortic stenosis	900
Fallot's tetralogy	1100
Patent ductus	1530
Ventricular septal defect/patent ductus	980
'Complex lesion'	980
Other:	
Anal fistula	1100
Dislocated hips/facial dysmorphism	1150
Malformed eyelid/ptosis	943
Hydrocele/fused digits	1269
Coloboma/abnormal ears	1200
Hypospadias	950
Hypertelorism/simian crease/spread toes	1830

DISCUSSION

The results of this study confirm and extend previous findings suggesting that introduction of a low phenylalanine diet from before conception reduces the harmful effects of maternal hyperphenylalaninaemia on fetal growth. However, the size of the advantage conferred by preconceptional treatment depended on the quality of phenylalanine control early in pregnancy. The 'therapeutic window' appeared to be narrow with some risk (though small) to the fetus even when maternal phenylalanine concentrations were no more than 2–3 times above the normal range.

The offspring of women who conceived whilst receiving a normal diet did not derive any benefit (at least so far as fetal growth or the frequency of malformations were concerned) from treatment started more than a few weeks after conception. Within each range of phenylalanine values there was a considerable variation in head

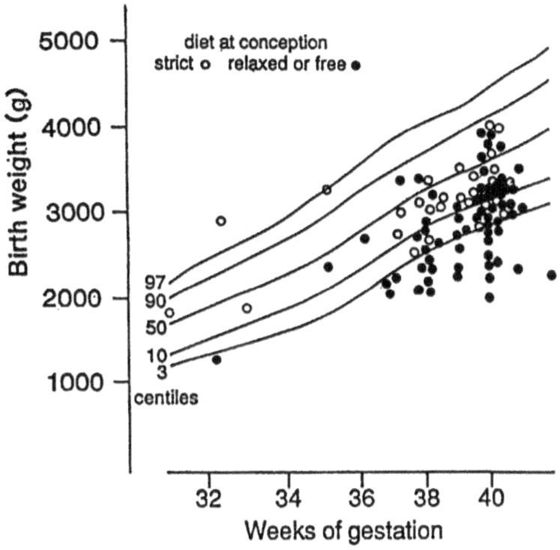

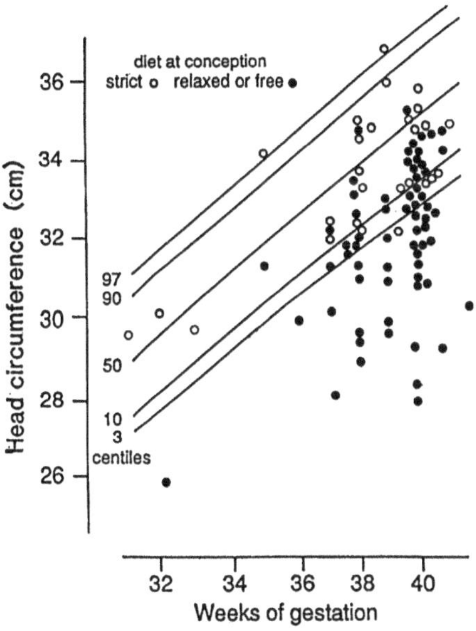

Figure 1 Birth weights (a) and head circumferences (b) plotted on boys centile charts (girls in proportionate centile positions)

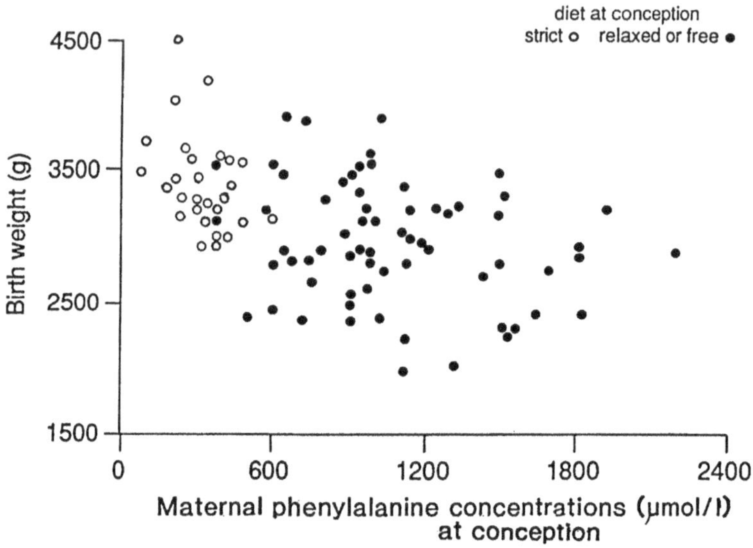

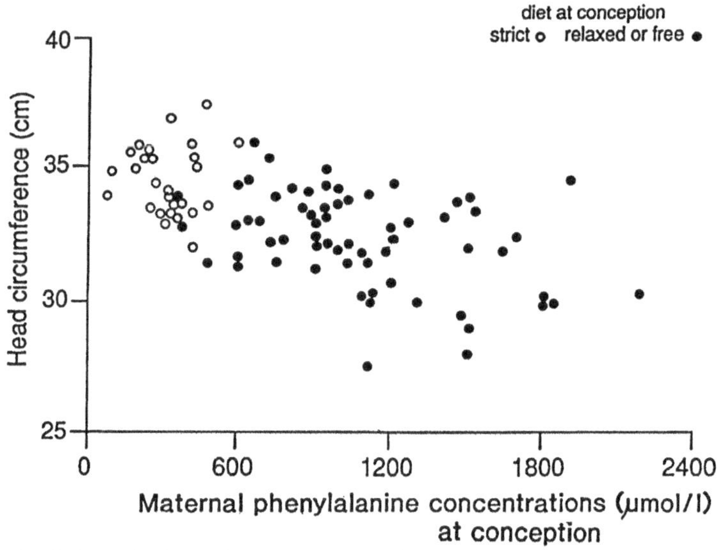

Figure 2 Birth weights (a) and head circumferences (b) plotted against maternal phenylalanine concentrations around the time of conception. Regression equations:
(a) Intercept = 3499.5, slope = −0.4763, $F = 25.49$, $p < 0.0001$
(b) Intercept = 35.15, slope = −0.0024, $F = 48.37$, $p < 0.0001$

circumference and birth weight but this variation was comparable to that seen in a normal population. Late treatment or no treatment did not preclude the birth of a clinically healthy infant, even in women with blood phenylalanine concentrations above 1200 μmol/L at conception. The offspring of untreated mothers appeared to belong to the same continuum as mothers who received treatment from before conception suggesting that fetal damage was to a large extent determined by the degree of hyperphenylalaninaemia around the time of conception.

On the basis of the results of this study we suggest that women with PKU should be advised to start a strict low phenylalanine diet before conception, and that the aim should be to control blood phenylalanine concentrations between 60 and 180 μmol/L. Such strict control runs the risk of causing hypophenylalaninaemia and biochemical monitoring needs to be both accurate and frequent. Women with biochemically mild forms of PKU should be treated if maternal phenylalanine concentrations are above 300 μmol/L.

ACKNOWLEDGEMENTS

We wish to thank the mothers and children who participated in the study and the paediatricians, biochemists, obstetricians and dietitians who have provided the data for the Register. We also wish to thank the Medical Research Council and Department of Health for financial support.

REFERENCES

Davidson, D. C., Isherwood, D. M., Ireland, J. T. and Rae, P. G. Outcome of pregnancy in a phenylketonuric mother after a low phenylalanine diet introduced from the ninth week of pregnancy. *Eur. J. Pediatr.* 137 (1981) 45–48

Drogari, E., Beasley, M. and Smith, I. Pregnancy in women with phenylketonuria (PKU): the influence of maternal phenylalanine concentrations at conception on birth weight and head circumference. In Therrell, B. L. (ed.) *Advances in Neonatal Screening*, Elsevier Science Publishers BV, New York, 1987a, pp. 175–176

Drogari, E., Smith, I., Beasley, M. and Lloyd, J. K. Timing of strict diet in relation to fetal damage in maternal phenylketonuria. *Lancet* 2 (1987b) 927–930

Fisch, R. O., Doeden, D., Lansky, L. L. and Anderson, J. A. Maternal phenylketonuria. Detrimental effects on embryogenesis and fetal development. *Am. J. Dis. Child.* 118 (1969) 847–858

Lenke, R. R. and Levy, H. L. Maternal phenylketonuria and hyperphenylalaninaemia. An international survey of the outcome of untreated and treated pregnancies. *N. Engl. J. Med.* 303 (1980) 1202–1208

Levy, H. L. and Waisbren, S. E. Effects of untreated maternal phenylketonuria and hyperphenylalaninaemia on the fetus. *N. Engl. J. Med.* 309 (1983) 1269–1274

Nielson, K. H., Wamberg, E. and Weber, J. Successful outcome of pregnancy in a phenylketonuric woman after low phenylalanine diet introduced before conception. *Lancet* 1 (1979) 1245

Rohr, F. J., Doherty, L. B., Waisbren, S. E. *et al.* New England Maternal PKU Project: Prospective study of untreated and treated pregnancies and their outcomes. *J. Pediatr.* 110 (1987) 391–398

Soeters, R. P., Sengers, R. C. A., van Dongen, P. W. J., Trijbels, J. M. F. and Eskes, T. K. A. B. Maternal phenylketonuria: comparison of two treated full term pregnancies. *Eur. J. Pediatr.* 145 (1986) 221–223

J. Inher. Metab. Dis. 13 (1990) 658–664

Maternal PKU Workshop

Maternal Phenylketonuria – the Irish Experience

E. NAUGHTEN and I. P. SAUL
The Children's Hospital, Temple Street, Dublin 1, Eire

Summary: The outcome of 48 pregnancies in 18 women with elevated phenylalanine was studied. The women were divided into two groups, diet and non-diet. All the women on diet had severe hyperphenylalaninaemia and only six were on the amino acid mixture at conception. In the non-diet group four women had concentrations of less than 1000 μmol/L and five had severe hyperphenylalaninaemia. Three deaths and one stillbirth occurred in the non-diet group. Microcephaly occurred in 24 children; 11 in the diet group and 13 in the non-diet group. There were five miscarriages in the non-diet group and one in the diet group. Diet is beneficial when started early but planned pregnancies, good motivation and compliance were difficult to achieve in this group of women despite every reasonable effort by the PKU clinic.

In the 33 years since Dent drew attention to the potential problem of mental handicap in children born to mothers with phenylketonuria (PKU), numerous reports have outlined problems of mental retardation, microcephaly and congenital heart disease (CHD) in such offspring. A consensus has emerged that diet is most beneficial when started before conception, but there is insufficient data to be able to state the phenylalanine level at which the fetus is safe. Mental handicap has been documented with maternal blood concentrations of phenylalanine between 180 and 600 μmol/L (Lenke and Levy, 1980). The average feto–maternal ratio for phenylalanine is 1.5:1, and the maternal value would need to be kept as close to the physiological range as possible to ensure a fetal phenylalanine concentration of less than 400 μmol/L.

In addition to optimal management, one of the problems confronting physicians dealing with maternal PKU is the detection of women at risk and the subsequent motivation to get them to adhere to diet. In Ireland there is a high incidence of phenylketonuria (1 in 4500; Cahalane, 1968) and institutions for the mentally handicapped have been surveyed to identify at-risk patients who were never screened neonatally (Chadwick *et al.*, 1977; O'Connor and Mulcahy, 1984). Although a maternal at-risk register was established in 1978, there has been difficulty in maintaining it.

PATIENTS

We now report the outcome in 48 pregnancies, including eight already reported previously (Murphy and Troy, 1979; Murphy *et al.*, 1985). Eleven mothers were known to be at risk. Two of these had been screened but one had been taken off diet at the age of 6 years in another hospital, and was not known to us until she presented in her second pregnancy; the second had poor home support and rebelled as a teenager. We have identified seven women retrospectively in addition to these because of abnormal offspring. Two women had phenylalanine concentrations checked by the obstetrician when the fetal bi-parietal diameter was noted to be abnormal, and paediatricians detected two mothers when children presented with microcephaly. There were two twin pregnancies born to one woman with the result that there were 50 offspring from 48 pregnancies.

TREATMENT

The data was gathered from hospital notes and obstetric units involved in the care of these women and from data collected in the metabolic unit. No mother was on strict preconception diet with satisfactorily low phenylalanine concentrations although a number were taking amino acid supplements with some protein restriction. A stricter diet was imposed or introduced during the first or second trimester and these patients represent the diet group: supplements were given either as Maxamum XP (Scientific Hospital Supplies) or Aminogran (Allen & Hanbury). All the diet group of mothers had severe PKU with mean plasma phenylalanine concentrations of 1540 μmol/L (range 850–2600). The non-diet group of mothers was a mixture of severe PKU patients whose pregnancies were untreated by diet, and patients with milder forms of hyperphenylalaninaemia whose pregnancies were also untreated. The mean plasma phenylalanine concentration for the group was 994 μmol/L (range 650–2600). Infant birth weights and head circumferences were corrected to term gestation using D. Gairdener and J. Pearson charts (1971). The third centile is 2 SD from the mean. Each woman had weekly blood tests, with the exception of the twin pregnancy where blood tests were carried out bi-weekly.

RESULTS

The diet group (median phenylalanine concentration 1540 μmol/L) resulted in 20 pregnancies with one miscarriage and one set of twins (Table 1). The twins both have

Table 1 Pregnancies in 18 women with phenylketonuria or hyperphenylalaninaemia

	Diet group	*Non-diet group*
Number of pregnancies	20	28
Number of miscarriages	1	5
Number of stillbirths	0	1
Deaths	0	3
Sets of twins	1	1
Surviving offspring	20	20
Head circumference > 3rd centile	9	5

congenital heart disease and diet commenced in the fifth month of pregnancy of a woman with a pre-diet concentration of 1040 μmol/L. All other women in this group had untreated phenylalanine concentrations greater than 1200 μmol/L pre-diet. Twenty children result from this group (median IQ 86, range 65–103).

The non-diet group (median phenylalanine concentration 994 μmol/L) produced 28 pregnancies including five miscarriages, one stillbirth and one set of twins (Table 1). There were three deaths – one of the twins and two babies with congenital heart disease. There were 20 surviving children.

Three women (sisters) with phenylalanine concentrations of less than 1000 (600–994 μmol/L) had four infants with microcephaly and three miscarriages. One woman who gave birth to a stillborn microcephalic infant is included in this group even though diet was attempted for 10 days before delivery at 35/36 weeks gestation. Two women from the non-diet group presented for diet after diagnosis and feature in both groups.

Twenty-four of the 48 pregnancies (50%) resulted in a microcephalic infant (< 3rd centile, Figure 1). Two out of five infants with congenital heart disease also had microcephaly. Three children died and two of these had congenital heart disease; 12 children were normal. Birth details were not available for five children.

Of the diet group, nine gave birth to infants with head circumferences > 3rd centile despite classical PKU and late (1st or 2nd trimester) establishment on diet. Six of these nine were on the synthetic amino acid drink but had high phenylalanine concentrations at conception. Only five of the non-diet group gave birth to infants with head circumference > 3rd centile and these women had phenylalanine concentrations less than 1000 μmol/L (see Figure 1).

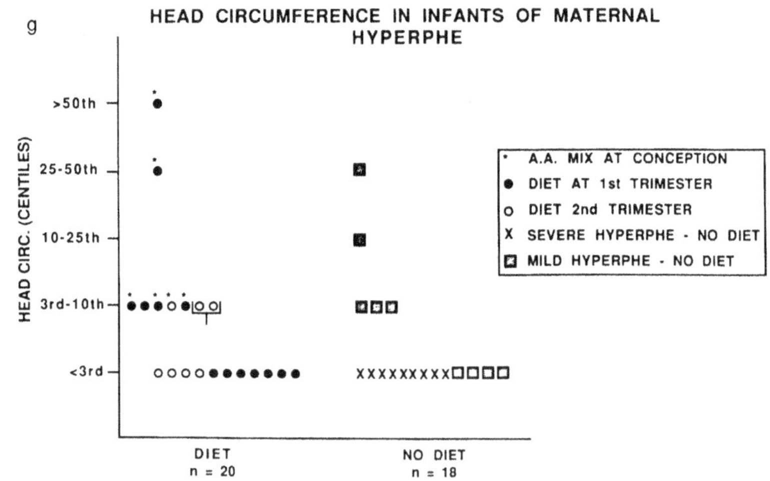

Figure 1 Head circumference in the diet and non-diet groups of women with hyperphenylalaninaemia and phenylketonuria.

Birth weight was > 3rd centile for all the mothers who started diet in the 1st trimester and in only three who started diet in the 2nd trimester. Only one of the non-diet group with phenylalanine > 1000 achieved a birth weight greater than the 25th centile compared to 10 in the diet group.

The group of six women with amino acid supplements at conception and who went on full diet later (and were therefore well nourished and replete with tyrosine) had a mean birth weight of 3470 g compared to 3500 g which is the expected mean for an Irish population. The offspring achieved a mean head circumference of 33.8 cm compared to an expected mean of 35 cm (Figure 2).

Preconception concentrations over 1300 μmol/L phenylalanine were associated with microcephaly, except in one baby whose head was between the 3rd and 10th centiles with a maternal phenylalanine concentration of 2600 μmol/L (Figure 3). Microcephaly also occurred at phenylalanine concentrations between 600 and 2600 μmol/L. The deaths and congenital heart disease occurred where the maternal phenylalanine concentrations were 800, 1000 and 1800 μmol/L respectively. There were no deaths in the diet group. The miscarriages occurred between phenylalanine concentrations of 897 to 2000 μmol/L.

The mean IQ of the mothers on diet was 71.36 (range 53–87), and the social class was 4 or 5 except for two mothers who were social class 2. Four of the 20 children from the diet group and five of the 20 children from the non-diet group attended special schools. Seven of the children from the diet group and 14 of the children from the non-diet group attend normal schools. Of the 14 of the non-diet group at normal school, ten are children of mothers with phenylalanine concentrations less than 1000 μmol/L. Ten children are still pre-school.

One mother is interesting in that her phenylalanine concentration is 800 μmol/L but on phenylalanine loading the blood levels rise above 1200 μmol/L and the urine is positive for phenylpyruvic acid. She has had a child with congenital heart disease

PREGNANCY OUTCOME			
DIET STATUS	NO. CASES Dub.	MEAN BW (g) Dub.	MEAN HC (cm) Dub.
Preconception – Strict	-	-	-
Preconception – Poor	6	3470	33.8
1st Trimester	8	3200	31.8
2nd-3rd Trimester	6	2567	31.6
No Diet (all)	18	2816	31.5
Expected		3500	35.0

Figure 2 Pregnancy outcome and diet status. Preconception poor diet: taking synthetic amino acid drink but with variable phenylalanine concentrations. Diet: synthetic drink plus low phenylalanine appropriate for gestation.

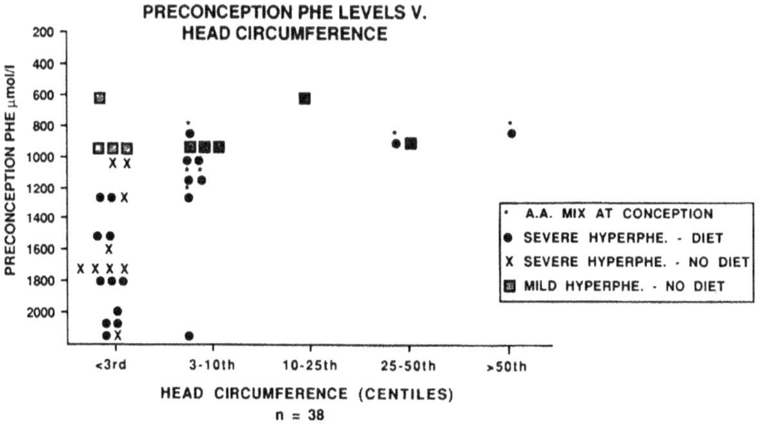

Figure 3 Preconception phenylalanine versus head circumference. Mild hyperphe: phenylalanine concentration less than 1000 µmol/L on normal diet. Severe hyperphe: phenylalanine concentration greater than 1000 µmol/L on normal diet. AA: amino acid mixture at conception.

who died; a child who has an IQ of 87 and a daughter who has an IQ of 80 who also has hyperphenylalaninaemia (phenylalanine tolerance = 800 mg daily).

DISCUSSION

Fetal wellbeing and size depend on maternal health, stature, blood pressure, presence or absence of smoking, alcohol, birth order, social class and placental function in addition to abnormal metabolism of amino acids such as phenylalanine and tyrosine. A clear statement on the optimal conditions for the fetus of a woman with PKU may not be possible until the numbers are large enough to allow correction for these other variables.

We identify three categories of women:

1. Those identified by newborn screening.
2. Those who were diagnosed late, e.g. were already in institutions or were older siblings of screened patients.
3. Those identified by their abnormal offspring.

Females from groups 2 and 3 will form a core group who are difficult to motivate or who are badly controlled on diet. Screened patients who come off diet may also prove difficult to manage as they may not present until already pregnant, despite education. The clinic in Dublin looks after almost all the individuals with phenylketonuria who are known but some will have come off diet despite the clinic advice to the contrary, as we have a 'diet for life' policy.

There is a high morbidity and mortality in this group of 48 pregnancies, highlighting the fact that currently the prescreen group of women – sibling and undetected – are the most difficult to identify and establish on diet before conception. Even where they are known to a clinic and are informed of the risks, in our experience they rarely present before six weeks; thirteen out of 20 pregnancies presented in the 1st trimester despite repeated contact and education. Taking the amino acid mixture may confer some protection (head circumference > 3rd centile in six women on the mixture despite poor phenylalanine concentrations) but motivating them to adhere to the restricted phenylalanine intake is labour intensive and involves the PKU clinic, public health nurses, family doctors and obstetric clinics.

Genetic counselling, family planning advice and clinic support have been given to all of these women but some remain greatly at risk and may not be capable of planning a pregnancy. Two women from the non-diet group are highly motivated and are now well controlled on diet. Only two women from the diet group have continued on full diet, but three others continue to take the full amino acid drink. Three husbands have been sterilized and two couples have separated.

The educational achievements of the children may fulfill the parents' criteria of normality as in the case of a mother with an IQ of 66 who had six children; one died following premature birth, his twin has an IQ of 80, a daughter has congenital heart disease, microcephaly and an IQ of 50; another daughter has an IQ of 64; and twins who both have congenital heart disease but IQs of 70+. In several homes the lack of stimulation is a further contributing factor to the childrens' poor performance and some of the children are considered at-risk because of the low parental IQ. Social services are involved in the care of three such families.

Identifiation of females at-risk is essential but the education, support, and work involved in maintaining diet control or achieving planned pregnancies should be not underestimated.

ACKNOWLEDGEMENTS

We would like to thank Dr S. Cahalane and his laboratory staff for their excellent service, our colleagues in the obstetric units and public health nurses for their help and co-operation, and Ms Deirdre Breen for typing this document. We would like to thank the paediatricians who referred cases to the clinic.

REFERENCES

Cahalane, S. Mass screening of newborns in Ireland. *Arch. Dis. Child.* 43 (1968) 141–144

Chadwick, G., Cahalane, S. *et al.* Maternal phenylketonuria in the Republic of Ireland. *Ir. Med. J.* 70 (1974) 612–614

Dent, C. E. Discussion of Armstrong, M. D. Relation of biochemical abnormality to development of mental defect in phenylketonuria. In *Aetiological Factors in Mental Retardation*, 23rd Ross Paediatric Research Conference, November 1956, Columbus, Ohio, p. 32

Lenke, R. and Levy, H. L. Maternal phenylketonuria and hyperphenylalaninaemia. *N. Engl. J. Med.* 303 (1980) 1202–1208

Murphy, D. and Troy, E. M. Maternal phenylketonuria. *Ir. J. Med. Sc.* 148 (1979) 310–313

Murphy, D., Saul, I. *et al.* Maternal phenylketonuria and phenylalanine restricted diet: studies of 7 pregnancies and of offsprings produced. *Ir. J. Med. Sc.* 154 (1985) 66–70

O'Connor, S. and Mulcahy, M. Maternal phenylketonuria in the Republic of Ireland. In Berg, J. M. (ed.), *Perspectives and Progress in Mental Retardation. Vol II – Biomedical Aspects*, pp. 85–92

J. Inher. Metab. Dis. 13 (1990) 665–671

Maternal PKU Workshop

Cognitive Development in Offspring of Untreated and Preconceptionally Treated Maternal Phenylketonuria

F. GÜTTLER, H. LOU, J. ANDRESEN, K. KOK, I. MIKKELSEN, K. B. NIELSEN and J. B. NIELSEN
The John F. Kennedy Institute, Gl. Landevej 7, DK-2600 Glostrup, Denmark

Summary: A survey is given of literature reports on the effect of performance in offspring from 26 maternal PKU pregnancies treated prior to conception. The survey includes two women who were referred to us for genetic counselling because they had both given birth to microcephalic, mentally retarded children. The women were discovered to suffer from unrecognized maternal PKU with fasting phenylalanine concentration of 1.1–1.5 mmol/L. A strict diet was introduced prior to planned pregnancy and after some months on diet (phenylalanine concentrations < 0.6 mmol/L) they became pregant again. Serum phenylalanine levels were monitored weekly throughout pregnancy, and adjustments in the diet were made to keep serum phenylalanine concentration within the range of 0.18–0.42 mmol/L. The outcome of the pregnancies were healthy children who have developed normally. Their IQs are 105 and 119 at ten and four years of age, respectively and their head circumferences are normal. Our data show that the effect of preconceptional dietary treatment was children with a normal performance, contrary to their older siblings born following untreated pregnancies. These results are in agreement with the survey of ten years' promising experiences with preconceptional treatment in maternal PKU. The data may help to motivate young PKU women to accept planned pregnancies and to encourage them to return to the strict diet, which has prevented them from being retarded.

Routine newborn screening for phenylketonuria (PKU) began in the mid-1960s. Early treated young women with PKU are no longer mentally retarded, and we suppose that most of them wish to have children. Without intervention, however, their children are very likely to become mentally retarded and microcephalic. Low birth weight and congenital heart disease are additional outcomes (Lenke and Levy, 1980; Levy and Waisbren, 1983; Lipson *et al.*, 1984; Drogari *et al.*, 1987; Levy, 1987). By the 1990s there will be about 2000 PKU women with normal intelligence of fertile age in the United Kingdom (Drogeri *et al.*, 1987) and at least 2800 women between the age of 16 and 26 are at risk of pregnancy in the United States (Friedman and Koch, 1988).

Fortunately there is reason to believe that this cause of second generation mental retardation can be prevented. Several studies suggest that low phenylalanine dietary treatment with control of the maternal biochemical abnormalities may prevent fetal damage. Normal offspring have been the outcome in some pregnancies, but several damaged offspring have come from others (Bush *et al.*, 1976; Smith *et al.*, 1979; Lenke and Levy, 1980; Drogari *et al.*, 1987; Levy, 1987; Rohr *et al.*, 1987). Factors such as maternal blood phenylalanine concentrations and the gestational age when treatment begins may be critical in determining the result. Current evidence obtained during the past ten years indicates that ideally treatment should begin prior to conception (Table 1) (Brenton *et al.*, 1981; Nielsen *et al.*, 1981; Murphy *et al.*, 1985; Brenton *et al.*, 1987; Drogari *et al.*, 1987; Levy, 1987; Rohr *et al.*, 1987; Lynch *et al.*, 1988).

One method of assessing the benefit of dietary treatment in maternal PKU is to compare non-phenylketonuric siblings from treated and untreated pregnancies (Levy *et al.*, 1982). There is only one reported case of a mother having more than one non-phenylketonuric offspring from treated pregnancies (Buist *et al.*, 1979) and in the study by Levy *et al.* (1982) the gestational age, when diet was initiated during treated pregnancies, was 10–18 weeks.

We have studied the outcome of preconceptional and gestational dietary treated pregnancies and untreated pregnancies in two women with PKU. Our results indicate that optimal benefits to the fetus may be obtained by dietary initiation before conception.

Table 1 IQ/DQ of offspring from 26 maternal PKU pregnancies treated prior to conception

	No.	*IQ/DQ*	*Age at testing*
Brenton *et al.* (1987)	4	106[a]	3 y 3 mon
		111	1 y 11 mon
		96	2 y 7 mon
		103	3 y 11 mon
Levy (1987)	13	100[b]	–
Lynch *et al.* (1988)	4	105[c]	5 y 8 mon
		110	2 y 9 mon
		85	4 y 9 mon
		95	11 mon
Murphy *et al.* (1985)	2	100[d]	2 y
		100	2 y 1 mon
Rohr *et al.* (1987)	1	89–90[e]	2 y
Present data	2	105[f]	9 y 11 mon
		119[g]	4 y

[a]Griffith [b]not indicated [c]Standford Binet [d]Merrill Palmer Scale [e]Bayley [f]WISC [g]WPPSI

MATERIAL

Literature survey

A survey was performed on the reported effects on performance in offspring from maternal PKU pregnancies treated before conception. Only recent reviews were selected.

Patients

Two women (US and KN) were referred to us for genetic counselling because they had given birth to microcephalic, mentally retarded children. Chromosome analyses and metabolic investigations of the children were normal, but it was discovered that their mothers were suffering from previously unrecognized PKU with fasting phenylalanine concentrations of 1.1–1.5 mmol/L (fluorimetric method).

RESULTS

The survey

Table 1 summarizes the reported IQ/DQ of offspring from 26 maternal PKU pregnancies treated prior to conception. The data indicate that the cognitive development of these children is within the normal range (IQ/DQ 85–119).

Family US

The mother (US) with unrecognized PKU had attended a special school for the subnormal, where she met her husband. Her IQ is within the borderline range and we suspect the same for her husband. He is a trained gardener and is permanently employed. She has been trained as a weaver. She manages her own household, and the family is socially well-adjusted. She is a 178 cm tall woman with fair complexion and blonde hair. No neurological abnormalities have been detected. When the family was referred to us for genetic counselling, their 4-year-old boy was obviously severely mentally retarded with microcephaly, myopia and obvious systolic murmur (Table 2). The mother and her husband wanted very much to have another baby. The husband proved by phenylalanine loading test to be a normal homozygote (Güttler, 1980). This has recently been confirmed by DNA haplotype investigations (unpublished data). A phenylalanine restricted dietary treatment was initiated in April 1978 and contraception was advised for the first month. After three months on diet, during which time the serum phenylalanine concentrations were kept below 0.6 mmol/L, the mother became pregnant. The diet contained initially 90 g of protein, equivalent to about 1.4 g/kg body weight. 60 g of protein were supplied in the form of a phenylalanine-free amino acid mixture. 30 g of protein were given as natural protein products. The phenylalanine tolerance was 15–17 mg/kg body weight/day. Serum phenylalanine values remained at 0.18–0.42 mmol/L throughout the pregnancy. In the second half of pregnancy the serum concentrations decreased despite increased phenylalanine intake. The phenylalanine tolerance increased parallel to the woman's

Table 2 Comparison of untreated pregnancies and pregnancies treated prior to conception in mothers with PKU

Mother	*Treatment*	*Infant data*			
		Head circumference at birth (cm)	*Birth weight* (g)	*Performance test IQ*	*Age at testing*
US	Untreated	microcephalic	2600	50	13 y
	Treated prior to conception	37	3500	105[b]	9 yr 11 mon
KN	Untreated	28	2060	73[c]	5 yr 2 mon
	Treated prior to conception	32[a]	2750[a]	119[c]	4 y

[a]Induced delivery at 37 weeks of gestation [b]WISC [c]WPPSI

weight gain, reflecting the growth of the uterus, placenta and fetus. Her weight gain of 1.5–2 kg/month in the second and third trimester is in accordance with international recommendations for pregnancy and was taken as an indication of the adequacy of the diet. The phenylalanine tolerance increased accordingly from 17 mg/kg/day to 22 mg/kg/day. Serum tyrosine concentrations were maintained at 0.04 mmol/L and at 16 weeks of gestation the diet was supplemented with 2 g of tyrosine per day. The daily caloric intake amounted to 2100–2500 kcal at the end of pregnancy. A standard mineral mixture and vitamin supplements were given in accordance with international recommendations. The diet was well tolerated and compliance was very good, with no known diet breaks. Serum phenylalanine concentrations were monitored weekly throughout pregnancy, and adjustments in the diet were made according to the phenylalanine level. The woman remained in her home throughout pregnancy, paying weekly visits to the Institute for blood tests and diet instructions. The biparietal diameter of the fetus was measured with ultrasound every second week from the 20th week on. It showed growth parallel to the standard curve just outside the upper border (2 standard deviations). The course of the curve seemed to indicate a large head and probably a slight miscalculation of term. This assumption was probably correct, as the woman went into spontaneous labour at 38 weeks' gestation.

The outcome of this pregnancy was a healthy boy of birth weight 3500 g, length 54 cm and head circumference 37 cm (Table 2). His Apgar score was 10 at 1 min. No malformations were found. Serum phenylalanine concentration in cord blood was 0.25 mmol/L. The phenylalanine concentration in amniotic fluid by the time of delivery was 0.07 mmol/L. The heel prick test showed that the phenylalanine level was normal in the baby on the second day of life. The boy has now been followed at the Kennedy Institute for 10 years; he is completely normal, height 137 cm, weight 29 kg, head circumference 55 cm and IQ (WISC) 105 (Table 2).

Family KN

The second mother with unrecognized PKU, KN, attended normal school for 10 years and was then trained as a shop assistant. She has resumed work after her last pregnancy. Her husband has permanent employment as an accountant. She is a 177 cm tall woman with fair complexion and blonde hair. No neurological abnormalities have been detected. When the family was referred to us for genetic counselling their 4-month-old girl was microcephalic, but with no other congenital malformations. At 5 years of age her IQ (WPPSI) was 73 (Table 2), and now, when she is 7, her IQ (WPPSI) is approximately 60. When the first child was two years of age KN and her husband wanted to have another baby and a strict diet was started, during which the phenylalanine concentrations were kept below 0.6 mmol/L. She became pregnant five months later and serum phenylalanine concentration remained at 0.18–0.42 mmol/L throughout the pregnancy. The pregnancy was monitored exactly as described for mother US. Seven weeks before term the biparietal diameter started to level off and during the next couple of weeks it remained stationary. Labour was induced and a normal boy was delivered at 37 weeks' gestation, with a birth weight of 2750 g, length 50 cm and head circumference 32 cm (Table 2). His Apgar score was 9 at 1 min. No malformations were noted. Serum phenylalanine concentration in cord blood was 0.36 mmol/L. The phenylalanine concentration was normal on the second day of life.

The boy has developed normally. The last control was performed at 4 years of age; weight 19.5 kg, length 107 cm, head circumference 49 cm, no neurological or other abnormalities, and IQ 119 (WPPSI) (Table 2).

DISCUSSION

The present survey of the effect on development in offspring from 26 maternal PKU pregnancies treated prior to conception covers preconceptional treatment in maternal PKU performed during the past ten years. The results are in agreement with the data obtained by a collaborative study mounted in the United Kingdom, Europe and Australia focussing on birth weights and head circumferences of infants born to women with PKU (Drogari *et al.*, 1987). This study, from the Institute of Child Health, London, showed normal birth weights and head circumferences in 17 infants born to mothers who by the time of conception received a strict low phenylalanine diet and had blood phenylalanine concentrations below 0.6 mmol/L. Some workers have reported borderline mental retardation, microcephaly, and other malformations in infants whose mothers did not start the diet until the first trimester (Smith *et al.*, 1979; Rohr *et al.*, 1987). The present survey combined with the data of Drogari and colleagues (1987) provides strong support for the view that only a strict diet started before conception is likely to prevent fetal damage.

The present results of preconceptional dietary treated and untreated pregnancies in the same women with PKU demonstrate that a strict diet started before conception, well controlled blood phenylalanine levels throughout the entire pregnancy and the quality of the diet are important factors in preventing fetal damage in maternal PKU. In the present study the diet was tolerated well, the co-operation was good and a close and personal contact with the dietition, doctor and laboratory was established. It is becoming increasingly obvious that optimal therapy for maternal PKU may be impossible unless the psychosocial environment of these young women is understood and their needs relative to the environment are met (Levy, 1987). We think that the psychological strain on the women during pregnancy was mitigated in the present study by the close and personal contact they had with the staff.

As some of the young women with PKU will have discontinued the diet, it is imperative that they learn about maternal PKU and receive information about the need to plan pregnancies and dietary reinstatement. Imparting this information to young women with PKU and their families requires contact between them and a programme which is knowledgeable about PKU and has the means to conduct appropriate follow-up measures. In recognition of this need at least four collaborative studies have begun, one combining centres in the United Kingdom and Australia, one combining centres in the United States and Canada, one combining centres in West Germany, and one combining centres in Scandinavia. There is reason to believe that fetal damage in offspring of women with PKU will be prevented in the future.

ACKNOWLEDGEMENTS

The study was supported by grants from NORDKEM, The Danish Medical Research Council, The Danish Health Insurance Foundation, Frantz Hoffmann's Memorial Fund, Emil and Inger Hertz Fund, Frode Nyegaard's Fund, P. Carl Petersen's Fund, and Stenild and Else Hjorth's Fund.

REFERENCES

Brenton, D. P., Cusworth, D. C., Garrod P., Krywawych, S., Lachelin, L., Liburn, M., Smith, I., Thornburn, R. and Wolff, O. H. Maternal phenylketonuria treated by diet before conception. In: Bickel, H. (ed.), *Maternal Phenylketonuria, Maizena, Frankfurt*, 1981, pp. 67–71

Brenton, D. P., Fraser, D., Haseler, M. E., Krywawych, S., Lachelin, G. C. I., Lilburn, M. and Stewart, A. Phénylcétonurie maternelle. *Arch. Fr. Pediatr.* 44 (1987) 667–670

Buist, R. N. M., Lis, E. W., Tuerck, J. M. and Murphy, D. Maternal phenylketonuria. *Lancet* 2 (1979) 589–591

Bush, R. T., Dukes, P. C., Progeny, pregnancy and phenylketonuria. *NZ Med. J.* 82 (1976) 226–229

Drogari, E., Beasley, M., Smith, I. and Lloyd, J. K. Timing of strict diet in relation to fetal damage in maternal phenylketonuria. *Lancet* 2 (1987) 927–930

Friedman, E. G. and Koch, R. Report from the Maternal PKU Collaborative Study. *Metabolic Currents* 1 (1988) 4–5

Güttler, F. Hyperphenylalaninemia: Diagnosis and classification of the various types of phenylalanine hydroxylase deficiency in childhood. *Acta Paediatr. Scand.* Suppl. 280 (1980) 1–80

Lenke, R. and Levy, J. Maternal phenylketonuria and hyperphenylalaninemia: an international survey of the outcome of untreated and treated pregnancies. *N. Engl. J. Med.* 303 (1980) 1202–1208

Levy, H. L. Maternal phenylketonuria. *Enzyme* 38 (1987) 312–320

Levy, H. and Waisbren, S. Effects of untreated maternal phenylketonuria and hyperphenylalaninemia on the fetus. *N. Engl. J. Med.* 309 (1983) 1269–1274

Levy, H. L., Kaplan, G. N. and Erickson, A. M. Comparison of treated and untreated pregnancies in a mother with phenylketonuria. *J. Pediatr.* 100 (1982) 876–880

Lipson, A., Beuhler, B., Bartley, J., Walsh, D., Yu, J., O'Halloran, M. and Webster, W. Maternal hyperphenylalaninemia fetal effects. *Eur. J. Pediatr.* 104 (1984) 216–220

Lynch, B. C., Pitt, D. B., Maddison, T. G., Danks, D. M. and Wraith, J. E. Maternal phenylketonuria: successful outcome in four pregnancies treated prior to conception. *Eur. J. Pediatr.* 148 (1988) 72–75

Murphy, D., Saul, I., Kirby, M. Maternal phenylketonuria and phenylalanine restricted diet. *Ir. J. Med. Sci.* 154 (1985) 66–70

Nielsen, K. B., Güttler, F., Weber, J. and Wamberg, E. Treatment of a phenylketonuric woman during planned pregnancy. In: Bickel, H. (ed.), *Maternal Phenylketonuria*, Maizena, Frankfurt, 1981, pp. 87–91

Rohr, F. J., Doherty, L. B., Waisbren, S. E., Bailey, I. V., Ampola, A. G., Benacerraf, B. and Levy, H. L. New England maternal PKU project. Prospective study of untreated and treated pregnancies and their outcomes. *J. Pediatr.* 110 (1987) 391–398

Smith, I., Erdohazia, M. and MacCartney, F. J. Fetal damage despite low-phenylalanine diet after conception in a phenylketonuric woman. *Lancet* 1 (1979) 17–19

Journal of Inherited Metabolic Disease

Aims and Scope of the Journal

The *Journal of Inherited Metabolic Disease* is the official scientific and clinical journal of the Society for the Study of Inborn Errors of Metabolism. The aim of this international and multidisciplinary journal is to provide otherwise unavailable information on inherited metabolic disorders covering clinical (medical, dental and veterinary), biochemical (including molecular genetics), genetic, experimental (including cell biology), theoretical, epidemiological, ethical and counselling aspects. Widespread and efficient communication between professional workers should improve the handling and understanding of inherited disorders.

The journal publishes papers, case and short reports, short communications, invited articles which are generally reviews, and book reviews. *Papers for submission* and correspondence should be written in English and sent to:

Dr. R. A. Harkness
Department of Clinical Biochemistry
Institute of Child Health
30 Guildford Street
London WC1N 1EH, UK

Acceptance of articles for publication is at the discretion of the editors. Authors are advised to consult a current issue of the journal before submission. It is a condition of acceptance that all articles have not been and will not be published elsewhere in substantially the same form. The submitting author must have circulated the article to and have secured agreement from all co-authors before submission of the article.

Detailed *Information for Authors* is published in issue no.1 of each volume of the journal, and in other issues as space permits, and is listed in the Contents.

Books for Review should be sent to Dr. Harkness at the above address.

Offprints. 25 offprints are provided free of charge. Authors will receive a form for ordering an extra 125 offprints with the proofs of their paper.

No page charges are levied on authors or their institutions.

Advertisements: As well as commercial advertisements, announcements of forthcoming scientific meetings and other material relevant to the journal can be included, at rates available from the publishers. All advertising is subject to the discretion of the editors.

Publication programme, 1990: Volume 13 (6 issues).
Subscriptions should be sent to: **Kluwer Academic Publishers Group, PO Box 322, 3300 AH Dordrecht, The Netherlands** or at **PO Box 358, Accord Station, Hingham, MA 02018-0358, USA**, or to any subscription agent.
Changes of mailing address should be notified together with your latest label.
Subscription prices, per volume (6 issues): Dfl 385.- plus postage: Dfl 30.- (Dfl 415.- per annum).
Subscription prices, per volume: US$193.50.
Second Class Postage paid at Rahway, NJ. USPS No. 757-750.
US Mailing Agent: Expediters of the Printed Word Inc., 2323 Randolph Avenue, Avenel, NJ 07001, USA.
Published by Kluwer Academic Publishers, PO Box 55, Lancaster, LA1 1PE, UK.
Postmaster: please send all address corrections to: *Journal of Inherited Metabolic Disease*, c/o Expediters of the Printed Word Inc., 2323 Randolph Ave, Avenel, NJ 07001, USA.

GPSR Compliance

The European Union's (EU) General Product Safety Regulation (GPSR) is a set of rules that requires consumer products to be safe and our obligations to ensure this.

If you have any concerns about our products, you can contact us on ProductSafety@springernature.com

In case Publisher is established outside the EU, the EU authorized representative is:

Springer Nature Customer Service Center GmbH
Europaplatz 3
69115 Heidelberg, Germany

Batch number: 10761599

Printed by Printforce, the Netherlands